Antioxidants: Chemical, Biological and Functional Properties

Antioxidants: Chemical, Biological and Functional Properties

Edited by Grace McCoy

hayle
medical

New York

Hayle Medical,
750 Third Avenue, 9th Floor,
New York, NY 10017, USA

Visit us on the World Wide Web at:
www.haylemedical.com

ISBN: 978-1-64647-107-2

Cataloging-in-Publication Data

Antioxidants : chemical, biological and functional properties / edited by Grace McCoy.
    p. cm.
Includes bibliographical references and index.
ISBN 978-1-64647-107-2
1. Antioxidants. 2. Chemical inhibitors. 3. Antioxidants--Physiological effect.
4. Antioxidants--Therapeutic use. I. McCoy, Grace.
RB170 .A58 2022
613.286--dc23

Table of Contents

Preface

Oxygen is a reactive molecule, which can damage living organisms by producing reactive species. To prevent this, organisms have antioxidant systems that prevent reactive species from being formed, or remove them before they damage the vital components of the cell. Since reactive oxygen species also tend to have important cellular functions, antioxidant systems do not entirely remove oxidants but keep them at an optimum level. Some of the reactive oxygen species produced in cells include hypochlorous acid, hydrogen peroxide and free radicals. This book includes some of the vital pieces of work being conducted across the world, on various topics related to antioxidants and their importance for human health. Most of the topics introduced herein cover the chemical, biological and functional properties of antioxidants. This book, with its detailed analyses and data, will prove immensely beneficial to professionals and students involved in this area at various levels.

After months of intensive research and writing, this book is the end result of all who devoted their time and efforts in the initiation and progress of this book. It will surely be a source of reference in enhancing the required knowledge of the new developments in the area. During the course of developing this book, certain measures such as accuracy, authenticity and research focused analytical studies were given preference in order to produce a comprehensive book in the area of study.

This book would not have been possible without the efforts of the authors and the publisher. I extend my sincere thanks to them. Secondly, I express my gratitude to my family and well-wishers. And most importantly, I thank my students for constantly expressing their willingness and curiosity in enhancing their knowledge in the field, which encourages me to take up further research projects for the advancement of the area.

Editor

Singlet Oxygen and Free Radical Reactions of Retinoids and Carotenoids

Ruth Edge [1] 🄳 **and T. George Truscott** [2,*]

[1] Dalton Cumbrian Facility, The University of Manchester, Westlakes Science and Technology Park, Moor Row, Cumbria CA24 3HA, UK; ruth.edge@manchester.ac.uk
[2] School of Chemical and Physical Sciences, Lennard-Jones Building, Keele University, Staffordshire ST5 5BG, UK
*   Correspondence: t.g.truscott@keele.ac.uk

Abstract: We report on studies of reactions of singlet oxygen with carotenoids and retinoids and a range of free radical studies on carotenoids and retinoids with emphasis on recent work, dietary carotenoids and the role of oxygen in biological processes. Many previous reviews are cited and updated together with new data not previously reviewed. The review does not deal with computational studies but the emphasis is on laboratory-based results. We contrast the ease of study of both singlet oxygen and polyene radical cations compared to neutral radicals. Of particular interest is the switch from anti- to pro-oxidant behavior of a carotenoid with change of oxygen concentration: results for lycopene in a cellular model system show total protection of the human cells studied at zero oxygen concentration, but zero protection at 100% oxygen concentration.

Keywords: carotenoids; xanthophylls; retinoids; lycopene; pro-/anti-oxidants; singlet oxygen; neutral free radicals; radical cations/anions; hydroxyl radical; hydrogen abstraction

1. Introduction

The C_{20} retinoids and C_{40} carotenoids play important roles in many diverse biological processes. The retinoids are major pigments associated with the eye and other aspects of human health (e.g., the skin) while the C_{40} carotenoids are not only involved in vision but also in photosynthesis and play a major role as anti-oxidants in human health [1]. In this review, we discuss the anti- and pro-oxidative reactions of the C_{20} retinoids. More extensively, we compare the anti-/pro-oxidant properties of the C_{40} hydrocarbon carotenoids (subsequently called "carotenoids") with those of the C_{40} oxygen-containing carotenoids (subsequently called xanthophylls). In biological systems there is some degree of "selectivity" between the carotenoids and the xanthophylls—thus, in the macula of the eye, there are no carotenoids but three xanthophylls (lutein, zeaxanthin and meso-zeaxanthin) [2] while in photosynthetic systems it is the hydrocarbon carotenoid, β-carotene which is the major carotenoid, although xanthophylls are also involved as accessory pigments [3]. Also, the treatment of the extreme photosensitivity associated with the disease of erythropoietic protoporphyria currently uses only β-carotene to ameliorate the damage due to singlet oxygen [4]—however, some xanthophylls have been considered (but more or less discounted) as skin colorants (artificial "tans") [5]. The roles of all three: the retinoids, the carotenoids and the xanthophylls, as both anti- and pro-oxidants, with respect to singlet oxygen and radical generation and quenching, are discussed.

2. The Retinoids

Retinoids have many roles in biological systems that do not involve anti- or pro-oxidant properties, such as roles in general growth, differentiation of epithelial tissues and in reproductive health. Nevertheless, there is some interest in such anti-/pro-oxidant activity, for example due to photosensitization, which is believed to involve singlet oxygen and free radical production. Topical retinoids are used to treat a wide range of dermatological disorders, however, advice to patients is that such drugs should only be used at nighttime to avoid the possibility of photosensitivity arising from activated oxygen species. The structures of several retinoids are shown below in Figure 1.

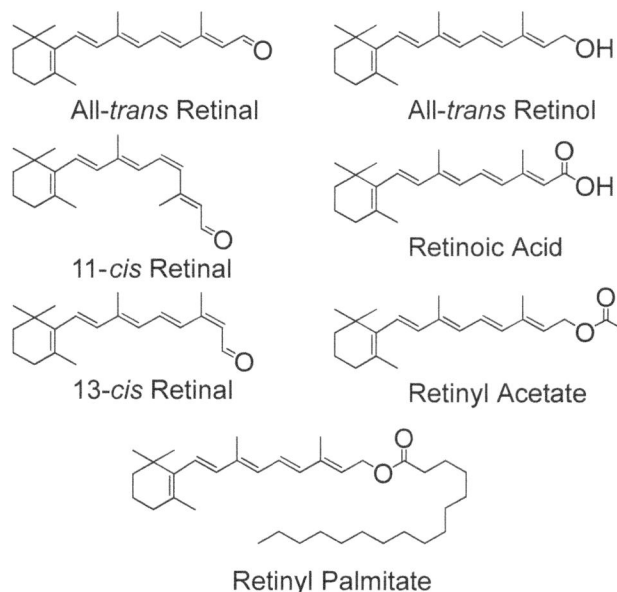

Figure 1. Chemical structures of several retinoids.

2.1. Triplet States and Singlet Oxygen ($^1O_2$)

All-*trans* retinal and other isomeric forms of retinal (see Figure 1) contain five conjugated carbon-carbon double bonds and a carbonyl group. The non-bonding electrons (n) on the oxygen lead to n-π^* excited states as well as the π-π^* excited states from the conjugated carbon–carbon double bonds. All-*trans* retinal is, of course, the key chromophore in vision, and laser flash photolysis has been used extensively to investigate the production of its triplet states and $^1O_2$. In addition, a simple, new method for estimating $^1O_2$ reactivity with retinoids and carotenoids, based on DBPF (1,3-Diphenylisobenzofuran)/UV-Vis (Ultra Violet-Visible) absorption spectroscopy in micellar solutions, has recently been proposed [6]. Pulsed laser studies show a significant production of triplet states and $^1O_2$ from all isomers of the retinals studied in non-polar solvents, including the all-*trans* isomer. Typical values for triplet and $^1O_2$ quantum yields being around 0.2–0.5, depending on the solvent, isomeric form and even laser excitation wavelength [7,8]. Note that a quantum yield value of 1.0 is equivalent to 100% yield. The solvent dependency (triplet yields being much lower in polar solvents than in non-polar solvents) allowed the ordering of the ^{1}n-π^*, $^1\pi$-π^*, ^{3}n-π^*, and $^3\pi$-π^* excited states to be determined. For the retinal isomers studied in polar, H-bonding or non-bonding solvents a state of $^1\pi$-π^* character, located below ^{3}n-π^*, appears to be the lowest excited singlet state. However, a ^{1}n-π^* state located above the $^3\pi$-π^*, is the lowest excited singlet state in non-polar, non H-bonding solvents, so that significant $^1O_2$ can be generated leading to photo-oxidative damage in, for example, CCl_4 and hydrocarbon solvents. In more polar environments the $^1O_2$ quantum yield is much lower [9], for example, in methanol values near 0.08 for all-*trans* retinal were reported via $^1O_2$ luminescence (these authors obtained rather similar results via steady-state techniques, which may be less accurate under some conditions). However, none of the other retinoids studied (see Figure 1) have such a high triplet quantum yield in any solvent. For the visual pigment models (retinal Schiff bases) there are claims of triplets being formed but with quantum yields in the region 0.01. Furthermore, Becker and co-workers suggest, at least in some solvents, that even this small yield of triplet state formation is due to minor hydrolysis of the Schiff base to produce a small amount of retinal [10].

Other retinoids, without a carbonyl group (see Figure 1) and hence no n-π^* states, have been studied and include retinol, retinyl acetate and retinoic acid. Triplet yields in the region 0.03 to near zero have been reported and reviewed previously, see, for example, [1]. Retinoic acid is of particular interest because of its use to treat leukemia and other cancers. However, such treatments lead to significant skin photosensitivity in at least some patients [11]. Laser flash photolysis studies have measured a triplet yield in hexane of 0.0013 for retinoic acid and this triplet was seen to be quenched by oxygen (presumably to generate $^1O_2$) very efficiently, k = 1.4×10^9 dm^3 mol^{-1} s^{-1}. Thus, despite the rather low triplet yield, there is still evidence of singlet oxygen formation. It seems reasonable to suggest the skin photosensitivity, at least to some extent, is related to $^1O_2$ and a trial to mitigate this, e.g., with β-carotene seems worthwhile.

Retinyl acetate and palmitate are frequently used to treat disease and are also components of cosmetics, and similar photophysical properties have been reported for retinyl acetate as for retinoic acid—typically, a triplet quantum yield of 0.025 and reaction rate constant with oxygen of 1×10^9 dm^3 mol^{-1} s^{-1} [12]. Once again, there is a low triplet yield but evidence of singlet oxygen formation.

2.2. Retinoid Radicals

As well as via triplets and $^1O_2$, retinoid-induced photosensitivity can also arise via radical formation and subsequent secondary processes [13]. Radical-based processes have been studied via laser flash photolysis and pulse radiolysis, however, the chemistry is complex and still not fully understood.

Certainly, while direct excitation of retinoic acid in methanol produces only the triplet (and presumably $^1O_2$, see above) for retinyl acetate, a species absorbing near 590 nm, other than the triplet, was also observed. Rosenfeld et al. [14] proposed this species as a carbenium ion. Lo et al. [12] reported the same transient, and in agreement with Rosenfeld's assignment, could see no solvated electron and no reaction with β-carotene (which would have been observed if photo-ionization was occurring)—the major process was proposed to be elimination of OCOCH$_3{}^-$

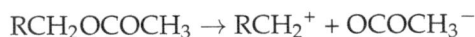

$$RCH_2OCOCH_3 \rightarrow RCH_2{}^+ + OCOCH_3{}^-$$

to produce the retinylic carbenium ion. When water mixed with methanol was used as the solvent, some degree of photo-ionization was also observed, suggesting a balance between photo-dissociation and photo-ionization of retinyl acetate depending on the micro environment. If the solvated electron is produced, a further complexity arises with the radical anion also being formed. Pulse radiolysis has suggested the radical anion itself will then dissociate by eliminating OH$^-$.

2.3. Radical Reactions

The superoxide radical anion ($O_2{}^{\bullet-}$) is generally regarded as unreactive while its conjugate acid, $HO_2{}^\bullet$, is much more reactive (the pK_a of $O_2{}^{\bullet-}/HO_2{}^\bullet$ is 4.7) and it is important not to claim reactivity for $O_2{}^{\bullet-}$ even at pH values near neutrality because this may simply be due to the small amounts of $HO_2{}^\bullet$ present at such pH values. Nevertheless, Collins et al. [15] used a cyclic voltammetry/computer simulation to obtain estimates of the rate constants for the reaction of all-*trans* retinol with $O_2{}^{\bullet-}$ and $HO_2{}^\bullet$ as $\approx 4 \times 10^5$ and $\geq 1.5 \times 10^8$ dm^3 mol^{-1} s^{-1}.

Rozanowska and colleagues [16] have reported pulse radiolysis studies of the interaction of retinal, retinol and retinoic acid with peroxyl radicals. The rationale for this work is that the assumed key process for their ability to inhibit lipid peroxidation, via the formation of carbon-centered radical adducts, is not sufficient to fully explain the high effectiveness of retinol and retinoic acid to inhibit lipid peroxidation, which can even exceed that of vitamin E. In order to further understand such protection, pulse radiolysis was used to generate peroxyl radicals and the reactions between the retinoids and peroxyl radicals were monitored in aqueous micelles. In all cases, at least two products were detected—the retinoid radical cation (absorbing near 590 nm) and species absorbing at shorter wavelengths, which are probably adducts of the retinoids with the peroxyl radicals. The subsequent processes of these "adducts" suggests that the mode of interaction of different retinoids with peroxyl radicals may vary.

Rozanowska et al. suggest the donation of an electron from the retinoid to the peroxyl radical:

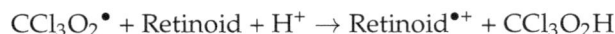

$$CCl_3O_2{}^\bullet + Retinoid + H^+ \rightarrow Retinoid^{\bullet+} + CCl_3O_2H$$

this provides an additional route for the anti-oxidant action of retinoids, provided that the formed radical cation is itself subsequently removed by a reducing species such as vitamin C—such a process for the carotenoids was observed [17].

El-Agamey and co-workers [18] reported kinetic studies of retinol addition radicals formed with various thiyl radicals, with and without oxygen, in an attempt to quantify the pro-oxidative effects of retinol. The reactions observed in methanol are neutral thiyl radical ($RS^\bullet$) additions to retinol and the estimated rate constants are the sum of the individual addition rate constants leading to the formation of various thiyl addition radicals. Typically, these were $2 - 8 \times 10^9$ dm^3 mol^{-1} s^{-1}, rather similar to that previously reported for β-carotene [19]. Oxygen addition reactions are important in understanding the anti-/pro-oxidation balance of retinoids and, if oxygen addition to the adducts is significant (to give R–CAR–OO$^\bullet$), then retinoids may well switch from being anti-oxidants to pro-oxidants. El Agamey et al. found that such oxygen addition processes for the thiyl-retinal neutral adducts are 10–1000 times larger (depending on the reactivity of the specific thiyl radical) than those reported for the carotenoids [20,21]. From these results, under the conditions studied by these workers, carotenoids may be the more potent anti-oxidants and, correspondingly the retinoids more potent pro-oxidants.

El-Agamey and Fukuzumi [22] used laser flash photolysis to study retinol in polar solvents (mainly methanol) and showed that 355 nm excitation leads to the formation of the retinol radical cation (λ_{max} = 580 nm) and the solvated electron. The electron then adding to the parent retinol to generate the corresponding radical anion (λ_{max} = 370 nm). In particular, the 580 nm species was proven to be the radical cation (and not the corresponding non-radical retinyl cation $RCH_2{}^+$). Using this identification of the absorption maximum for the retinol radical cation, El-Agamey and co-workers have studied the reactivity of this radical cation with a very wide range of organic and biological molecules [23]. The systems studied included C_{40} carotenoids, vitamins C and E, amino acids and natural and synthetic phenols, neurotransmitters such as catechols and various phenols. Their results, comparing rate constants with those of $CCl_3O_2{}^\bullet$, showed that the reactivity of the retinol radical cation is greater or similar to that of $CCl_3O_2{}^\bullet$, i.e., retinol radical cation is an extremely powerful oxidizing species and can be expected to cause bio-damage. However, their results also showed that the presence of vitamins E and C, C_{40} carotenoids, and naturally occurring phenols (e.g., L-dopa, vanillin and reservatrol) can inhibit the potentially damaging effects of the retinol radical cation by reducing it to retinol.

3. Carotenoids

The anti-/pro-oxidant roles of carotenoids and xanthophylls (representative structures shown in Figures 2 and 3, below) are of particular interest to photosynthesis and vision. In photosynthesis their roles include protection of the reaction centers and the antenna complex. In vision the xanthophylls protect the macula from light-induced damage via a simple blue light filtering mechanism and, probably, also via quenching of reactive oxygen species, such as free radicals and singlet oxygen. Much interest has centered on the beneficial and possible deleterious effects of using both carotenoids and xanthophylls as dietary supplements against diseases such as cancer and age-related macular degeneration, which is the major cause of blindness in older people in the western world.

Carotenoids are one of the most common pigments found in nature, being responsible for the red/yellow colors of many leaves, fruits and fish. Epidemiological work has associated their dietary intake with a reduced risk of degenerative diseases but supplement trials have suggested pro-oxidant abilities.

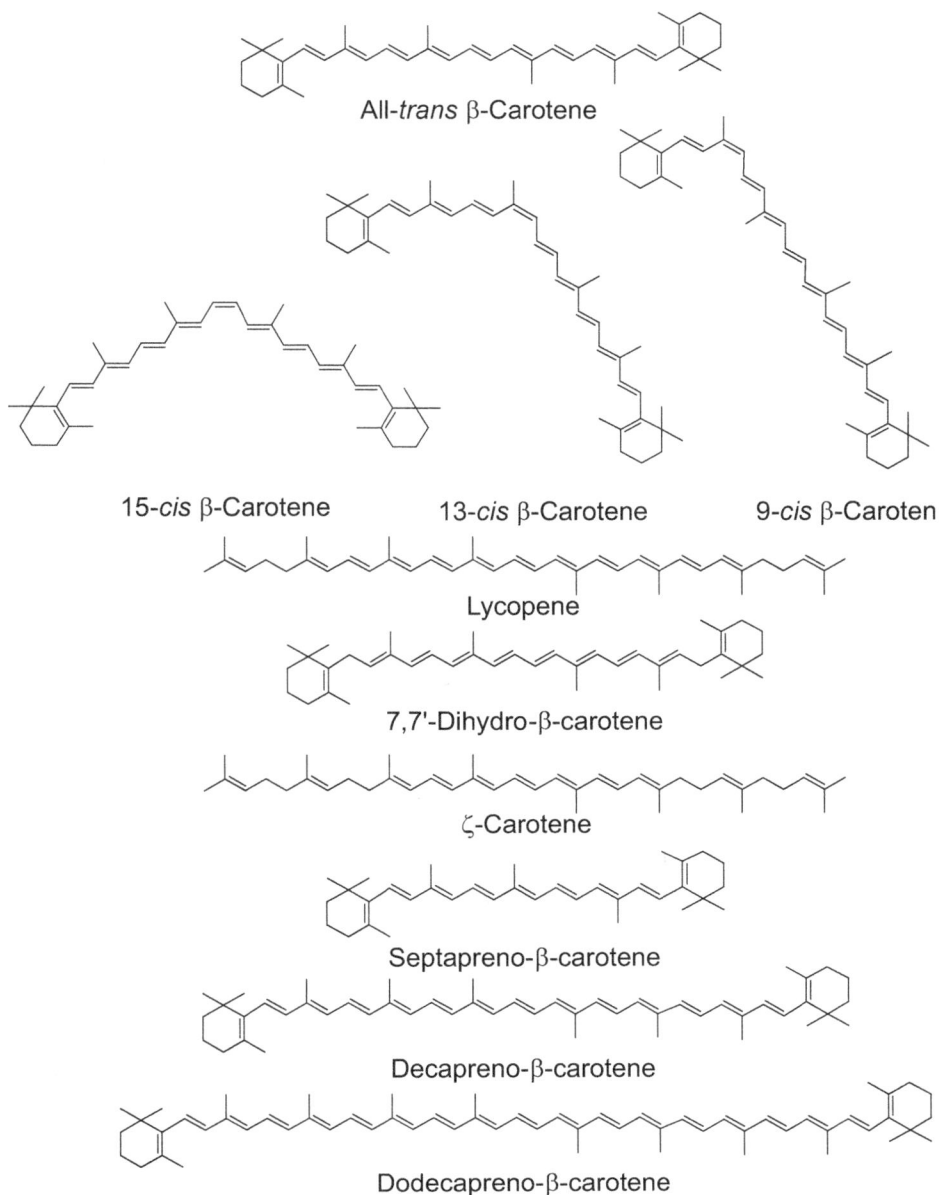

Figure 2. Chemical structures of typical carotenoids; *cis* isomers have been given for β-carotene only.

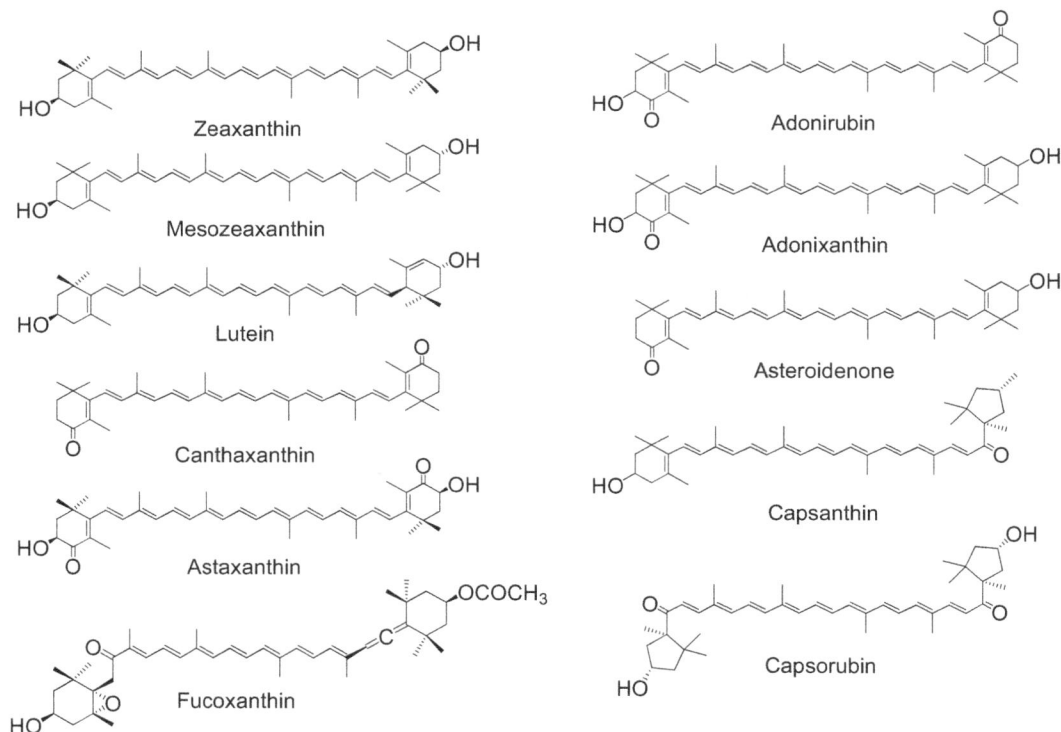

Figure 3. Chemical structures of typical xanthophylls.

3.1. Carotenoids and Singlet Oxygen

Ground state molecular oxygen is a triplet state with the two unpaired electrons being in the degenerate pair of π^* orbitals. The two lowest electronic excited states of oxygen in the gas phase are both singlet states and it is the lowest lying that is commonly termed singlet oxygen ($^1O_2$) [24].

Singlet oxygen can be produced in a number of ways, e.g., peroxide decomposition, high frequency discharge and via energy transfer from the excited state of a photosensitizer to ground state molecular oxygen [24], which is the most common method. The relatively low energy level of $^1O_2$ (E = 0.98 eV or 94.5 kJ mol^{-1}) means that a wide range of sensitizers have a high enough energy in both their singlet and triplet states to convert molecular oxygen to its excited state, $^1O_2$. Typical in vivo sensitizers are porphyrins, chlorophylls and riboflavin, which can lead to a variety of deleterious effects, including DNA damage and lipid peroxidation [25,26]. Other sensitizers include dyes such as rose bengal and eosin, which are often used in organic solvents or in ex vivo cell suspensions to produce $^1O_2$.

Once produced $^1O_2$ is capable of oxidizing many cellular substrates, especially in the skin and eyes, where photo-production can occur [27,28], but it has a limited lifetime and, if no reaction occurs, will decay back to the ground state either radiatively or by solvent-induced non-radiative deactivation. The non-radiative process dominates in solution and so the $^1O_2$ lifetime is strongly influenced by the solvent vibrational frequencies, varying from a few microseconds to several milliseconds (compared with a half-life of 45 min in the gas phase [29]). The radiative component of the deactivation of $^1O_2$ (phosphorescence) has a maximum around 1270 nm and this decay is often used for monitoring $^1O_2$ and determining quenching rate constants of antioxidants.

In fluid systems/solvents carotenoids quench $^1O_2$ physically via collisional energy transfer, and there have been studies of both their quenching abilities and of their protection against $^1O_2$-mediated photo-oxidation reactions.

Foote and Denny [30] were the first to show inhibition of photosensitized oxidation by β-carotene and that it was due to its ability to efficiently quench $^1O_2$. Farmilo and Wilkinson [31] showed that (electron exchange) energy transfer quenching is the principal mechanism of carotenoid $^1O_2$ quenching, producing the carotenoid triplet state. Chemical quenching (which destroys the carotenoid) only occurs as a much slower process leading to mainly carotene endoperoxides [32–34].

As noted above, many carotenoids have been studied with regard to their $^1O_2$ quenching ability in organic solvents and it has been shown that ability increases with increasing number of conjugated double bonds and, therefore, increasing wavelength of the $\pi\pi^*$ absorption maximum [35,36]. For the biologically important C_{40} carotenoids the triplet energy is below that of $^1O_2$ and all quench at near-diffusion-controlled rates of around 1×10^{10} dm^3 mol^{-1} s^{-1}. Longer chain carotenoids, such as decapreno-β-carotene and dodecapreno-β-carotene, have quenching rate constants approximately double those of the C_{40} carotenoids. While shorter chain ones show a lower quenching, e.g., lutein, with 10 double bonds, quenching at a rate half that of β-carotene (or zeaxanthin, both with 11 double bonds) and septapreno-β-carotene (9 double bonds) having a quenching rate constant around one tenth that of β-carotene in benzene [36]. Lycopene is a more efficient quencher than β-carotene (and all other C_{40} carotenoids) in organic solvents and the reason for this has been suggested to be structural (although the difference is less marked in benzene compared a mixed solvent system containing ethanol, chloroform and water) [36,37] (see Table 1, below). There is a loss of planarity in β-carotene and other C_{40} carotenoids and xanthophylls with terminal six membered rings. This creates twisting of the rings due to steric hindrance, leading to an effective reduction in the conjugated chain length, which is not present in lycopene [38].

Table 1. Comparison of the $^1O_2$ quenching rate constants for lycopene and β-carotene in a range of environments.

Carotenoid	$k_q/10^9$ dm^3 mol^{-1} s^{-1}				
	DPPC Liposomes [39]		Micelles [36]	Benzene [36]	Ethanol:Chloroform:Water 50:50:1 [37]
	*	†			
Lycopene	2.4	2.3	2.0	17.0	31.0
β-Carotene	2.3	2.5	2.4	13.0	14.0

* = Water soluble $^1O_2$-generation by rose Bengal; † = Lipid soluble $^1O_2$-generation by 4-(1-pyrene)butyric acid; DPPC: dipalmitoyl phosphatidylcholine.

The functional groups of the xanthophylls do show a limited effect on the quenching activity, with a recent paper [40] showing those xanthophylls containing two carbonyl groups (astaxantin, capsorubin and its diacetate) to have the best scavenging ability in acetonitrile, while those containing one carbonyl group (capsanthin and its diacetate) are better able to scavenge than those with none at all. However, this is the opposite of previous research on three asymmetric xanthophylls [41,42] where adonirubin, with two carbonyl groups, showed a lower quenching rate constant for $^1O_2$ in both benzene and deuterated methanol compared with adonixanthin and asteroidenone (both containing only one carbonyl group). This apparent disparity suggests further studies are needed.

Studies using organic solvents have also looked at the quenching abilities of *cis* carotenoids and, in benzene, they quench $^1O_2$ less efficiently than the all-trans isomer with the rate constants decreasing for β-carotene as the *cis* bond moves away from the center of the molecule, e.g., from 13.5×10^9 dm^3 mol^{-1} s^{-1} for the all-trans isomer to 8.99×10^9 dm^3 mol^{-1} s^{-1} for the 9-*cis* isomer [36]. A time-resolved resonance Raman study has indicated that all β-carotene isomers share a common triplet state, twisted about the central carbon–carbon double bond compared with the ground state [43]. A recent study in hexane has shown that *cis* isomers are produced after reaction of the all-*trans* isomers with $^1O_2$ for both lycopene and β-carotene and that lycopene can prevent β-carotene isomerization [44].

Studies have also been undertaken using primarily aqueous media, such as micelles [6,36] and liposomes [39,45,46] where the quenching rate constants are still found to be high ($>10^8$ dm^3 mol^{-1} s^{-1}). In the liposome studies the quenching ability was independent of the site of generation (i.e., whether the $^1O_2$ was generated by a water or lipid soluble photosensitizer). There was a marked difference in quenching ability for the xanthopylls in liposomes compared to micelles, where the rate constants fell by up to 50 times (for lutein) in liposomes, whereas the quenching rate constant for β-carotene in liposomes was close to that in micellar solution. A significant concentration effect on $^1O_2$ quenching was also observed for xanthophylls in the liposomes (especially for zeaxanthin), suggesting aggregation lowers quenching efficiency. It is also interesting to note that, unlike in organic solvents, the difference between the quenching abilities of lycopene and β-carotene is virtually non-existent in mixed micelles of Triton-X 100 and Triton-X 405 and in dipalmitoyl phosphatidylcholine (DPPC) liposomes (see Table 1, above). Note that lycopene is virtually insoluble in Triton-X 100 micelles alone, so was not studied in this media [6].

One of the liposome studies, in dimyristoyl phosphatidylcholine (DMPC) [46] also monitored inhibition of $^1O_2$-induced lipid peroxidation and showed that inhibition by β-carotene, canthaxanthin and astaxanthin was similar but that the inhibition by lycopene was 10-fold less. A more recent study has also shown inhibition of $^1O_2$-induced plasma lipid oxidation by β-carotene and fucoxanthin [47], with fucoxanthin being the better inhibitor, despite the $^1O_2$ quenching rate constant of fucoxanthin being reported to be lower than that of β-carotene [48].

Cellular studies have shown differing results; carotenoids efficiently quench $^1O_2$ in isolated photosystem II reaction centers [49] and can also protect ex vivo lymphocytes from $^1O_2$-induced damage [50–52], though the decrease in $^1O_2$ lifetime is more easily observed for lymphoid cells which have been incubated with carotenoids and then washed [50,51], rather than when individuals have taken the carotenoids orally over several weeks [51,52].

Additionally, a recent study [53] using microscopy to observe the time-resolved $^1O_2$ luminescence in single HeLa cells has shown no change in the lifetime of intracellular $^1O_2$ in the presence of β-carotene, even in D_2O where the $^1O_2$ lifetime is significantly lengthened (15–40 μs) compared to water (~3 μs) [54]. Thus, these workers suggest that the protective effects of β-carotene observed in their cell environment may be due to radical trapping and not direct $^1O_2$ quenching, and they propose this is due to a very low diffusion rate within the high viscosity intra-cellular environment. The $^1O_2$ lifetime in a single cell in water is around 3 μs, which is similar to the lifetime in pure water of 3.1–4.2 μs [55]. This and the D_2O effect on its lifetime in a single cell also suggests a low diffusion rate, otherwise it would be quenched more effectively by endogenous quenchers such as lipids and proteins.

3.2. Carotenoid and Xanthophyll Radicals

Free radicals, of course, are characterized by an unpaired electron. When a free radical interacts with a carotenoid several possible modes of reaction arise and these depend mainly on the nature of the free radical. The situation is, therefore, much more complex than the quenching of $^1O_2$ by carotenoids.

Many of the studies of the generation and reactivities of carotenoid radical cations, and anions, up to 2015 have been reported in several reviews [56–58].

One of the most well studied species is the carotenoid radical cation obtained via abstraction of an electron from the carotenoid by an oxidizing free radical.

$$CAR + R^\bullet \rightarrow CAR^{\bullet+} + R^-$$

Typical examples of the strongly oxidizing free radicals that lead to this electron transfer process are: chlorinated peroxyl radicals, such as $CCl_3O_2^\bullet$, nitrogen dioxide ($NO_2^\bullet$ arylperoxyl radicals, sulfonyl radicals ($RSO_2^\bullet$) and dibromine radical anion ($Br_2^{\bullet-}$). However, as we will discuss below, the strongly oxidizing hydroxyl radical ($OH^\bullet$) mainly adds to the carotenoid rather than producing the carotenoid radical cation. Furthermore, $CCl_3O_2^\bullet$, and possibly $NO_2^\bullet$, may give both the radical cation and also add to the carotenoid.

Radical anions ($CAR^{\bullet-}$) can be generated from sufficiently reducing radicals, for example, via addition of the solvated electron (e^-) to the carotenoid (CAR):

$$CAR + e^- \rightarrow CAR^{\bullet-}$$

The properties and reactivity of several carotenoid radical anions, including the reactivity of carbonyl containing carotenoid anions with water, have been reviewed previously [42] and some others are briefly mentioned below. However, the radical anions are not thought to be as biologically important as the radical cations. Quenching of oxidizing free radicals, which can arise via normal metabolic processes or via environmental hazards, such as smoking and air pollution, is of considerable biological importance and therefore, the carotenoid radical cations have been studied much more extensively than the carotenoid radical anions.

The radical cations (CAR$^{\bullet+}$) can be generated in various ways, such as via pulse radiolysis [59–61], flash photolysis [62–64], and electrochemically [65,66]. Pulse radiolysis is also a convenient method to generate and characterize the radical anions. These techniques are well established and have allowed the one-electron oxidation potentials of several carotenoids to be measured in aqueous micellar solution—they are typically near 1000 mV, so that carotenoid radical cations, are rather strong oxidizing agents [60,61] themselves. This data shows that carotenoid radical cations may oxidize important bio-substrates such as cysteine, tyrosine and tryptophan and also allowed electron transfer between one carotenoid and the radical cation of another to be observed for many pairs of carotenoids. Therefore, we were able obtain the relative one-electron oxidation potentials of several important carotenoids showing that lycopene has the lowest potential (i.e., is the most easily oxidized of the dietary carotenoids). This may lead to lycopene being the "sacrificial" carotenoid in vivo, when there is a mixture of carotenoids present, and may well be related to the health benefits often claimed for dietary lycopene as we have previously discussed [56].

Another important result, discussed in previous reviews, for example [58], arises from pulse radiolysis studies showing that carotenoid radical cations are converted back to the parent carotenoid by water-soluble antioxidants such as ascorbic acid. Therefore, a potentially damaging pro-oxidant effect due to the high reduction potential of carotenoid radical cations will be removed by ascorbic acid. Smokers have low levels of ascorbic acid, and free radicals from cigarette smoke can reach the lungs. It has been shown that, for heavy smokers, a high concentration of β-carotene can have a damaging effect, and a speculation is that this may be due to these smoke-based free radicals (e.g., $NO_2^{\bullet}$) reacting with β-carotene to generate the β-carotene radical cation, which can then damage biomolecules.

Recent results from Skibsted and co-workers [63,64] are consistent with the above reactions of β-carotene radical cation with tyrosine and tryptophan, regenerating the parent β-carotene. Interestingly, Skibsted used pH conditions where the redox potentials (the standard reduction potentials) were the same for tyrosine and tryptophan (the reduction potential for β-carotene radical cation is independent of pH in the region studied). These workers found that tyrosine reacted an order of magnitude faster than tryptophan and speculate that this may account for tyrosine, rather than tryptophan, as the protein moiety reacting with β-carotene in the protective mechanism, which operates in the photosynthetic reaction center. As Skibsted points out, the driving force in these reactions depends on the "local" pH and in proteins the reverse reaction between a tyrosine radical and β-carotene may also be important.

In their most recent work [64] Skibsted and co-workers have extended their studies of the regeneration of β-carotene from its radical cation to eugenol and isoeugenol—naturally occurring phenols that may well be important in the stability of carotenoids in various food products. The redox potentials are 0.75 V and 0.66 V (vs. SHE) for eugenol and isoeugenol respectively however the corresponding rate constants for the "repair" of β-carotene are 4.3×10^9 dm^3 mol^{-1} s^{-1} and 7.2×10^8 dm^3 mol^{-1} s^{-1}. Therefore, even though isoeugenol is the most reducing it reacts faster with the βCAR$^{\bullet+}$. Skibsted explains this result in terms of the so-called "inverted region" of Marcus theory.

A recent review [67] has highlighted a significant apparent disagreement concerning the fate of β-carotene radical cation. El-Agamey and co-workers [68] studied the effect of pH on the decay of the β-carotene radical cation (HCAR$^{\bullet+}$) while the extensive work of Kispert and co-workers used advanced electron paramagnetic resonance techniques and optical measurements beside electrochemical and theoretical studies [67,69–71]. The Kispert group showed that proton loss from β-carotene radical cation leads to the neutral carotenoid radical (CAR$^\bullet$)

$$HCAR^{\bullet+} \rightarrow CAR^\bullet + H^+$$

with an absorption maximum around 750 nm. In their studies, Kispert et al. form the radicals on silicate-based matrices [67,69–71]. Proton loss from the radical cation to produce a neutral species was identified using both electron paramagnetic resonance and optical detection. It should be noted that this work established the optical absorption spectrum for the neutral species without using transient absorption spectroscopy. This assignment of the neutral species in the absence of oxygen was confirmed via studies of the effect of pH and this species was linked to a previously unassigned peak reported from spectral studies of Photosystem II (PSII) [69]. The Kispert group speculate that in PS II itself photoprotection can arise both by the loss of the excess vibrational energy of the radical cation and by quenching of excited chlorophyll by the carotenoid proton loss neutral radical. However, El-Agamey [68] used laser flash photolysis to generate the β-carotene radical cation and study its transient absorption in aqueous Triton-X micelles. They observed the decay of the radical cation as a function of pH and conclude that such neutral radicals of β-carotene show no absorption at wavelengths above 550 nm.

The work of El-Agamey concerns β-carotene in Triton X100 "solutions" while that of Kispert concerns a very different microenvironment with the carotene radicals stabilized on silica-alumina or molecular sieves. Therefore, for example, diffusional processes may be more important in the solution studies of El-Agamey, while they will be unimportant in the organized microenvironments. While this may account for the different results and conclusions, clearly more work is needed to understand these apparently contradictory, but important, observations.

El-Agamey and McGarvey have extended their research on the microenvironment of carotenoids using pulsed laser studies of micro-emulsions [72]. These preparations allow the water/cyclohexane ratio to be changed, so that the polarity of the microenvironment of the carotenoid can be varied, and this in turn was found to affect the ratio of the carotenoid radical cation to other, probably neutral radicals, formed. The authors used 266 nm pulsed laser excitation of air-saturated solutions to generate the peroxyl radicals from both water soluble 4-acety-4-phenylpiperidene hydrochloride and lipid soluble 1,1-diphenylacetone. They studied two carotenoids, zeta-carotene and 7,7'dihydro-β-carotene and both led to the formation of the corresponding radical cation and another, unidentified, species absorbing also in the near infra-red but at somewhat shorter wavelengths (possible an ion pair or radical cation isomer) called NIR1 with wavelengths in the 650–750 nm region. Two important findings were (i) the nature of the peroxyl precursor used (water soluble or lipid soluble) had little or no influence on the yields and kinetics of the transient species formed from the reaction of the two carotenoids with the different peroxyl radicals and (ii) the ratio of the radical cation formed to NIR1 varied significantly with the environment polarity, this suggesting that the micro-emulsion composition will have a great impact on the pro-oxidant/anti-oxidant activity of carotenoids.

We have previously reviewed the generation, and reactivity of carotenoid radical anions [42]. As mentioned, these are of less relevance to biological processes than the radical cations. There are many differences between the anions and cations. For example, β-carotene radical anions react with oxygen at near diffusion-controlled rates (for several isomers in hexane) presumably to generate the superoxide radical anion, while there is no reaction between β-carotene radical cations and oxygen:

$$CAR^{\bullet-} + O_2 \rightarrow CAR + O_2^{\bullet-}$$

Interestingly, the corresponding reaction of oxygen with lycopene radical anion is 10 times slower $(1 \times 10^8 \ dm^3 \ mol^{-1} \ s^{-1})$ whereas there is little difference between the rates of $^1O_2$ quenching by lycopene and β-carotene as discussed earlier.

It is also worth noting the difference in protonation/deprotonation between the carotenoid radical cations and anions. The radical anions of carbonyl containing xanthophylls ($HCAR=O^{\bullet-}$) react with water and methanol to generate a neutral radical in which the carbonyl oxygen is protonated [73].

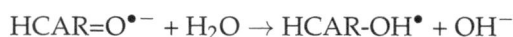

$$HCAR=O^{\bullet-} + H_2O \rightarrow HCAR\text{-}OH^{\bullet} + OH^-$$

Of course, this is quite a different species to the neutral radical generated by deprotonation of a carotenoid radical cation, discussed above:

$$HCAR^{\bullet+} \rightarrow CAR^{\bullet} + H^+$$

Therefore, as also discussed above, neutral carotenoid radicals can arise from deprotonation of the corresponding radical cation or protonation of the corresponding radical anion. However, another important route to neutral carotenoid radicals is via radical addition to a carotenoid.

A well-studied series of carotenoid radical adducts concerns carotenoids reacting with sulfur containing radicals, thiyl ($RS^{\bullet}$) and thiyl sulfonyl ($RSO_2^{\bullet}$), e.g.,

$$CAR + RS^{\bullet} \rightarrow RS\text{-}CAR^{\bullet}$$

Much of this early work has come from the groups of Willson (e.g., [74]) and Skibsted and Mortensen (e.g., [75]) and has been reviewed previously [41].

An extension of this work comes from the studies of El-Agamey and McGarvey who have observed [20] the first direct reversible oxygen addition to a carotenoid-derived carbon-centered neutral radical. These workers used phenylthiyl radicals ($PhS^{\bullet}$) to add to 7,7′dihydro-β-carotene (and to β-carotene). The corresponding adduct PhS-77DH$^{\bullet}$ being sufficiently long-lived (no endo- or epoxidation processes occurring) to allow the rate of reversible oxygen addition to be observed for the first time. Typical addition rate constants are in the region of 10^4 dm^3 mol^{-1} s^{-1} but are about 7 times slower for β-carotene compared to 7,7′dihydro-β-carotene (presumably related to the different conjugated chain lengths).

There has been recent interest in the reactions (trapping) of the important radical OH$^{\bullet}$ with carotenoids. Nishino and co-workers have used electro-spray ionization, time-of-flight mass spectrometry and Electron Spin Resonance (ESR) spectroscopy to study the products of several carotenoids reacting with OH$^{\bullet}$ [33,40]. In all cases carotenoid epoxides were formed with a single oxygen atom adding across the 5,6 double bond of the carotenoid ring rather than on to the polyene chain. By contrast $^1O_2$ added as two oxygen atoms forming various endoperoxides.

As noted above the strongly oxidizing hydroxy radical (OH$^{\bullet}$), reduction potential 2.31 V vs. SHE (Standard Hydrogen Electrode) at pH 7 [76], mainly adds to carotenoids to give neutral radical adducts rather than undergoing electron transfer to produce carotenoid radical cations. Additionally, hydrogen atom abstraction by OH$^{\bullet}$, also yielding a carotenoid neutral radical, has been observed [77].

It is also well established that, once formed, neutral radicals can add molecular oxygen forming peroxyl radicals and, as first shown by Burton and Ingold [78] this can lead to a switch from anti-oxidant to pro-oxidant behavior of carotenoids.

A similar mechanism was suggested by Boehm and co-workers to explain their recent observation of a substantial effect of oxygen concentration on the protection of human cells against γ-radiation by lycopene [79]. In this study, human volunteers either took a high lycopene diet or near zero lycopene and the extracted blood lymphoid cells were exposed to high energy γ-radiation from a ^{60}Co source. Cell membrane destruction, leading to immediate cell death, was measured via cell staining with eosin. Under normal atmospheric conditions and at the radiation doses studied (up to 5000 Gy) the lycopene protected the cells by a factor of 4–5 compared to the unprotected cells (no lycopene in the diet). However, a really dramatic effect of oxygen concentration was observed. At near zero oxygen there was virtually total cell protection by the lycopene (no cell damage due to the high energy γ-radiation) whereas at 100% oxygen the lycopene gave no protection whatsoever. It was suggested that the molecular mechanism for this oxygen effect was related to the observations of Burton and Ingold [78] in non–biological conditions. Therefore, the proposed mechanisms involved, for example, cell protection via scavenging of the reactive OH$^\bullet$ by lycopene (either by addition or hydrogen abstraction) followed by oxygen addition to give a reactive peroxyl neutral radical. The reactive peroxyl radical then causes the cell membrane destruction.

Whatever the precise molecular mechanism (e.g., involving one or more neutral lycopene radicals followed by oxygen addition) this huge difference in cell protection, due to oxygen concentration, may (with appropriate clinical techniques) lead to a mitigation of damage caused by radiation treatment of tumors. From a simplistic point of view (and following a high lycopene diet), flushing the tumor with oxygen should have no effect on the radiation therapy while flushing the non-necrotic regions, with say nitrogen, may led to significant protection against the unwanted radiation damage.

This oxygen addition reaction may also offer an alternative explanation for the damaging effect of high doses of β-carotene in heavy smokers (increase in lung cancers) discussed above. If the NO$_2^\bullet$ (or other radicals) present in cigarette smoke can also add to β-carotene (as well as oxidize it), then the high concentration of oxygen in the lungs will increase the likelihood of oxygen addition to the neutral radical adducts, producing a reactive carotenoid peroxyl radical. However, since it seems likely that the NO$_2^\bullet$ adduct (if formed) is short-lived, this may not be an important process [74], but, of course, it could be important for other radicals present in cigarette smoke.

Mildly oxidizing radicals, such as alkylperoxyl radicals, frequently react with carotenoids via adduct formation and/or hydrogen abstraction and generate a neutral carotenoid radical.

Hydrogen abstraction from a carotenoid to a free radical leads, of course, to the same carotenoid neutral radical as deprotonation of the corresponding radical cation

$$HCAR \rightarrow CAR^\bullet + H^\bullet$$

$$HCAR^{\bullet+} \rightarrow CAR^\bullet + H^+$$

and, as noted above there is interest in such neutral radicals because of their possible formation in PSII [67,69–71].

The detection of neutral radicals following hydrogen atom abstraction is not easy, but, as mentioned above, has been reported by Chen et al. [77] for OH$^\bullet$ reacting with β-carotene. This identification was based on an extremely weak and short-lived transient detected at 750 nm with a lifetime of around 150 ns—the assignment is partly based on the wavelength being in the region where neither the radical cation or radical adducts absorb.

The most recent study of hydrogen abstraction [80] concerned the extremely slow (over 10's of hours) reaction of an aroxy radical—2,6 di-t-butyl-4-(4′-methoxyphenyl)phenoxy (AO$^\bullet$, a rather stable radical used as a model for radicals of biological interest)—with fatty acids and with 6 carotenoids. The hydrogen abstraction rate constants were reported for astaxanthin (1), β-carotene (2), lycopene (3), capsanthin (4), zeaxanthin (5) and lutein (6). These rate constants increased in the order $1 < 2 < 3 < 4 < 5 < 6$ with values ranging from 8.3×10^{-4} dm^3 mol^{-1} s^{-1} for lutein to 2.2×10^{-4} dm^3 mol^{-1} s^{-1} for β-carotene. No value was given for the extremely slow reaction with astaxanthin. These values for the allylic hydrogen abstractions from the 6 carotenoids were explained in terms of the structures of the carotenoids and, in particular, the differing types of hydrogen atoms (based on their positions relative to π-electrons) in the parent carotenoid. It must be noted that the spectral changes reported in this work are very tiny indeed, typically from the data given, an absorption reduction of 0.025 for β-carotene after 22 h reaction time with AO$^\bullet$.

While more work on this potentially important route to neutral carotenoid radicals is worthwhile progress is hindered by the difficulties in detection of such radicals—the transient from OH$^\bullet$ reacting with β-carotene and the carotenoid spectral changes reported after reaction with AO$^\bullet$ being good examples of this problem.

4. Conclusions

The near infrared emission and subsequent decay of singlet oxygen is not difficult to study. Furthermore, the carotenoid/xanthophyll and retinoid radical cations are also not difficult to detect and study in appropriate solvents (the spectral properties, absorption and emission bands have virtually no experimental problems associated with spectral overlap). As a result, much is now understood of the reaction of carotenoids protective ability against photo-damage via singlet oxygen and also of the properties of carotenoid/xanthophyll and retinoid radical cations. These radical cations themselves are rather strongly oxidizing species and are able to oxidize other important bio-substrates. Regeneration of a parent C_{40} (dietary) carotenoid from the corresponding radical cation by reducing agents such as ascorbic acid has been reported. It has been suggested that detrimental effects of carotenoid radical cations (generated via environment pollutants, for example) on human health may arise when concentrations of reductants such as ascorbic acid are low. The other radicals of carotenoids, the neutral radicals formed via hydrogen abstraction processes or via radical addition, are more difficult to study for spectral and kinetic reasons. While a carotenoid radical cation does not react with oxygen, a neutral radical or a neutral radical adduct can add molecular oxygen to generate peroxyl radicals, which are likely to be damaging species.

Acknowledgments: The authors thank Fritz Boehm (Photobiology Research, IHZ, Berlin) for useful discussions.

References

1. Bensasson, R.V.; Land, E.J.; Truscott, T.G. *Excited States and Free Radicals in Biology and Medicine*; Oxford University Press: Oxford, UK, 1993; pp. 201–227.
2. Zhao, D.-Y.; Wintch, S.W.; Ermakov, I.V.; Gellermann, W.; Bernstein, P.S. Resonance Raman measurement of macular carotenoids in retinal, choroidal, and macular dystrophies. *Arch. Opthalmol.* **2003**, *121*, 967–972. [CrossRef] [PubMed]
3. Frank, H.A.; Cogdell, R.J. Carotenoids in photosynthesis. *Photochem. Photobiol.* **1996**, *63*, 257–264. [CrossRef] [PubMed]
4. Mathews-Roth, M.M. Treatment of erythropoietic protoporphyria with beta-carotene. *Photo-dermatology* **1984**, *1*, 318–321. [CrossRef] [PubMed]
5. Garone, M., Jr.; Howard, J.; Fabrikant, J. A review of common tanning methods. *J. Clin. Aesthet. Dermatol.* **2015**, *8*, 43–47. [PubMed]
6. Mukai, K.; Ouchi, A.; Azuma, N.; Takahashi, S.; Aizawa, K.; Nagaoka, S. Development of a singlet oxygen absorption capacity (SOAC) assay method. Measurements of the SOAC values for carotenoids and α-tocopherol in an aqueous Triton X-100 micellar solution. *J. Agric. Food Chem.* **2017**, *65*, 784–792. [CrossRef] [PubMed]
7. Bensasson, R.V.; Land, E.J. Intersystem crossing efficiencies of retinal isomers in different solvents measured by laser flash absorption spectrophotometry. *Nouv. J. Chim.* **1978**, *2*, 503–507.
8. Bensasson, R.V.; Land, E.J.; Truscott, T.G. *Flash Photolysis and Pulse Radiolysis*; Pergamon Press: Oxford, UK, 1983; pp. 67–92.
9. Dillon, J.; Gaillard, E.R.; Bilski, P.; Chignell, C.F.; Reszka, K.J. The photochemistry of the retinoids as studied by steady-state and pulsed methods. *Photochem. Photobiol.* **1996**, *63*, 680–685. [CrossRef] [PubMed]
10. Becker, R.S.; Freedman, K.; Lenoble, C. Photophysical and photochemical behavior of 11-*cis*-retinal and its Schiff base in a micelle. *J. Phys. Chem.* **1986**, *90*, 4334–4336. [CrossRef]
11. Ferguson, J.; Johnson, B.E. Photosensitivity due to retinoids: Clinical and laboratory. *Br. J. Dermatol.* **1986**, *115*, 275–283. [CrossRef]
12. Lo, K.K.N.; Land, E.J.; Truscott, T.G. Primary intermediates in the pulsed irradiation of retinoids. *Photochem. Photobiol.* **1982**, *36*, 139–145. [CrossRef]
13. Tolleson, W.H.; Cherng, S.-H.; Xia, Q.; Boudreau, M.; Yin, J.J.; Wamer, W.G.; Howard, P.C.; Yu, H.; Fu, P.P. Photodecomposition and phototoxicity of natural retinoids. *Int. J. Environ. Res. Public Health* **2005**, *2*, 147–155. [CrossRef] [PubMed]

14. Rosenfeld, T.; Alchalal, A.; Ottolenghi, M. Primary photoprocesses in retinol. *Chem. Phys. Lett.* **1973**, *20*, 291–297. [CrossRef]

15. Collins, C.M.; Leventis, N.; Sotiriou-Leventis, C. Relative reactivity of vitamin A versus a mixture of β-carotene geometric isomers with electrochemically generated superoxide and hydroperoxyl radicals. *Electrochimica Acta* **2001**, *47*, 567–576. [CrossRef]

16. Różanowska, M.; Cantrell, A.; Edge, R.; Land, E.J.; Sarna, T.; Truscott, T.G. Pulse radiolysis study of the interaction of retinoids with peroxyl radicals. *Free Radic. Biol. Med.* **2005**, *39*, 1399–1405. [CrossRef] [PubMed]

17. Böhm, F.; Edge, R.; Land, E.J.; McGarvey, D.J.; Truscott, T.G. Carotenoids enhance vitamin E antioxidant efficiency. *J. Am. Chem. Soc.* **1997**, *119*, 621–622. [CrossRef]

18. El-Agamey, A.; Fukuzumi, S.; Naqvi, K.R.; McGarvey, D.J. Kinetic studies of retinol addition radicals. *Org. Biomol. Chem.* **2011**, *9*, 1459–1465. [CrossRef] [PubMed]

19. Aveline, B.M.; Kochevar, I.E.; Redmond, R.W. Photochemistry of the nonspecific hydroxyl radical generator, N-hydroxypyridine-2(1H)-thione. *J. Am. Chem. Soc.* **1996**, *118*, 10113–10123. [CrossRef]

20. El-Agamey, A.; McGarvey, D.J. First direct observation of reversible oxygen addition to a carotenoid-derived carbon-centered neutral radical. *Org. Lett.* **2005**, *7*, 3957–3960. [CrossRef] [PubMed]

21. El-Agamey, A.; McGarvey, D.J. The reactivity of carotenoid radicals with oxygen. *Free Radic. Res.* **2007**, *41*, 295–302. [CrossRef] [PubMed]

22. El-Agamey, A.; Fukuzumi, S. Laser flash photolysis study on the retinol radical cation in polar solvents. *Org. Biomol. Chem.* **2011**, *9*, 6437–6446. [CrossRef] [PubMed]

23. El-Agamey, A.; Melø, T.B.; Sliwka, H.-R. Exploring the reactivity of retinol radical cation toward organic and biological molecules: A laser flash photolysis study. *J. Photochem. Photobiol. B Biol.* **2017**, *170*, 33–39. [CrossRef] [PubMed]

24. Gorman, A.A.; Rodgers, M.A.J. Singlet molecular oxygen. *Chem. Soc. Rev.* **1981**, *10*, 205–231. [CrossRef]

25. Piette, J. Biological consequences associated with DNA oxidation mediated by singlet oxygen. *J. Photochem. Photobiol.* **1991**, *11*, 241–260. [CrossRef]

26. Girotti, A.W. Photodynamic lipid peroxidation in biological systems. *Photochem. Photobiol.* **1990**, *51*, 497–509. [CrossRef] [PubMed]

27. Minami, Y.; Yokoyama, K.; Bando, N.; Kawai, Y.; Terao, J. Occurance of singlet oxygen oxygenation of oleic acid and linoleic acid in the skin of live mice. *Free Radic. Res.* **2008**, *42*, 197–204. [CrossRef] [PubMed]

28. Davies, M.J.; Truscott, R.J.W. Photo-oxidation of proteins and its role in cataractogenesis. *J. Photochem. Photobiol. B Biol.* **2001**, *63*, 114–125. [CrossRef]

29. Badger, R.M.; Wright, A.C.; Whitlock, R.F. Absolute intensities of the discrete and continuous absorption bands of oxygen gas at 1.26 and 1.065 μ and the radiative lifetime of the $^1\Delta_g$ state of oxygen. *J. Chem. Phys.* **1965**, *43*, 4345–4350. [CrossRef]

30. Foote, C.S.; Denny, R.W. Chemistry of singlet oxygen. VII. Quenching by β-carotene. *J. Am. Chem. Soc.* **1968**, *90*, 6233–6235. [CrossRef]

31. Farmilo, A.; Wilkinson, F. On the mechanism of quenching of singlet oxygen in solution. *Photochem. Photobiol.* **1973**, *18*, 447–450. [CrossRef] [PubMed]

32. Fiedor, J.; Fiedor, L.; Haeβner, R.; Scheer, H. Cyclic endoperoxides of β-carotene, potential pro-oxidants, as products of chemical quenching of singlet oxygen. *Biochim. Biophys. Acta* **2005**, *1709*, 1–4. [CrossRef] [PubMed]

33. Nishino, A.; Yasui, H.; Maoka, T. Reaction and scavenging mechanism of β-carotene and zeaxanthin with reactive oxygen species. *J. Oleo Sci.* **2017**, *66*, 77–84. [CrossRef] [PubMed]

34. Liebler, D.C. Antioxidant reactions of carotenoids. *Ann. N. Y. Acad. Sci.* **1993**, *691*, 20–31. [CrossRef] [PubMed]

35. Oliveros, E.; Braun, A.M.; Aminian-Saghafi, T.; Sliwka, H.R. Quenching of singlet oxygen (1Δg) by carotenoid derivatives: Kinetic analysis by near infra-red luminescence. *New J. Chem.* **1994**, *18*, 535–539.

36. Edge, R.; McGarvey, D.J.; Truscott, T.G. The carotenoids as antioxidants—A review. *J. Photochem. Photobiol. B Biol.* **1997**, *41*, 189–200. [CrossRef]

37. Di Mascio, P.; Kaiser, S.; Sies, H. Lycopene as the most efficient biological carotenoid singlet oxygen quencher. *Arch. Biochem. Biophys.* **1989**, *274*, 532–538. [CrossRef]

38. Weedon, B.C.L.; Moss, C.P. Structure and nomenclature. In *Carotenoids: Isolation and Analysis*; Britton, G., Liaaen-Jensen, S., Pfander, H., Eds.; Birkhäuser: Basel, Switzerland, 1995; Volume 1A, pp. 27–70.

39. Cantrell, A.; McGarvey, D.J.; Truscott, T.G. Singlet oxygen quenching by dietary carotenoids in a model membrane environment. *Arch. Biochem. Biophys.* **2003**, *412*, 47–54. [CrossRef]

40. Nishino, A.; Yasui, H.; Maoka, T. Reaction of paprika carotenoids, capsanthin and capsrubin, with reactive oxygen species. *J. Agric. Food Chem.* **2016**, *64*, 4786–4792. [CrossRef] [PubMed]

41. Burke, M. Pulsed Radiation Studies of Carotenoid Radicals and Excited States. Ph.D Thesis, Keele University, Staffordshire, UK, April 2001.

42. Edge, R.; Truscott, T.G. Properties of carotenoid radicals and excited states and their potential role in biological systems. In *Carotenoids. Physical, Chemical, and Biological Functions and Properties*; Landrum, J.T., Ed.; CRC Press: Boca Raton, FL, USA, 2010; pp. 283–307.

43. Teraoka, J.; Hashimoto, H.; Matsudaira, S.; Koyama, Y. Resonance Raman spectra of excited triplet states of β-carotene isomers. *Chem. Lett.* **1985**, *14*, 311–314. [CrossRef]

44. Heymann, T.; Heinz, P.; Glomb, M.A. Lycopene inhibits the isomerization of β-carotene during quenching of singlet oxygen and free radicals. *J. Agric. Food. Chem.* **2015**, *63*, 3279–3287. [CrossRef] [PubMed]

45. Fukuzawa, K. Singlet oxygen scavenging in phospholipid membranes. *Methods Enzymol.* **2000**, *319*, 101–110. [PubMed]

46. Fukuzawa, K.; Inokami, Y.; Tokumura, A.; Terao, J.; Suzuki, A. Rate constants for quenching singlet oxygen and activities for inhibiting lipid peroxidation of carotenoids and α-tocopherol in liposomes. *Lipids* **1998**, *33*, 751–756. [CrossRef] [PubMed]

47. Morita, M.; Naito, Y.; Yoshikawa, T.; Niki, E. Rapid assessment of singlet oxygen-induced plasma lipid oxidation and its inhibition by antioxidants with diphenyl-1-pyrenylphosphine (DPPP). *Anal. Bioanal. Chem.* **2016**, *408*, 265–270. [CrossRef] [PubMed]

48. Sachindra, N.M.; Sato, E.; Maeda, H.; Hosokawa, M.; Niwano, Y.; Kohno, M.; Miyashita, K. Radical scavenging and singlet oxygen quenching activity of marine carotenoid fucoxanthin and its metabolites. *J. Agric. Food Chem.* **2007**, *55*, 8516–8522. [CrossRef] [PubMed]

49. Telfer, A.; Dhami, S.; Bishop, S.M.; Phillips, D.; Barber, J. β-Carotene quenches singlet oxygen formed in isolated photosystem II reaction centers. *Biochemistry* **1994**, *33*, 14469–14474. [CrossRef] [PubMed]

50. Böhm, F.; Haley, J.; Truscott, T.G.; Schalch, W. Cellular bound β-carotene quenches singlet oxygen in man. *J. Photochem. Photobiol. B Biol.* **1993**, *21*, 219–221. [CrossRef]

51. Tinkler, J.H.; Böhm, F.; Schalch, W.; Truscott, T.G. Dietary carotenoids protect human cells from damage. *J. Photochem. Photobiol. B Biol.* **1994**, *26*, 283–285. [CrossRef]

52. Boehm, F.; Edge, R.; Burke, M.; Truscott, T.G. Dietary uptake of lycopene protects human cells from singlet oxygen and nitrogen dioxide—ROS components from cigarette smoke. *J. Photochem. Photobiol. B Biol.* **2001**, *64*, 176–178. [CrossRef]

53. Bosio, G.N.; Breitenbach, T.; Parisi, J.; Reigosa, M.; Blaikie, F.H.; Pedersen, B.W.; Silva, E.F.F.; Martire, D.O.; Ogilvy, P.R. Antioxidant β-carotene does not quench singlet oxygen in mammalian cells. *J. Am. Chem. Soc.* **2013**, *135*, 272–279. [CrossRef] [PubMed]

54. Da Silva, E.F.F.; Pedersen, B.W.; Breitenbach, T.; Toftegaard, R.; Kuimova, M.K.; Arnaut, L.G.; Ogilvy, P.R. Irradiation- and sensitizer-dependent changes in the lifetime of intracellular singlet oxygen produced in a photosensitized process. *J. Phys. Chem. B* **2012**, *116*, 445–461. [CrossRef] [PubMed]

55. Wilkinson, F.; Helman, W.P.; Ross, A.B. Rate constants for the decay and reactions of the lowest electronically excited singlet state of molecular oxygen in solution. An expanded and revised compilation. *J. Phys. Chem. Ref. Data* **1995**, *24*, 663–1021. [CrossRef]

56. Böhm, F.; Edge, R.; Truscott, T.G. Interactions of dietary carotenoids with activated (singlet) oxygen and free radicals: Potential effects for human health. *Mol. Nutr. Food Res.* **2012**, *56*, 205–216. [CrossRef] [PubMed]

57. Álvarez, R.; Vaz, B.; Gronemayer, H.; de Lera, A.R. Functions, therapeutic applications, and synthesis of retinoids and carotenoids. *Chem. Rev.* **2014**, *114*, 1–125. [CrossRef] [PubMed]

58. Boehm, F.; Edge, R.; Truscott, T.G.; Witt, C. Photoprotection and radiation protection by dietary carotenoids. In *Carotenoids—Nutrition, Analysis and Technology*; Kaczor, A., Baranska, M., Eds.; John Wiley & Sons: Chichester, UK, 2016; pp. 43–58.

59. Land, E.J.; Lafferty, J.; Roach, A.C.; Sinclair, R.S.; Truscott, T.G. Absorption spectra of radical ions of polyenes of biological interest. *J. Chem. Soc. Faraday Trans.* **1977**, *73*, 416–429.

60. Edge, R.; Land, E.J.; McGarvey, D.J.; Burke, M.; Truscott, T.G. The reduction potential of the β-carotene$^{\bullet+}$/β-carotene couple in an aqueous micro-heterogeneous environment. *FEBS Lett.* **2000**, *471*, 125–127. [CrossRef]

61. Burke, M.; Edge, R.; Land, E.J.; McGarvey, D.J.; Truscott, T.G. One-electron reduction potentials of dietary carotenoid radical cations in aqueous micellar environments. *FEBS Lett.* **2001**, *500*, 132–136. [CrossRef]

62. Tinkler, J.H.; Tavender, S.M.; Parker, A.W.; McGarvey, D.J.; Mulroy, L.; Truscott, T.G. An investigation of carotenoid radical cations and triplet states by laser flash photolysis and time-resolved resonance Raman spectroscopy: Observation of competitive energy and electron transfer. *J. Am. Chem. Soc.* **1996**, *118*, 1756–1761. [CrossRef]

63. Cheng, H.; Han, R.-M.; Lyu, M.-K.; Zhang, J.-P.; Skibsted, L.H. Regeneration of β-carotene from the radical cation by tyrosine and tryptophan. *J. Phys. Chem. B* **2015**, *119*, 6603–6610. [CrossRef] [PubMed]

64. Chang, H.-T.; Cheng, H.; Han, R.-M.; Wang, P.; Zhang, J.-P.; Skibsted, L.H. Regeneration of β-carotene from radical cation by eugenol, isoeugenol, and clove oil in the Marcus theory inverted region for electron transfer. *J. Agric. Food Chem.* **2017**, *65*, 908–912. [CrossRef] [PubMed]

65. Mairanovsky, V.G.; Engovatov, A.A.; Ioffe, N.T.; Samokhvalov, G.I. Electron-donor and electron-acceptor properties of carotenoids: Electrochemical study of carotenes. *J. Electroanal. Chem.* **1975**, *66*, 122–137. [CrossRef]

66. Focsan, A.L.; Pan, S.; Kispert, L.D. Electrochemical study of astaxanthin and astaxanthin n-octanoic monoester and diester: Tendency to form radicals. *J. Phys. Chem. B* **2014**, *118*, 2331–3229. [CrossRef] [PubMed]

67. Focsan, A.L.; Magyar, A.; Kispert, L.D. Chemistry of carotenoid neutral radicals. *Arch. Biochem. Biophys.* **2015**, *572*, 167–174. [CrossRef] [PubMed]

68. El-Agamey, A.; El-Hagrasy, M.A.; Suenobu, T.; Fukuzumi, S. Influence of pH on the decay of β-carotene radical cation in aqueous Triton X-100: A laser flash photolysis study. *J. Photochem. Photobiol. B Biol.* **2015**, *146*, 68–73. [CrossRef] [PubMed]

69. Focsan, A.L.; Kispert, L.D. Radicals formed from proton loss of carotenoid radical cations: A special form of carotenoid neutral radical occurring in photoprotection. *J. Photochem. Photobiol. B Biol.* **2017**, *166*, 148–157. [CrossRef] [PubMed]

70. Gao, Y.; Shinopoulos, K.E.; Tracewell, C.A.; Focsan, A.L.; Brudvig, G.W.; Kispert, L.D. Formation of carotenoid neutral radicals in Photosystem II. *J. Phys. Chem. B* **2009**, *113*, 9901–9908. [CrossRef] [PubMed]

71. Magyar, A.; Bowman, M.K.; Molnar, P.; Kiapert, L. Neutral carotenoid radicals in photoprotection of wild-type *Arabidopsis thaliana*. *J. Phys. Chem. B* **2013**, *117*, 2239–2246. [CrossRef] [PubMed]

72. El-Agamey, A.; McGarvey, D.J. Peroxyl radical reactions with carotenoids in microemulsions: Influence of microemulsion composition and the nature of peroxyl radical precursor. *Free Radic. Biol. Med.* **2016**, *90*, 75–84. [CrossRef] [PubMed]

73. El-Agamey, A.; Edge, R.; Navaratnam, S.; Land, E.J.; Truscott, T.G. Carotenoid radical anions and their protonated derivatives. *Org. Lett.* **2006**, *8*, 4255–4258. [CrossRef] [PubMed]

74. Everett, S.A.; Patel, K.B.; Maddix, S.; Kundu, S.C.; Willson, R.L. Scavenging of nitrogen dioxide, thiyl, and sulfonyl free radicals by the nutritional antioxidant β-carotene. *J. Biol. Chem.* **1996**, *271*, 3988–3994. [CrossRef] [PubMed]

75. Mortensen, A.; Skibsted, L.H. Kinetics of photobleaching of β-carotene in chloroform and formation of transient carotenoid species absorbing in the near infrared. *Free Radic. Res.* **1996**, *25*, 355–368. [CrossRef]

76. Koppenol, W.H. Generation and thermodynamic properties of oxyradicals. In *CRC Critical Reviews in Membrane Lipid Oxidation*, 2nd ed.; Vigo-Pelfrety, C., Ed.; CRC Press: Boca Raton, FL, USA, 1989; Volume 1, pp. 1–13.

77. Chen, C.-H.; Han, R.-M.; Liang, R.; Fu, L.-M.; Wang, P.; Ai, X.-C.; Zhang, J.-P.; Skibsted, L.H. Direct observation of the β-carotene reaction with hydroxyl radical. *J. Phys. Chem. B* **2011**, *115*, 2082–2089. [CrossRef] [PubMed]

78. Burton, G.W.; Ingold, K.U. beta-Carotene: An unusual type of lipid antioxidant. *Science* **1984**, *224*, 569–573. [CrossRef] [PubMed]

79. Boehm, F.; Edge, R.; Truscott, T.G.; Witt, C. A dramatic effect of oxygen on protection of human cells against γ-radiation by lycopene. *FEBS Lett.* **2016**, *590*, 1086–1093. [CrossRef] [PubMed]

80. Mukai, K.; Yoshimoto, M.; Ishikura, M.; Nagaoka, S. Kinetic study of the aroxyl-radical-scavenging activity of five fatty acid esters and six carotenoids in toluene solution: Structure-activity relationship for the hydrogen abstraction reaction. *J. Phys. Chem. B* **2017**, *121*, 7593–7601. [CrossRef] [PubMed]

2

Inhibitory Effects of Solvent-Partitioned Fractions of Two Nigerian Herbs (*Spondias mombin* Linn. and *Mangifera indica* L.) on α-Amylase and α-Glucosidase

Oluwafemi Adeleke Ojo [1,2,*] (iD), Adeola Agnes Afon [1], Adebola Busola Ojo [3] (iD),
Basiru Olaitan Ajiboye [1] (iD), Babatunji Emmanuel Oyinloye [1,4] (iD) and Abidemi Paul Kappo [4] (iD)

[1] Phytomedicine, Biomedical Toxicology and Diabetes Research Laboratories, Department of Biochemistry,
Afe Babalola University, Ado-Ekiti 360001, Nigeria; adeolabunmi24@gmail.com (A.A.A.);
ajiboyebo@abuad.edu.ng (B.O.A.); babatunjioe@abuad.edu.ng (B.E.O.)

[2] Department of Biochemistry, University of Ilorin, Ilorin 240222, Nigeria

[3] Department of Medical Biochemistry, Afe Babalola University, Ado-Ekiti 360001, Nigeria;
ojoab@abuad.edu.ng

[4] Biotechnology and Structural Biology (BSB) Group, Department of Biochemistry and Microbiology,
University of Zululand, KwaDlangezwa 3886, South Africa; kappoA@unizulu.ac.za

*   Correspondence: ojooa@abuad.edu.ng

Abstract: Therapies directed towards controlling hyperglycemia, the hallmark of type-2 diabetes mellitus, go a long way in managing diabetes and its related complications. Reducing glucose level through the inhibition of the relevant carbohydrate hydrolyzing enzymes is one among many routes in the management of diabetes. This study investigates the *in vitro* enzyme inhibitory and antioxidant properties of solvent-partitioned fractions of *Spondias mombin* and *Mangifera indica* leaves; which are used extensively in the treatment of diabetic patients locally. The leaves of *S. mombin* and *M. indica* were extracted with methanol and fractionated to obtain *n*-hexane (HF), ethyl acetate (EAF), *n*-butanol (BF), and aqueous (AF) fractions successively. The α-amylase and α-glucosidase inhibitory activities of fractions of *S. mombin* and *M. indica* leaves were investigated while the antioxidant activity of each fraction was analyzed using iron chelating and ABTS (2,2′-azino-bis(3-ethylbenzothiazoline)-6-sulphonic acid) radical scavenging assay. Our findings indicated that the ethyl acetate fraction of *M. indica* leaves contained a considerably higher ($p < 0.05$) amount of total phenolic, flavonoids, metal ion, and ABTS radical scavenging activity than the ethyl acetate fractions of *S. mombin*. Furthermore, the ethyl acetate fraction of *M. indica* had a considerably higher ($p < 0.05$) inhibitory effect on α-glucosidase ($IC_{50} = 25.11 \pm 0.01$ μg mL^{-1}), and α-amylase ($IC_{50} = 24.04 \pm 0.12$ μg mL^{-1}) activities than the *S. mombin* fraction. Hence, the inhibitory activities of *S. mombin* and *M. indica* leaves suggest that they are a potential source of orally active antidiabetic agents and could be employed to formulate new plant-based pharmaceutical and nutraceutical drugs to improve human health.

Keywords: *Spondias mombin*; *Mangifera indica*; α-amylase; α-glucosidase; antioxidant activity

1. Introduction

Diabetes mellitus (DM) is a major public health problem. The projected prevalence among adults in 2015 was 8.8%, affecting about 415 million adults. The prevalence of diabetes has been predicted to increase to about 10.4% by 2040 [1]. The recent exponential increase in the prevalence of this chronic disease requires a multiple therapeutic approach in the search of a real solution for diabetes and this includes the development of other alternative or complementary medications. Evidence from traditional prescription and scientific investigation reveals optimum therapeutic efficacy of medicinal plants with a good margin of safety. Since medicinal plants form a major part of human food, it is worthwhile to evaluate their inhibitory activity against hyperglycemia [2,3].

Hyperglycemia is considered the major basis for many problems in the diabetic state. Meanwhile, carbohydrates are the main sources of blood glucose and inhibition of relevant enzymes such as α-amylase and α-glucosidase associated with non-insulin dependent diabetes mellitus is vital in preventing sudden increase in blood glucose. Hence, the inhibition of theses enzymes is the reason why the digestion process of carbohydrates can be retarded and the absorption rate of glucose from the gut decreased to result in an extreme low level of blood glucose. As it was previously mentioned, the ability to maintain low blood glucose level is the hallmark of the treatment of diabetes. Although, this may be accomplished via the use of a standard therapy regimen such as biguanides and insulin secretagogues, the inhibition of α-amylase and α-glucosidase is another key therapeutic approach to be explored in order to improve glycemic control [4,5]. Additional searches for plant-based antidiabetic components would be valuable as revealed by their prominent role in some of the presently accessible orthodox drugs [6].

Spondias mombin L. (Anarcadiaceae) is called "Hog plum", "*Iyeye*" and "*Olosan*" (Yoruba) [7]. It is a tree with giant panicles of little white flowers, frequent in farmland and villages, particularly within the forest region in addition to the savannah. In traditional practice, *S. mombin* is employed in curing duodenal disorders, gonorrhoea, diabetes, psychiatric disorders, and for the removal of the placenta in childbirth. In addition, it is used as an antidiarrheal agent [8], and as an antimicrobial agent as well as for the healing of wounds [9–11]. Iweala and Oludare, also reported the hypoglycemic effects, as well as the biochemical and histological changes of the ethanolic extract of *Spondias mombin* in alloxan-induced diabetic rats [12]. Pelandjuaic acid, ellagitannins, caffeoyl esters, and anacardic acid are reported to be present in *S. mombim* [13–15].

Mangifera indica L. (Anacardiaceae) called "Mango", "*Mangoro*" (Yoruba) is a perennial tree prevalent in rural and semi-urban parts of Nigeria. It is one of the vital tropical plants marketed in the world [16]. It is grown largely in several parts of Africa, particularly in the western parts of Nigeria, where it is valued for its edible fruits. There are numerous conventional uses for the bark, roots, and leaves of *M. indica* throughout the globe. *M. indica* is used therapeutically to cure several ailments such as asthma, cough, diarrhea, dysentery, leucorrhoea, jaundice, pain, and malaria. Phytochemical studies from different parts of *M. indica* have revealed the presence of phenolic constituents, triterpenes, flavonoids, phytosterol, and polyphenols [17]. *M. indica* is believed to possess several therapeutic uses including analgesic, anti-inflammatory, antimicrobial as well as immune-stimulant, antioxidant and antilipidemic applications [18,19]. Ethanol extract of *M. indica* peel has been investigated and reported to inhibit α-amylase and α-glucosidase activities, and to ameliorate diabetes related biochemical parameters in streptozotocin (STZ)-induced diabetic rats [20]. Previous studies have reported extraction of different chemical compounds such as phenolic acid 6-alkenyl-salicylic acid, anarcardic acid, chlorogenic acid, ellagic acid, betulin, coumaroyl, quercetin, and gallic acid from *S. mombin*, which exhibited different biological activities including antidiabetic, anti-inflammatory and anti-oxidant effects [15,21–24]. On the other hand, studies have reported that bioactive compounds identified from *M. indica* leaves include quercetin and chlorogenic acid which possess anti-oxidant, anti-inflammatory, and antidiabetic activities [25]. The current study aimed to investigate the *in vitro* enzyme inhibitory activities and antioxidant properties of the *S. mombin* and *M. indica* leaf solvent-partitioned fractions as potential therapeutic sources, which may be helpful in attaining the normoglycemic state in the diabetic condition.

2. Materials and Methods

2.1. Chemicals

All chemical agents and standards were of analytical grade reagents unless otherwise stated. Folin–Ciocalteu's reagent and methanol were purchased from Merck (Darmstadt, Germany). ABTS radical cation (2,2'-azino-bis(3-ethylbenzothiazoline)-6-sulphonic acid), DTNB (5,5-dithio-bis (2-nitrobenzoic) acid), acarbose, α-amylase, and α-glucosidase were purchased from Sigma-Aldrich (Steinheim, Germany).

2.2. Plant Material and Extraction Procedure

Fresh leaves of *S. mombin* and *M. indica* were obtained from Ibadan in Nigeria in September 2017. Fresh leaves of *S. mombin* and *M. indica* were identified and documented by Mr. Odewo from Forestry Research Institute of Nigeria (FRIN) with Forest Herbarium Ibadan: FHI 111312 and FHI 111313, respectively as the herbarium number deposited. The fresh leaves were air-dried at normal room temperature and humidity for three weeks and ground to powder using a mechanical blender. To obtain methanol extracts, 100 g of air-dried leaves were soaked with 800 mL of methanol and 200 mL of water for 48 h [26]. The methanol extract obtained was concentrated using a rotary evaporator and stored until use.

2.3. Solvent-Partitioned Fractionation of Crude Methanol Extracts

Methanol leaves extract of *S. mombin* (9 g) and *M. indica* (15.5 g) was solubilized in 200 mL of distilled water and sequentially extracted with solvents of increasing polarity (hexane, ethyl acetate, and *n*-butanol). Methanol extract was partitioned between *n*-hexane (2 × 200 mL) and water to obtain an *n*-hexane fraction (HF) and an aqueous portion. The aqueous portion obtained was further partitioned by ethyl acetate (2 × 200 mL) to obtain an ethyl acetate fraction (EAF) and an aqueous portion. The aqueous portion obtained was further partitioned by *n*-butanol (2 × 200 mL) to obtain an *n*-butanol fraction (BF) and a residual aqueous fraction (AF).

2.4. α-Amylase Inhibitory Activity of Fractions of S. mombin and M. indica Leaves

Alpha-amylase activity was assessed concurring to the protocol described by [27] with slight modification by [28]. A volume of 300 µL of *S. mombin* and *M. indica* leaf fractions (HF, EAF, BF, AF) at different concentrations (10–150 µg mL^{-1}) was incubated with 500 µL of porcine pancreatic amylase (2 U mL^{-1}) in 100 mmol L^{-1} phosphate buffer (pH 6.8) at 37 °C for 20 min. Three hundred µL of 1% starch dissolved in 100 mmol L^{-1} phosphate buffer (pH 6.8) was then added to the mixture and incubated at 37 °C for 1 h. One mL of dinitrosalicylic acid (DNS) color was then added to the solution and boiled for 10 min. The absorbance of the ensuing mixture was read at 540 nm and the enzyme inhibitory activity was calculated as percentage of control sample without inhibitors. Acarbose was used as standard.

$$\alpha - \text{amylase inhibition } (\%) = \frac{A_{540\text{control}} - A_{540\text{sample}}}{A_{540\text{control}}} \times 100$$

$A_{540\text{control}}$: Absorbance of control at 540 nm; $A_{540\text{sample}}$: Absorbance of sample at 540 nm

2.5. α-Glucosidase Inhibitory Activity of Fractions of S. mombin and M. indica Leaves

Alpha-glucosidase inhibitory activity was determined in line with the protocol by [29], with small alterations by [30]. Briefly, 300 µL of *S. mombin* and *M. indica* leaf fractions (HF, EAF, BF, AF), at varying concentrations (10–150 µg mL^{-1}), was mixed with 500 µL of 1.0 U mL^{-1} α-glucosidase solution in 100 mmol L^{-1} phosphate buffer (pH 6.8) at 37 °C for 15 min. Afterwards, 300 µL of p-nitrophenyl-α-D-glucopyranoside (pNPG) solution (5 mmol L^{-1}) in 100 mmol L^{-1} phosphate buffer (pH 6.8) was added and then the solution was further mixed at 37 °C for 20 min. Absorbance of the free p-nitrophenol was read at 405 nm and then the inhibitory activity was expressed as percentage of a the control sample. Acarbose was used as standard.

$$\alpha - \text{glucosidase inhibition } (\%) = \frac{A_{405control} - A_{405sample}}{A_{405control}} \times 100$$

$A_{405control}$: Absorbance of control at 405 nm; $A_{405sample}$: Absorbance of sample at 405 nm

2.6. Estimation of Total Phenol Content

S. mombin and *M. indica* phenol content of the leaf fractions (HF, EAF, BF, AF) was estimated as described by [31]. In short, 200 µL fractions (HF, EAF, BF, AF) dispersed in 10% dimethylsulfoxide (DMSO) (240 µg mL^{-1}) was incubated with 1.0 mL of Folin Ciocalteau (diluted 10 times) and 800 µL of 0.7 mol L^{-1} Na$_2$CO$_3$ for 30 min. Absorbance was read at 765 nm and all readings were in triplicate with results expressed as mg gallic acid equivalents (GAE)/100 g dry fractions.

2.7. Estimation of Flavonoid Content

S. mombin and *M. indica* leaf fractions (HF, EAF, BF, AF) were estimated for flavonoid content using the procedure described by [32]. Briefly, 0.5 mL of suitably diluted sample was mixed with 0.5 mL methanol, 50 µL 10% AlCl$_3$, 50 µL 1 M potassium acetate, and 1.4 mL water, and incubated at room temperature for 30 min. Absorbance of the solution was read at 415 nm. All experiments were in triplicate.

2.8. Evaluation of Antioxidant Activities of Fractions of S. mombin and M. indica Leaves

2.8.1. Iron (Fe^{2+}) Chelation

The metal chelating property of *S. mombin* and *M. indica* leaf fractions (HF, EAF, BF, AF) was determined by employing an altered procedure of [33]. Freshly prepared 500 µmol L^{-1} FeSO$_4$ (150 µL) was mixed to the solution comprising 168 µL of 0.1 mol L^{-1} Tris-HCl (pH 7.4), 218 µL saline, the aqueous extract (10–150 µL), and the fractions. The solution was incubated for 5 min, with addition of 13 µL of 0.25% (*w/v*) of 1,10-phenanthroline. Ethylenediaminetetraacetic acid (EDTA) was used as standard. Absorbance was read at 510 nm.

2.8.2. Estimation of 2,2-Azino-bis3-ethylbenthiazoline-6sulphonic acid (ABTS) Radical Scavenging Ability

S. mombin and *M. indica* leaf fractions (HF, EAF, BF, AF) were assessed primarily based on the ability to scavenge ABTS using the protocol delineated by [34]. The ABTS was produced by reacting 7 mM ABTS aqueous solution with K$_2$S$_2$O$_8$ (2.45 mM) in the dark for 16 h and altering the absorbance at 734 nm. Afterward, 200 µL of suitable dilution of extracts and fractions was added to 2.0 mL ABTS solution. Vitamin C was used as standard. Absorbances were read at 734 nm after 15 min.

2.9. Data Analysis

Results were expressed as the mean ± standard error of mean (SEM) of triplicates [35] from independent samples. Level of significance was set to $p < 0.05$. These analyses were presented using one-way analysis of variance (ANOVA) using SPSS version 21.0 (IBM Corporation, NY, USA).

3. Results

3.1. Inhibitory Effect of Various Fractions of S. mombin and M. indica Leaves against α-Amylase

Figure 1 shows the inhibition percentage of α-amylase by various fractions of crude methanol extract of *S. mombin*, *M. indica* leaves and standard drug acarbose. The *M. indica* fractions had appreciable *in vitro* inhibitory activity against α-amylase in a fashion, with the ethyl acetate fraction ($IC_{50} = 24.04 \pm 0.12$ μg mL^{-1}) showing a considerably better ($p < 0.05$) α-amylase inhibitory activity than *S. mombim* leaf ($IC_{50} = 28.12 \pm 0.48$ μg mL^{-1}) fractions. However, acarbose had the highest activity against α-amylase as shown by the IC_{50} (22.08 ± 0.03 μg mL^{-1}).

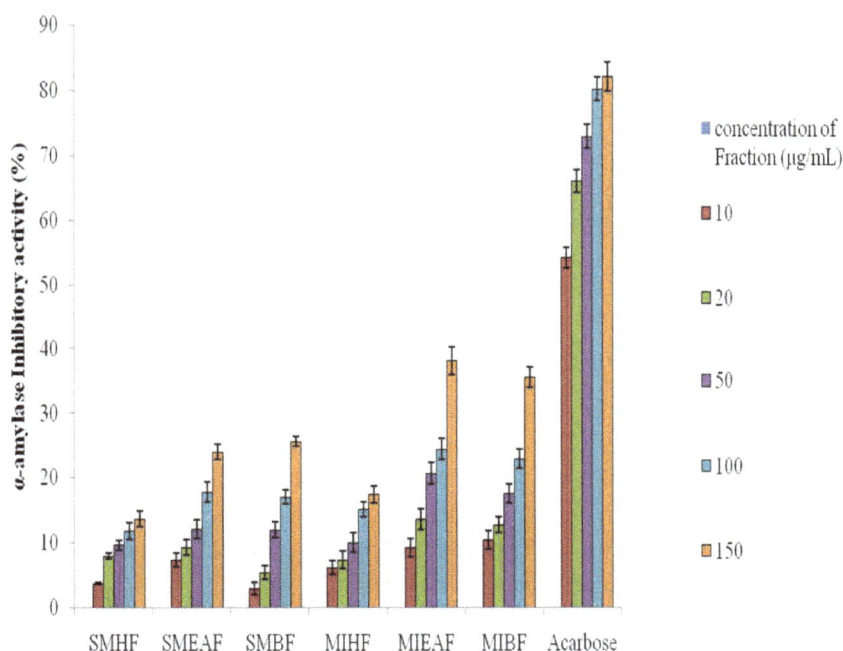

Figure 1. Alpha-amylase inhibitory activity of fractions of *S. mombin* and *M. indica* leaves. Legends: SMHF: *S. mombin* n-hexane fraction; SMEAF: *S. mombin* ethyl acetate fraction; SMBF: *S. mombin* n-butanol fraction; MIHF: *M. indica* n-hexane fraction; MIEAF: *M. indica* ethyl acetate fraction; MIBF: *M. indica* n-butanol fraction.

3.2. Inhibitory Effect of Various Fractions of S. mombin and M. indica Leaves against α-Glucosidase

Figure 2 shows the percentage inhibition of α-glucosidase by various fractions of crude methanol extract of *S. mombin* and *M. indica* leaves. The *M. indica* fractions inhibited α-glucosidase activities in vitro. The ethyl acetate fraction displays a better inhibition of α-glucosidase activity compared to other fractions. Notably, the inhibitory activity of the ethyl acetate fraction of *M. indica* ($IC_{50} = 25.11 \pm 0.01$ μg mL^{-1}) was considerably higher ($p < 0.05$) than *S. mombim* ($IC_{50} = 12.05 \pm 0.02$ μg mL^{-1}) fraction as indicated by their IC_{50} values. However, acarbose had a better inhibitory activity against α-glucosidase than *S. mombin* and *M. indica* leaves.

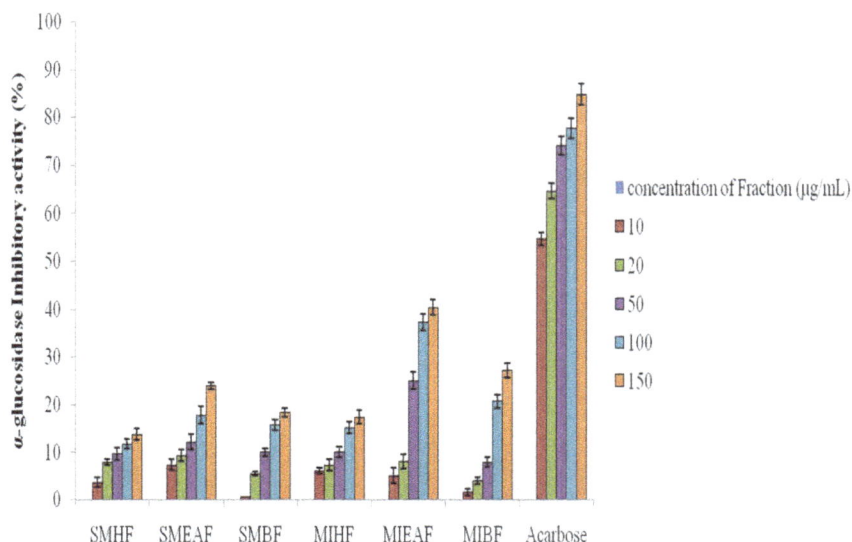

Figure 2. Alpha-glucosidase inhibitory activities of fractions of *S. mombin* and *M. indica* leaves. Legends: SMHF: *S. mombin* *n*-hexane fraction; SMEAF: *S. mombin* ethyl acetate fraction; SMBF: *S. mombin* *n*-butanol fraction; MIHF: *M. indica* *n*-hexane fraction; MIEAF: *M. indica* ethyl acetate fraction; MIBF: *M. indica* *n*-butanol fraction.

3.3. Total Phenolics and Total Flavonoids Content of Fractions of S. mombin and M. indica Leaves

Table 1 reveals the total phenolics, total flavonoids, by various fractions of crude aqueous extract of *S. mombin* and *M. indica* leaves. The ethyl acetate fraction of *M. indica* leaves (193.49 ± 18.64 mg GAE/100 g) had considerably ($p < 0.05$) higher phenol content than *S. mombin* ethyl acetate fraction (33.44 ± 1.57 mg GAE/100 g). Also, the ethyl acetate fraction of *M. indica* (52.35 ± 1.23 mg AAE/100 g) had appreciably ($p < 0.05$) higher flavonoids (Table 1) than *S. mombin* ethyl acetate fraction (19.86 ± 2.89 mg QUE (Quercetin equivalents)/100 g).

Table 1. Total phenolic and total flavonoid content of fractions of *Spondias mombin* and *Mangifera indica* leaves.

Parameters/Fractions	SMHF	SMEAF	SMBF	MIHF	MIEAF	MIBF
Total Phenolic (mg GAE/100 g)	5.23 ± 0.31	33.44 ± 1.57	7.73 ± 1.73	8.10 ± 2.69	193.49 ± 18.64	47.73 ± 2.21
Total Flavonoid (mg QUE/100 g)	3.36 ± 1.41	19.86 ± 2.89	5.75 ± 0.88	4.21 ± 0.85	52.35 ± 1.23	17.01 ± 0.44

Values are given as mean $\pm$ standard error of mean (SEM) ($n = 3$). QUE: Quercetin equivalents; GAE: Gallic acid equivalents; SMHF: *S. mombin* *n*-hexane fraction; SMEAF: *S. mombin* ethyl acetate fraction; SMBF: *S. mombin* *n*-butanol fraction; MIHF: *M. indica* *n*-hexane fraction; MIEAF: *M. indica* ethyl acetate fraction; MIBF: *M. indica* *n*-butanol fraction.

3.4. Metal Ion Chelating Ability of Fractions of S. mombin and M. indica Leaves

The metal ion chelating property of various fractions of *S. mombin* and *M. indica* leaves is displayed in Figure 3. This demonstrated that the ethyl acetate fraction of *S. mombin* ($IC_{50} = 21.76 \pm 0.02$ µg mL^{-1}) had a considerably ($p < 0.05$) higher metal chelating property than *M. indica* ($IC_{50} = 21.82 \pm 0.05$ µg mL^{-1}), ethyl acetate fractions. However, EDTA had a metal-ion chelating ability better than the fractions.

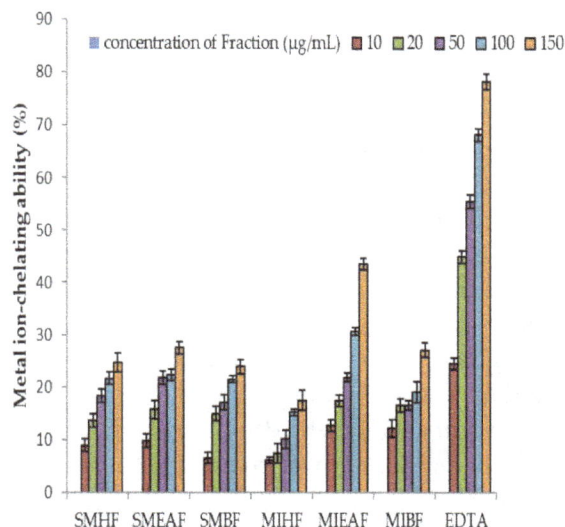

Figure 3. Metal ion chelating property of fractions of *S. mombin* and *M. indica* leaves. Legends: SMHF: *S. mombin* n-hexane fraction; SMEAF: *S. mombin* ethyl acetate fraction; SMBF: *S. mombin* n-butanol fraction; MIHF: *M. indica* n-hexane fraction; MIEAF: *M. indica* ethyl acetate fraction; MIBF: *M. indica* n-butanol fraction; EDTA: ethylenediaminetetraacetic acid.

3.5. Antioxidant Capacity of Fractions of S. mombin and M. indica Leaves

The free radical scavenging ability of the various fractions of *S. mombin* and *M. indica* leaves was consequently evaluated using the abstemiously steady ABTS radical and is displayed in Figure 4. Results showed that the ethyl acetate fraction of *M. indica* (IC_{50} = 54.88 ± 0.01 µg mL^{-1}) quenched ABTS radical (20–100 µg mL^{-1}) better than *S. mombin* ethyl acetate leaves (IC_{50} = 17.15 ± 0.02 µg mL^{-1}), fractions as indicated by their IC_{50} values. However, vitamin C scavenged ABTS radical better than the fractions.

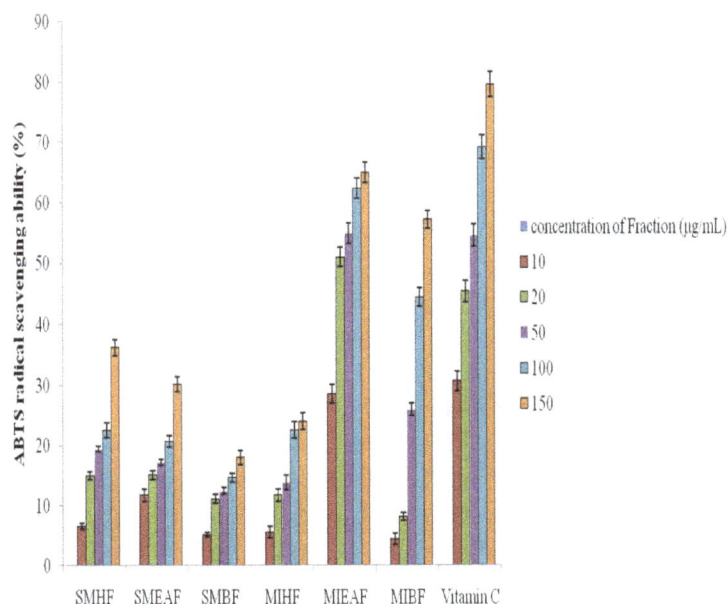

Figure 4. ABTS (2,2'-azino-bis(3-ethylbenzothiazoline)-6-sulphonic acid) radical scavenging ability of fractions of *S. mombin* and *M. indica* leaves. Legends: SMHF: *S. mombin* n-hexane fraction; SMEAF: *S. mombin* ethyl acetate fraction; SMBF: *S. mombin* n-butanol fraction; MIHF: *M. indica* n-hexane fraction; MIEAF: *M. indica* ethyl acetate fraction; MIBF: *M. indica* n-butanol fraction.

4. Discussion

Although several scientific studies have reported the antioxidant and antidiabetic activities of numerous medicinal plants including *M. indica* and *S. mombin* [36–41], to the best of our knowledge, this is the first report that directly compares the inhibitory effects of solvent-partitioned fractions of *M. indica* and *S. mombin* on α-amylase and α-glucosidase. There are several therapeutic approaches for managing diabetes mellitus; one way to achieve controlled blood glucose levels is to delay glucose absorption via inhibition of relevant carbohydrate hydrolyzing enzymes, such as α-amylase and α-glucosidase, found in the small intestine. The present study showed that *S. mombin* and *M. indica* leaves (HF, EAF, BF, AF) fractions inhibit α-amylase and α-glucosidase activities. The inhibition of carbohydrate metabolizing enzymes like α-amylase and α-glucosidase retards the absorption and digestion of starch and later suppresses postprandial symptom. The inhibitory properties of *S. mombin* and *M. indica* leaf fractions may suggest its usefulness as an oral antidiabetic drug for the management of high blood sugar in patients with these syndromes. Inhibitions of these enzymes interrupt macromolecule digestion and overall extend the breakdown time inflicting a reduction in the degree of glucose ingestion and thus plummeting postprandial blood sugar [30]. Better medical output may be derived from α-amylase and α-glucosidase inhibitors with mild inhibitory activity against α-amylase and strong inhibitory activity against α-glucosidase [42]. The inhibition of α-glucosidase, together with α-amylase by ethyl acetate fractions of *M. indica* and *S. mombin*, is considered to be an effective strategy for the control of diabetes by diminishing the absorption of glucose [42,43]. Remarkably, in this study, the ethyl acetate fractions of *M. indica* and *S. mombin* validated these properties and hence could be considered for therapeutic approach to retard postprandial hyperglycemia.

Recently, phenolic compounds have attracted great interest for their potential use in the development of new nutraceuticals or pharmaceuticals products due to their remarkable anti-oxidant, anti-inflammatory or antibacterial activities. Although, the protective effects of polyphenols could be in a concentration-dependent manner, recently there has been accumulating evidence in support of the hypothesis that a high-concentration of polyphenols can mechanistically cause adverse effects through pro-oxidative action and negatively affect cell growth, causing toxicity [43]. Several of the present antioxidants show mutagenic and genotoxic responses in cells reflecting their oxidant activity [44,45]. Flavonoids are major classes of phenolics and many studies have documented their biological and pharmacological activities [46,47]. The phenolic contents of *M. indica* and *S. mombin* fractions were determined respectively and the ethyl acetate fraction of *M. indica* leaves had higher total phenolic and flavonoid content than *S. mombin* fractions.

Metal ion chelating ability is important since it reduces the concentration of transition metals [48]. By chelating Fe^{2+}, the generation of hydroxyl radicals in the Fenton reaction may be attenuated and thus prevent damage to biomolecules. Accumulation of iron has been reported to cause an elevation in the generation of free radicals and development of oxidative stress [49,50].

Rice-Evans [51] reported that compounds with phenolic content could play an important role in eliminating radicals. The ABTS· scavenging property of the leaf might be due to the donating ability of the phenolics present in the fractions [52–54]. The antioxidant capacity of the leaves can be linked to their bioactive compounds, mainly antioxidant polyphenols, because of their ability to scavenge free radicals [55]. On this note, we suggest that the phenolic acids present in the fractions of *M. indica* and *S. mombin* could contribute to the fraction antioxidant activity. Hence, the results might be explained by the higher total phenolic content found in the fraction of *M. indica* and *S. mombin*. Similar findings were reported by other researchers, who found a strong correlation between radical scavenging ability and total phenolic contents of different samples [56]. However, the ethyl acetate fraction of *M. indica* and *S. mombin* leaf revealed the highest radical reducing ability of all other fractions.

5. Conclusions

Conclusively, our results demonstrate that the fractions from *S. mombin* and *M. indica* leaves exert an inhibitory activity against α-amylase and α-glucosidase. This study recommends the use of these plants for further in vivo studies to determine their potential in the management of diabetes. In addition, the data obtained compliments the conventional use of *S. mombin* and *M. indica* in the management of diabetes.

Author Contributions: O.A.O. designed the study, A.A.A. and A.B.O. carried out the study, A.B.O. wrote the manuscript, O.A.O., B.E.O., and B.O.A. carried out analysis and interpretation of data, B.O.A. assisted with and supervised the manuscript writing, B.E.O. did the first proof reading and A.P.K. The second proof reading. A.P.K. supported the manuscript preparation, made conceptual contributions on data analysis, manuscript drafting, provided administrative support, and critically revised the manuscript. The authors have read and approved the final manuscript.

Funding: Research reported in this article was supported by the South African Medical Research Council (SAMRC) through funding received from the South African National Treasury (Grant Number: PC 57009). Its contents are solely the responsibility of the authors and do not necessarily represent the official views of the South African Medical Research Council.

References

1. Cefalu, W.T.; Buse, J.B.; Tuomilehto, J.; Fleming, G.A.; Ferrannini, E.; Gerstein, H.C.; Bennett, P.H.; Ramachandran, A.; Raz, I.; Rosenstock, J.; et al. Update and next steps for Real-World Translation of Interventions for Type 2 Diabetes Prevention: Reflections from a Diabetes Care Editors' Expert Forum. *Diabetes Care.* **2016**, *39*, 1186–1201. [CrossRef] [PubMed]

2. Ogunyinka, B.I.; Oyinloye, B.E.; Osunsanmi, F.O.; Kappo, A.P.; Opoku, A.R. Comparative study on proximate, functional, mineral, and antinutrient composition of fermented, defatted, and protein isolate of Parkia biglobosa seed. *Food Sci Nutr.* **2017**, *5*, 139–147. [CrossRef] [PubMed]

3. Ojo, O.A.; Ojo, A.B.; Ajiboye, B.O.; Oyinloye, B.E.; Imiere, O.; Adeyonu, O. Ameliorative potentials of *Blighia sapida* K.D. Koenig bark against pancreatic-cell dysfunction in alloxan-induced diabetic rats. *J. Complement. Integr. Med.* **2017**, *14*, 20160145. [CrossRef] [PubMed]

4. Kumar, S.; Narwal, S.; Kumar, V.; Prakash, O. A-glucosidase inhibitors from plants: A natural approach to treat diabetes. *Pharmacogn. Rev.* **2011**, *5*, 19–29. [CrossRef] [PubMed]

5. Telagari, M.; Hullatti, K. In-vitro α-amylase and α-glucosidase inhibitory activity of *Adiantum caudatum* Linn. and *Celosia argentea* Linn. extracts and fractions. *Indian J. Pharmacol.* **2015**, *47*, 425–429. [PubMed]

6. Shirwaikar, A.; Rajendran, K.; Punitha, I.S. Antidiabetic activity of alcoholic stem extract of *Coscinium fenestratum* in streptozotocin-nicotinamide induced type 2 diabetic rats. *J. Ethnopharmacol.* **2005**, *97*, 369–374. [CrossRef] [PubMed]

7. Ezuruike, U.F.; Prieto, J.M. The use of plants in the traditional management of diabetes in Nigeria: Pharmacological and toxicological considerations. *J. Ethnopharmacol.* **2014**, *155*, 857–924. [CrossRef] [PubMed]

8. Iwu, M.M. *Handbook of African Medicinal Plants*; CRC Press: Boca Raton, FL, USA, 1993; p. 435.

9. Oliver-Bever, B. *Medicinal Plants in Nigeria; Being a Course of Four Lectures Delivered in April 1959 in the Pharmacy Department of the Nigerian College of Arts, Science and Technology, Ibadan*; Ibadan University press: Ibadan, OY, Nigeria, 1960; p. 760.

10. Kokwaro, J.O. *Medicinal Plants of East Africa*; East/Africa Literature Bureau: Nairobi, Kenya, 1976; p. 384.

11. Abo, K.A.; Ogunleye, V.O.; Ashidi, J.S. Antimicrobial potential of *Spondias mombin, Croton zambesicus* and *Zygotritonia crocea. Phytother. Res.* **1999**, *13*, 494–497. [CrossRef]

12. Iweala, E.J.; Oludare, F.D. Hypoglycemic effect, biochemical and histological changes of *Spondias mombin* Linn and *Parinari polyandra* Benth seeds ethanolic extracts in Alloxan-induced diabetic rats. *J. Pharmacol. Toxicol.* **2011**, *6*, 101–110. [CrossRef]

13. Corthout, J.; Pieters, L.A.; Claeys, M.; Vanden Berghe, D.A.; Vlietinck, A.J. Antiviral ellagitannins from *Spondias mombin. Phytochemistry* **1991**, *30*, 1129–1130. [CrossRef]

14. Corthout, J.; Pieters, L.; Claeys, M.; Vanden Berghe, D.; Vlietinck, A. Antiviral caffeoyl esters from *Spondias mombin. Phytochemistry* **1992**, *31*, 1979–1981. [CrossRef]

15. Corthout, J.; Pieters, L.; Claeys, M.; Geerts, S.; Vanden Berghe, D.; Vlietinck, A. Antibacterial and molluscicidal phenolic acids from *Spondias mombin. Planta Med.* **1994**, *60*, 460–463. [CrossRef] [PubMed]

16. Rymbai, H.; Srivastav, M.; Sharma, R.; Patel, C.R.; Singh, A.K. Bioactive compounds in mango and their roles in human health and plant defence—A review. *J. Hortic. Sci. Biotechnol.* **2013**, *88*, 369–379. [CrossRef]

17. Núñez Sellés, A.J.; Vélez Castro, H.T.; Agüero-Agüero, J.; González-González, J.; Naddeo, F.; De Simone, F.; Rastrelli, L. Isolation and Quantitative Analysis of Phenolic Antioxidants Free Sugar and Polyols from Mango (*Mangifera indica* Linn) Stem Bark Aqueous Decoction Used in Cuba as a Nutritional Supplement. *J. Agric. Food Chem.* **2002**, *50*, 762–766. [CrossRef] [PubMed]

18. Islam, M.R.; Mannan, M.A.; Kabir, M.H.B.; Islam, A.; Olival, K.J. Analgesic, anti-inflammatory and antimicrobial effects of ethanol extract of mango leaves. *J. Bangladesh Agric. Univ.* **2010**, *8*, 239–244. [CrossRef]

19. Martínez, G.; Delgado, R.; Pérez, G.; Garrido, G.; Núñez Sellés, A.J.; León, O.S. Evaluation of the in vitro antioxidant activity of *Mangifera indica*: Extract (Vimang). *Phytother. Res.* **2004**, *14*, 424–427. [CrossRef]

20. Gondi, M.; Prasada Rao, U.J.S. Ethanol extract of mango (*Mangifera indica* L.) peel inhibits α-amylase and α-glucosidase activities, and ameliorates diabetes related biochemical parameters in streptozotocin (STZ)-induced diabetic rats. *J. Food Sci. Technol.* **2015**, *52*, 7883–7893. [CrossRef] [PubMed]

21. Coates, N.J.; Gilpin, M.L.; Gwynn, M.N.; Lewis, D.E.; Milner, P.H.; Spear, S.R.; Tyler, J.W. SB-202742 a novel beta-lactamase inhibitor isolated from *Spondias mombin*. *J. Nat. Prod.* **1994**, *57*, 654–657. [CrossRef] [PubMed]

22. Ayoka, A.O.; Owolabi, R.A.; Bamitale, S.K.; Akomolafe, R.O.; Aladesanmi, J.A.; Ukponmwan, E.O. Effect of Fractionated Extracts and Isolated Pure Compounds of *Spondias mombin* (*L. Anacardiaceae*) Leaves on Novelty-Induced Rearing and Grooming Behaviours in Mice. *Afr. J. Tradit. Complement. Altern. Med.* **2013**, *10*, 244–255. [CrossRef] [PubMed]

23. Cabral, B.; Siqueira, E.M.S.; Bitencourt, M.A.O.; Lima, M.C.J.S.; Lima, A.K.; Ortmann, C.F.; Chaves, V.C.; Fernandes-Pedrosa, M.F.; Rocha, H.A.O.; Scortecci, K.C.; et al. Phytochemical study and anti-inflammatory and antioxidant potential of *Spondias mombin* leaves. *Rev. Bras. Farmacogn.* **2016**, *26*, 304–311. [CrossRef]

24. Elufioye, T.O.; Obuotor, E.M.; Agbedahunsi, J.M.; Adesanya, S.A. Anticholinesterase constituents from the leaves of *Spondias mombin* L. (Anacardiaceae). *Biologics* **2017**, *11*, 107–114. [CrossRef] [PubMed]

25. Alshammaa, D. Preliminary Screening and Phytochemical Profile of *Mangifera indica* Leave's Extracts, Cultivated in Iraq. *Int. J. Curr. Microbiol. Appl. Sci.* **2016**, *5*, 163–173. [CrossRef]

26. Ojo, O.A.; Oloyede, O.I.; Tugbobo, O.S.; Olarewaju, O.I.; Ojo, A.B. Antioxidant and inhibitory effect of scent leaf (*Ocimum gratissimum*) on Fe^{2+} and sodium nitroprusside induced lipid peroxidation in rat brain in vitro. *Adv. Biol. Res.* **2014**, *8*, 8–17.

27. Shai, L.J.; Masoko, P.; Mokgotho, M.P.; Magano, S.R.; Mogale, A.M.; Boaduo, N.; Eloff, J.N. Yeast alpha glucosidase inhibitory and antioxidant activities of six medicinal plants collected in Phalaborwa, South Africa. *S. Afr. J. Bot.* **2010**, *76*, 65–470. [CrossRef]

28. Ojo, O.A.; Ojo, A.B.; Ajiboye, B.O.; Olayide, I.; Fadaka, A.O. *Helianthus annuus* Leaf Ameliorates Postprandial Hyperglycaemia by inhibiting carbohydrate hydrolyzing enzymes associated with Type-2 diabetes. *Iran. J. Toxicol.* **2016**, *7*, 17–22. [CrossRef]

29. Ademiluyi, A.; Oboh, G. Soybean phenolic-rich extracts inhibit key-enzymes linked to type 2 diabetes (α-amylase and α-glucosidase) and hypertension (angiotensin I converting enzyme) in vitro. *Exp. Toxicol. Pathol.* **2013**, *65*, 305–309. [CrossRef] [PubMed]

30. Ojo, O.A.; Ajiboye, B.O.; Olayide, I.; Fadaka, A.O.; Olasehinde, O.R. Ethyl acetate fraction of bark of *Bridelia ferruginea* Benth. inhibits carbohydrate hydrolyzing enzymes associated with type 2 diabetes (α-glucosidase and α-amylase). *Adv. Biores.* **2016**, *7*, 126–133.

31. Mcdonald, S.; Prenzier, P.D.; Autokiwich, M.; Robards, K. Phenolics content and antioxidant activity of olive oil extracts. *Food Chem.* **2001**, *73*, 73–84. [CrossRef]

32. Meda, A.; Lamien, C.E.; Romito, M.; Millogo, J.; Nacoulma, O.G. Determination of the total phenolic, flavonoid and praline contents in Burkina Fasan honey, as well as their radical scavenging activity. *Food Chem.* **2005**, *91*, 571–577. [CrossRef]

33. Puntel, R.L.; Nogueira, C.W.; Rocha, J.B.T. Krebs cycle intermediates modulate Thiobarbituric Acid Reactive Species (TBARS) production in rat brain in vitro. *Neurochem. Res.* **2005**, *30*, 225–235. [CrossRef] [PubMed]

34. Re, R.; Pellegrini, N.; Proteggente, A.; Pannala, A.; Yang, M.; Rice-Evans, C. Antioxidant activity applying an improved ABTS radical cation decolorization assay. *Free Radic. Biol. Med.* **1999**, *26*, 1231–1237. [CrossRef]

35. Zar, J.H. *Biostatistical Analysis*; Prentice-Hall Inc.: Upper Saddle River, NJ, USA, 1984.

36. Ajiboye, B.O.; Ojo, O.A.; Adeyonu, O.; Imiere, O.; Olayide, I.; Fadaka, A.; Oyinloye, B.E. Inhibitory effect of key enzymes relevant to acute type-2-diabetes and antioxidative activity of ethanolic extract of *Artocarpus heterophyllus* stem bark. *J. Acute Dis.* **2016**, *5*, 423–429. [CrossRef]

37. Fred-Jaiyesimi, A.A.; Wilkins, M.R.; Abo, K.A. Hypoglycaemic and amylase inhibitory activities of leaves of *spondias mombin* Linn. *Afr. J. Med. Med. Sci.* **2009**, *38*, 343–349. [PubMed]

38. Prashanth, D.; Padmaja, R.; Samiulla, D.S. Effects of certain plant extracts on alpha amylase activity. *Fitoterapia* **2001**, *72*, 179–181. [CrossRef]

39. Bhuvaneshwari, J.; Khanam, S.; Devi, K. In Vitro enzyme inhibition studies for antidiabetic activity of mature and tender leaves of Mangifera indica var. Totapuri. *Res. Rev. J. Microbiol. Biotechnol.* **2014**, *3*, 36–41.

40. Ganogpichayagrai, A.; Palanuvej, C.; Ruangrungsi, N. Antidiabetic and anticancer activities of *Mangifera indica* cv. Okrong leaves. *J. Adv. Pharm. Technol. Res.* **2017**, *8*, 19–24. [PubMed]

41. Moke, E.G.; Ilodigwe, E.E.; Okonta, J.M.; Emudainohwo, J.O.T.; Ajaghaku, D.L.; Erhirhie, O.E.; Chinwuba, P.; Ahante, E. Antidiabetic activity and toxicity evaluation of aqueous extracts of *Spondias mombin* and *Costus afer* on Wistar rats. *Br. J. Pharm. Res.* **2015**, *6*, 333–342.

42. Ibrahim, M.; Koorbanally, N.; Islam, M.D. Antioxidative activity and inhibition of key enzymes linked to type-2 diabetes (α-glucosidase and α-amylase) by *Khaya senegalensis*. *Acta Pharm.* **2014**, *64*, 311–324. [CrossRef] [PubMed]

43. Mohamed, E.L.H.; Siddiqui, M.J.A.; Ang, L.F.; Sadikun, A.; Chan, S.H.; Tan, S.C.; Asmawi, M.Z.; Yam, M.F. Potent α-glucosidase and α-amylase inhibitory activities of standardized 50% ethanolic extracts and sinensetin from Orthosiphonstamineus Benth as anti-diabetic mechanism. *BMC Complement. Altern. Med.* **2012**, *12*, 176. [CrossRef] [PubMed]

44. Spanou, C.; Stagos, D.; Aligiannis, N.; Kouretas, D. Influence of potent antioxidant leguminosae family plant extracts on growth and antioxidant defense system of Hep2 cancer cell line. *J. Med. Food* **2010**, *13*, 149–155. [CrossRef] [PubMed]

45. Ojo, O.A.; Oloyede, O.I. Extracts of *Ocimum gratissimum* leaves inhibits Fe^{2+} and sodium nitroprusside induced oxidative stress in rat liver. *J. Pharm. Sci. Innov.* **2016**, *5*, 85–89. [CrossRef]

46. Hoensch, H.P.; Oertel, R. The value of flavonoids for the human nutrition: Short review and perspectives. *Clin. Nutr. Exp.* **2015**, *3*, 8–14. [CrossRef]

47. Ojo, O.A.; Oloyede, O.I.; Olarewaju, O.I.; Ojo, A.B. In Vitro Antioxidant Activity and Estimation of Total Phenolic Content in Ethyl Acetate Extract of *Ocimum gratissimum*. *Pharmacologyonline* **2013**, *3*, 37–44.

48. Tabert, M.H.; Liu, X.; Doty, R.L.; Serby, M.; Zamora, D.; Pelton, G.H.; Marder, K.; Albers, M.W.; Stern, Y.; Devanand, D.P. A 10-item smell identification scale related to risk for Alzheimer's disease. *Ann. Neurol.* **2005**, *58*, 155–160. [CrossRef] [PubMed]

49. Duh, P.D.; Tu, Y.Y.; Yen, G.C. Antioxidant activity of water extract of Harng Jyur (*Chrysenthemum morifolium* Ramat). *Lebnes Wiss Technol.* **1999**, *32*, 269–277. [CrossRef]

50. Oyetayo, F.L.; Ojo, O.A. *Dennettia tripetala* seeds inhibiting ferrous sulfate-induced oxidative stress in rat tissues in vitro. *Oxidants. Antioxi. Med. Sci.* **2017**, *6*, 35–39. [CrossRef]

51. Rice-Evans, C.A.; Miller, N.M.; Paganda, G. Structure–antioxidant activity relationships of flavonoids and phenolic acids. *Free Radic. Biol. Med.* **1996**, *20*, 933–956. [CrossRef]

52. Amic, D.; Davidovic-Amic, D.; Beso, D.; Trinajstic, N. Structure radical scavenging activity relationship of flavonoids. *Croatia. Chem. Acta.* **2003**, *76*, 55–61.

53. Oboh, G.; Puntel, R.L.; Rocha, J.B.T. Hot pepper (*Capsicum annuum*, *Tepin* and *Capsicum Chinese*, Hernero) prevent Fe^{2+}-induced lipid peroxidation in brain: In Vitro. *Food Chem.* **2007**, *102*, 178–185. [CrossRef]

54. Bhandarkar, A.P.; Bhat Rohith, A.; Vinodraj, K.; Shetty Manjunath, S.; Shenoy Ganesh, K. In vitro evaluation of antioxidant activity of *Spondias mombim* leaf extract: Discovering future avenues for an affordable and efficient antioxidant. *Int. Res. J. Pharm.* **2015**, *6*, 164–168. [CrossRef]

55. Mandic, A.L.; Dilas, S.M.; Cetkovic, G.S.; Canadanovic-Brunet, J.M.; Vesna, T.T. Polyphenolic composition and antioxidant activities of grape seed extract. *Int. J. Food Prop.* **2008**, *11*, 713–726. [CrossRef]

56. Khan, H.; Jan, S.A.; Javed, M.; Shaheen, R.; Khan, Z.; Ahmad, A.; Safi, S.Z.; Imran, M. Nutritional composition, antioxidant and antimicrobial activities of selected wild edible plants. *J. Food Biochem.* **2016**, *40*, 61–70. [CrossRef]

3

Selenium and Selenoproteins in Gut Inflammation

Shaneice K. Nettleford [1,2] **and K. Sandeep Prabhu** [1,2,*]

[1] Center for Molecular Immunology and Infectious Disease and Center for Molecular Toxicology and Carcinogenesis, The Pennsylvania State University, University Park, PA 16802, USA; sjn5208@psu.edu

[2] Department of Veterinary and Biomedical Sciences, The Pennsylvania State University, University Park, PA 16802, USA

* Correspondence: ksprabhu@psu.edu

Abstract: Inflammatory bowel disease (IBD), characterized by severe flares and remissions, is a debilitating condition. While the etiology is unknown, many immune cells, such as macrophages, T cells and innate lymphoid cells, are implicated in the pathogenesis of the disease. Previous studies have shown the ability of micronutrient selenium (Se) and selenoproteins to impact inflammatory signaling pathways implicated in the pathogenesis of the disease. In particular, two transcription factors, nuclear factor-κB (NF-κB), and peroxisome proliferator activated receptor (PPAR)γ, which are involved in the activation of immune cells, and are also implicated in various stages of inflammation and resolution, respectively, are impacted by Se status. Available therapies for IBD produce detrimental side effects, resulting in the need for alternative therapies. Here, we review the current understanding of the role of NF-κB and PPARγ in the activation of immune cells during IBD, and how Se and selenoproteins modulate effective resolution of inflammation to be considered as a promising alternative to treat IBD.

Keywords: IBD; NF-κB; PPARγ; immune cells; innate lymphoid cells

1. Introduction

Inflammatory Bowel Disease (IBD), is a generalized term that encompasses Crohn's disease and ulcerative colitis. Characterized by relapses and remissions, IBD patients experience debilitating symptoms varying from abdominal pain to rectal bleeding and anemia [1]. While ulcerative colitis is restricted to the colon, Crohn's disease affects any portion of the gastrointestinal tract [2]. IBDs result from dysregulated immune responses to the intestinal microbiota due to genetic predispositions [2,3]. The emerging evidence suggests that there is a genetic component, in addition to environmental influences and microbial factors along with immune responses involved in the pathogenesis of these inflammatory disorders [3]. The dysbiosis of the microbiota contributes to the pathogenesis of IBD. There is a decrease in the diversity of the microbiota during IBD, especially anaerobic bacteria including, but not limited to, *Lactobacillus*, *Escherichia* and *Bacteroides* [4]. As it pertains to immune responses, transcription factors and nuclear receptors including, but not limited to, nuclear factor-kappa B, NF-κB, and peroxisome proliferator-activated receptor gamma, PPARγ, have been implicated in the pathogenesis of IBDs [4,5].

Currently, IBDs are incurable. Treatments for the diseases are aimed at alleviating the debilitating symptoms to ensure long term remission. To treat inflammation, a characteristic of IBDs, anti-inflammatory steroids and immunosuppressants are often used [1]. In extreme cases, resection of parts of the bowel is performed as an alternative means of treatment [1]. However, these anti-inflammatory and immunosuppressive agents are somewhat ineffective in a percentage (20%) of the patients who use them and can result in deleterious side effects associated with infections arising from the inhibition of the immune system [6,7] that is accompanied by poor resolution or wound healing. Thus, there is a need for new therapeutics that lack any detrimental side effects, while enhancing the pathways of resolution and immune regulatory networks mitigating inflammation.

Selenium (Se) is an essential micronutrient that exists in the form of selenocysteine (Sec), the 21st amino acid, upon its incorporation into selenoproteins via the tRNA[Sec] encoded by *Trsp* [8]. A few epidemiological studies indicate Se levels in patients of both ulcerative colitis and Crohn's disease to be reduced [9,10]. There is a decrease in selenoprotein P (SEPP1) in the serum, as well as decrease in the activity of glutathione peroxidase in Crohn's Disease patients [9,11]. Similarly, selenoprotein S (SelenoS) and selenoprotein K (SelenoK) have been implicated in inflammation and IBD [12–14]. In fact, it has been reported that there is an increase in the production of inflammatory cytokines, with a decrease in the expression of SelenoS [13]. Interestingly, in the absence of SelenoK, the opposite is observed, with a decrease in inflammatory cytokines. These differences could be context-dependent and need to be further investigated. Along with a decrease in Se levels, there is an increase in prostaglandin E_2 (PGE$_2$) in the plasma of patients with ulcerative colitis [15]. A few experimental models of IBD and associated colon cancer suggest Se and selenoproteins to play a key role in inflammatory tumorigenesis and inflammatory microenvironment [16,17]. Previous studies from our laboratory has reported that Se, in the form of selenoproteins, can shunt the arachidonic acid pathway from the production of more pro-inflammatory mediators such as PGE$_2$ and interleukin (IL)-1β to more anti-inflammatory mediators such as prostaglandin D_2 (PGD$_2$) and its cyclopentenone metabolites, Δ^{12}-prostaglandin J$_2$ (Δ^{12}-PGJ$_2$) and 15-deoxy-$\Delta^{12,14}$-prostanglandin J$_2$ (15d-PGJ$_2$), in macrophages [18]. Additional studies from our laboratory have also demonstrated that the symptoms resulting from chemically-induced colitis, with dextran sodium sulfate (DSS), is alleviated in the colon of mice that have been supplemented with Se, characterized by increased colon length, decreased pro-inflammatory cytokines such as IL-1β, tumor necrosis factor alpha (TNFα) and interferon gamma (IFNγ) and increased anti-inflammatory markers such as arginase 1 (Arg1) [19]. Thus, Se supplementation mitigates inflammation, while increasing pro-resolutory pathways, suggesting that Se may be a potential therapeutic candidate for IBD. As such, this review will present a number of studies where the role of NF-κB and PPARγ play in the pathogenesis of IBD, the effect of Se on NF-κB and PPARγ in many cell types, and provide insight into the potential use of Se as a treatment for IBD.

2. NF-κB

Nuclear Factor-kappa B, a rel family of transcription factors, consisting of five subunits, namely RelA (p65), RelB, c-Rel, NF-κB1 (p105) and NF-κB2 (p100), plays an important role in a number of biologically important functions such as regulating stress response, immune responses, and inflammation [20,21]. These transcription factors can lead to the activation or repression of certain genes [21]. Under unstimulated conditions, NF-κB is inactivated and bound to members of the IκB family of proteins that prevent active NF-κB from nuclear translocation [22]. However, upon cellular stimulation through ligands such as lipopolysaccharide (LPS) and cytokines, there is a dissociation of the IκB proteins from NF-κB, through the action of the IκB kinase (IKK), consisting of the regulatory subunit NF-κB essential modulator (NEMO), IKKα (IKK1) and IKKβ (IKK2), resulting in the phosphorylation of IκB followed by its ubiquitin-dependent degradation by the proteasome. Such a dissociation of IκB from the NF-κB dimer exposes the nuclear localization sequence in NF-κB dimers to translocate into the nucleus and bind to promoters in target genes [21,23]. Under normal conditions in the gut, NF-κB activation is required for preserving the homeostatic conditions of the intestinal epithelial cells and, thus, the epithelial integrity [24].

It has been suggested that NF-κB is crucial for maintaining the integrity of the epithelium, but the studies conducted are somewhat contradictory. For instance, Pasparakis reported that the NF-κB signaling in the intestinal epithelium was an integral part of maintaining the homeostatic environment of the gut [25]. It was observed that mice that lack NEMO in the epithelium experienced colitis even in the absence of any form of epithelial injury. Further studies found that mice experienced increased intestinal epithelial cell death, which could act as a trigger of colitis, since the commensal bacteria could breach the epithelial barrier due to this disturbance [25,26]. However, usage of mice that lack IKK2, spontaneous colitis was not observed. It was subsequently found that this difference between the NEMO and IKK2 knock out mice was a result of the partial inhibition of the NF-κB canonical pathway in the IKK2 knock out mice, which was completely inhibited in NEMO knock out. Therefore, it is possible that there are some compensatory mechanisms in the NF-κB canonical pathway by IKK1 in IKK2 knock out mice.

Studies have shown that there is a correlation between the levels of NF-κB in the gut and the severity of IBD. Han et al., conducted studies using Crohn's disease patients, particularly those scheduled for resection surgery [4]. It was found that prior to surgery, histological scores conducted on colon samples revealed a correlation between NF-κB levels and histological score, where higher levels of NF-κB led to a greater histological score [4]. Currently, therapies for IBDs are aimed at blocking the NF-κB pathway [4]. Murine studies have shown that successful inhibition of NF-κB alleviates IBDs. Use of *Wasabia japonica*, a plant abundant in phytochemicals, in DSS-induced colitis inhibited the activation of NF-κB, the secretion of pro-inflammatory cytokines and prevented the onset of colitis at high dosages [27]. Similarly, Nimbolide, a phytochemical isolated from the Neem (*Azadirachta indica*) tree, alleviated both acute and chronic colitis induced in mice and inhibited NF-κB activation in macrophages [28].

Being a redox-sensitive transcription factor, NF-κB is also regulated by selenoproteins. Previous studies from our laboratory show that upon Se supplementation, following LPS stimulation, NF-κB activation was inhibited in macrophages through the inhibition of the phosphorylation of IκBα [29]. The ability of Se to negatively regulate NF-κB activation was dependent on the production of the arachidonic acid metabolite, 15d-PGJ$_2$ [29]. The cyclopentenone moiety present in 15d-PGJ$_2$ was a key factor in the inhibition of IKK2 that involved the formation of a covalent Michael reaction adduct of 15d-PGJ$_2$ with essential Cys in the kinase domain of IKK2 leading to decreased kinase activity [29,30]. Studies further demonstrated that Michael electrophiles (such as 15d-PGJ$_2$) could also interact with essential Cys residues in p65 and p50 to interfere in their binding to their cognate binding sites on the DNA [31]. While such a redox modulation was likely to be the underlying mechanism of Se in macrophages, other mechanisms involving the direct interaction of Se with Cys cannot be ruled out. Christensen et al. reported a decrease in NF-κB activity in prostate cancer cells, which they hypothesized could have been due to the inhibition of NF-κB through the direct interaction of Se with cysteine thiol in NF-κB [32]. Zhu et al. used Se nanoparticles coated with *Ulva lactuca* polysaccharide (ULP) to treat mice subjected with DSS-induced colitis [33]. They found that there was decreased pathology, characterized by decreased weight loss, lower disease activity index scores, and greater colon length in the mice given the Se nanoparticle compared to mice who were not given the treatment. The authors also found that there was inhibition of NF-κB activation in the mice subjected to DSS and administered the Se nanoparticle [33].

When the epithelial barrier is disturbed as in ulcerative colitis and Crohn's Disease, immune cells become increasingly activated, resulting in the production of pro-inflammatory cytokines such as IL-6, IFNγ, and TNFα by epithelial cells, lymphocytes, and macrophages [34]. As such, NF-κB has been implicated in the etiology of IBD. Patients suffering from IBD episodes present increased activation of NF-κB produced by innate immune cells, such as macrophages, in addition to epithelial cells in the gut [34]. In fact, the activation of NF-κB in macrophages is accompanied by the production of IL-12, which is involved in the differentiation of naïve T cells into T-helper (Th1) cells [35]. It is well established that the T-cell receptor (TCR) and cluster of differentiation 28 (CD28) co-stimulation can lead to the translocation of NF-κB into the nucleus of the cell. It follows that upon stimulation of the TCR, 3-phosphoinositide–dependent protein kinase-1 (PDK1) becomes activated, leading to the formation of the CARMA1-BCL10-MALT1 complex, which activates the IKK complex leading to the subsequent activation of NF-κB [23]. It has also been shown that NF-κB modulates the activation of various CD4$^+$ T cell subsets [23]. CD4$^+$ T cells are key players in adaptive immune responses that is accompanied by their differentiation into Th1, Th2, and Th17 cells. While Th1 and Th2 cells are involved in host defense against intracellular pathogens and allergic and anti-parasitic responses, respectively, Th17 cells play a pivotal role in host defense against extracellular pathogens, including fungi [23,36]. Of importance to this review is that both Th1 and Th17 are key in shaping the intestinal immune responses [37,38].

Innate lymphoid cells (ILCs) represent another important group of immune cells localized to the mucosal surfaces and respond to the secreted molecules from the epithelium, which are involved in mounting intestinal immune responses as well as maintaining a homeostatic environment within the intestine [36,39]. ILCs are categorized into three groups based on the transcription factor that is key in their development and the cytokines produced. It has recently been shown that ILC3s can be activated in an NF-κB dependent manner, through the action of IL-18, resulting in the production of IL-22 [39]. Interestingly, both T helper cells and ILCs are implicated in the pathogenesis of IBD. It has been observed that there is an increase in the Th1 inducing cytokine, IL-12, in patients suffering from Crohn's Disease [40]. Similarly, in ulcerative colitis and Crohn's disease patients, an increase in the expression of the Th17 cytokine IL-17A is seen [41,42]. Patients suffering from IBDs have increased expression of the ILC3 cytokines, IL-17A and IL-22, in addition to high expression of retinoic acid receptor-related orphan receptor gamma (ROR-γt) transcription factor in the gut mucosa [43].

As discussed earlier, given that uncontrolled T cell activation and biased differentiation towards Th1 and Th17 cells, as well as ILC3 activation, are suggested to be one of the key causative factors in the development of IBD, the ability of Se to downregulate NF-κB activation could potentially impact such pathways. This could be effected through multiple mechanisms. First, the ability of Se to impact IL-6 and transforming growth factor beta (TGF-β) along with IL-23 could affect Th17 differentiation. IL-23 can also stimulate γδ T cells, invariant natural killer T (iNKT) cells, and intestinal innate-like sentinel T cells that promote Th17 differentiation [44–46]. The cytokines, TGF-β (only in murine) and IL-6 that are important for Th17 differentiation are driven by NF-κB [47,48]. IL-6 can also induce NF-κB in the intestinal epithelial cells to exert a positive loop leading to an inflammatory milieu. Secondly, the inability of NF-κB to be activated through the dissociation and degradation of IκB from the complex results in decreased Th1 activation [20]. Therefore, one can hypothesize that Se could affect this process, potentially leading to a biased response towards anti-inflammatory Th2 pathway leading to further downregulation of NF-κB activation. Finally, within the inflammatory milieu, IL-6, TNFα, and other NF-κB target genes can induce the production of PGE_2 [49]. Increased PGE_2 in patients with active colitis versus those in remission coupled with a reciprocal increase in PGD_2 in the latter group suggests that switching of eicosanoid pathways from pro-inflammatory prostaglandins to anti-inflammatory bioactive lipid mediators could help resolve and sustain the remission of colitis in patients [50]. More importantly, PGE_2 can also induce IL-23 leading to the increased Th17 differentiation. Thus, the ability of Se to resolve gastrointestinal (GI) inflammation via the decreased PGE_2 via Th17 differentiation is an attractive hypothesis that is currently being tested in our laboratory. As ILC3s are activated by NF-κB through the action of IL-18, again, it is plausible that Se levels can potentiate the disease. Inhibiting the production of IL-18 by either dendritic cells or macrophages through Se could result in the blockade of NF-κB activation in this context. Similarly, it is probable that Se directly inhibiting the dissociation of IκB proteins from NF-κB could result in the downregulation of NF-κB, and thus, decrease the ability of NF-κB to activate ILC3 and trigger secretion of IL-17A and IL-22.

Since oxidative stress can result in the development of IBD through destruction of the mucosal barrier of the gastrointestinal tract, it is possible selenoproteins acting as antioxidants can ameliorate the symptoms of IBD [51]. In fact, glutathione peroxidase 2 (GPx2), which is abundant in the gut, has been shown to be protective against oxidative stress during inflammation and experimental models of IBD [52,53]. SEPP1, which has both reductase and peroxidase activities, has been reported to be decreased during IBD [54]. The oxidative stress experienced during IBD can lead to the activation of NF-κB, thus selenoproteins such as GPx2 and SEPP1 can act to reduce this stress, which could lead to a decrease in the activation of NF-κB. Interestingly, thioredoxin reductase 1 (Txnrd1) can also reduce the oxidative stress during IBD as well as impact the gut microbiome through reduction of tetrathionate, which bacteria such as *Salmonella* are able to utilize as a means as outgrowing other bacteria in the gut, to thiosulfate [55]. Thus, presenting another means through which Se, through various selenoproteins can help to alleviate IBD by decreasing oxidative stress as well as diversify the microbiota.

While studies suggest a pro-inflammatory role of NF-κB, it could be argued that NF-κB is also essential for maintaining homeostasis in the intestinal epithelial cells, which could be ablated upon its inhibition. However, in the case of IBD, where NF-κB is highly activated, it is possible that Se supplementation may serve as a treatment imparting beneficial functions by decreasing NF-κB activation and creating a homeostatic environment in the gut. Needless to say, further studies are needed to ascertain if this is the case and to what extent the baseline NF-κB activity might be required for homeostasis as the ability of other transcription factors to counter NF-κB could also play an important role.

3. PPARγ

Peroxisome proliferator-activated receptor gamma, PPARγ, a nuclear hormone receptor, is involved in the biosynthesis and metabolism of lipids [56,57]. PPARs, also termed lipid sensors, carry out their functions through activation by endogenous ligands that includes fatty acid metabolites [58]. PPARγ, along with other PPARs, has an anti-inflammatory function when activated by exogenous ligands, such as thiazolidinediones (rosiglitazone and pioglitazone). Of interest to this review is the ability of eicosanoids such PGD_2 metabolites, Δ^{12}-prostaglandin J_2 (Δ^{12}-PGJ_2) and 15d-PGJ_2, which serve as endogenous ligands for PPARγ, to lead to the activation of PPARγ. Activated PPARγ, can effectively regulate downstream target genes via diverse mechanisms. Interaction of PPARγ, with its heterodimeric partner, retinoid X receptor-α (RXRα) precedes its binding to peroxisome proliferator response elements (PPREs) within the promoters of downstream target genes [59]. Another mechanism of repression of inflammatory pathways involves the ability of PPARγ: RXRα to interfere in the binding of NF-κB by a process known as "squelching" that could depend on the ability to recruit a nuclear receptor corepressor-I (NCoRI) complex that causes inhibition of expression of pro-inflammatory mediators [5,60,61].

Like NF-κB, PPARγ has been implicated in the regulation of colonic inflammation. In fact, it is a key receptor that is abundantly expressed in the epithelial cells of the colon, second to adipose tissue [62]. While it has been reported that there is increased expression of NF-κB during IBD, in the context of PPARγ, the opposite is observed. Interestingly, a greater decrease of PPARγ is observed in patients suffering from ulcerative colitis when compared to patients who suffer from Crohn's disease [5]. While the majority of the information on the role of PPARγ during resolution of inflammation has been mostly restricted to macrophages, PPARγ has been demonstrated to also influence the T cell activation, in that it acts as a negative regulator of T cells following activation, through its inhibition of nuclear factor of activated T cells (NFAT), a transcription factor involved in the regulation of IL-2, which is important for T cell proliferation [63,64]. On the other hand, PPARγ can also influence regulatory T cells (T_{regs}) by increasing their differentiation.

There are several clinical and pre-clinical studies that report the mechanism underlying the role and effects of PPARγ in inflammatory disease. Dubuqouy et al., conducted studies using human subjects, where colon biopsies obtained from two patient groups revealed a decrease in PPARγ mRNA expression in both ulcerative colitis and Crohn's disease samples, with a greater decrease in patients suffering from ulcerative colitis [65]. Interestingly, the expression of PPARγ or lack thereof was mostly confined to the epithelial cells and was correlated to the activity of ulcerative colitis [65]. Desreumaux et al., also demonstrated that there is increased susceptibility to 2,4,6-trinitrobenzenesulfonic acid (TNBS)-induced colitis in PPARγ heterozygous mice compared to their wild type counterparts [66]. Administration of a PPARγ agonist attenuated the experimental colitis. In fact, Choo et al., reported that 2-hydroxyethyl 5-chloro-4,5-didehydrojasmonate (J11-Cl), a PPARγ agonist, reduced the symptoms of

DSS-induced colitis, increased the activity of PPARγ and increased the expression of anti-inflammatory cytokines [67]. Similarly, Bassaganya-Riera et al., demonstrated that conjugated linoleic acid (CLA), another PPARγ agonist, was able to induce the expression of PPARγ and inhibit TNFα expression and NF-κB activation during colitis [68].

Our laboratory has shown a crucial role for Se in the activation of PPARγ and its ligands, which are derived from the arachidonic acid (AA) pathway of cyclooxygenase metabolism, in macrophages. Treatment of the macrophage like Abelson leukemia virus transformed cell line (RAW264.7 macrophages) and bone marrow-derived macrophages with Se resulted in the upregulation of hematopoietic PGD2 synthase (HPGDS) and its product PGD_2 as well as its non-enzymatic metabolites, Δ^{12}-PGJ_2 and 15d-PGJ_2, which are agonists of PPARγ and inhibitors of NF-κB activation [18]. Activation of PPARγ by these endogenous cyclopentenone prostaglandins (CyPGs) was shown to activate the expression of HPGDS through the binding of PPARγ to the PPREs present in the proximal promoter of murine HPGDS [18]. Additionally, our laboratory has shown that Se supplementation leads to the upregulation of 15-hydroxyprostaglandin dehydrogenase (15-PGDH), the enzyme that oxidizes PGE_2, and a subsequent decrease in PGE_2 during DSS-induced colitis leading to the resolution of inflammation [19]. Other studies from our laboratory have shown that 15-PGDH is regulated by PPARγ, in that it can be increased by PPARγ leading to the resolution of inflammation. While the increased 15-PGDH catabolically inactivates PGE_2, the products of PGE_2 oxidation, 13,14-dihydro-15-keto-PGE_2 via its dehydrated product 13,14-dihydro-15-keto-PGA_2, could potentially increase the activation of PPARγ thus, forming a feedback loop of control of NF-κB via activation of PPARγ. This is an attractive hypothesis that remains to be completely tested.

While there are not many studies that focus on the effect of Se and PPARγ on inflammatory bowel diseases and the mechanism through which Se acts, one can make conjectures based on the available data using murine models of IBD [67,68]. Since PPARγ is decreased in IBDs such as ulcerative colitis and Crohn's disease and it has been shown that Se can increase both PPARγ and its ligand 15d-PGJ_2 [5,13], it is plausible that under supplemented Se status, the disease would be significantly decreased. This effect could be mediated in a number of ways. It could be that the upregulation of PPARγ inhibits the activation of NF-κB in a number of cell types including intestinal epithelial cells, macrophages and dendritic cells, thus preventing the production of pro-inflammatory cytokines that are involved in the pathology of IBD. It has been shown that PPARγ can regulate T cell activation [63]. When activated T cells were treated with 15d-PGJ_2 or ciglitazone, IL-2 expression was significantly inhibited [69]. Thus, it is possible that PPARγ could inhibit the differentiation of Th1 cells or the cytokine producing capabilities of these cells. Interestingly, the expression of T_{regs} during IBD is not uniform. For instance, there is decreased T_{regs} circulating in the peripheral blood of active IBD patients compared to inactive IBD patients. However, it was reported that there is increased T_{regs} in the intestinal mucosa of active IBD patients [70]. T_{regs} are defined by their expression of FoxP3, a transcription factor expressed by and that is important for the development as well as the function of T_{regs} [60]. However, T_{regs} are not the only cell type that express this, since FoxP3 is also observed on activated effector T cells [71]. Thus, activated effector T cells expressing FoxP3 could account for the increase in T_{regs} observed in the intestinal mucosa. It has been shown that PPARγ increases the expression of Foxp3$^+$ T_{regs}, suggesting that during IBD this could lead to greater numbers of FoxP3$^+$ T_{regs} in the colon, where it is needed to suppress the actions of the activated effector T cells. Thus, Se could exert its effects through activation of PPARγ by inhibiting certain pathways or immune cell functions, which could impact cell specific functions to lead to the active resolution of inflammation in the gut.

4. Complications of IBD

Complications can arise as a result of the continuous injury and repair taking place in the gut during IBD. Intestinal fibrosis, occurring in patients suffering from both ulcerative colitis and Crohn's disease, results in strictures and obstructions in the gut [72]. The cytokine milieu of the gut during IBD can contribute to the development of intestinal fibrosis, which include, but are not limited to IL-1β, TNFα, IL-22 and IL-17. PPARγ is able to prevent the development of fibrotic cells in the gut through antagonizing a number of pathways [71]. For instance, PPARγ disrupts the transforming growth factor beta/mothers against decapentaplegic homolog 3 (TGF-β/SMAD3) pathway, which is involved in the formation of fibrotic tissues in a number of organs including the intestine, thus preventing the differentiation and activation of myofibroblasts [73,74]. It can then be speculated that Se can have an effect on intestinal fibrosis, through the actions of selenoproteins or through PPARγ. In fact, it has been reported that other forms of fibrosis such as cardiac fibrosis, resulted from a deficiency in Se.

Colorectal cancer (CRC) is also another complication of IBD. In fact, sufferers of IBD have an increased risk of developing colorectal cancer. Clinical trials using selenium as supplementation reported a decrease in the number of colorectal cancer cases when patients administered a placebo were compared to patients administered Se [75]. Oxidative damage to DNA can result in the generation of tumors, in which case selenoproteins antioxidant properties can decrease the risk of CRC [75]. Thus, Se and selenoproteins are can be used as chemopreventative agents, especially since Se is involved in regulating apoptosis and proliferation in the intestinal epithelium.

5. Conclusions

The etiology of IBD is multifaceted. Immune responses brought about by the activation of transcription factors and nuclear receptors are implicated in the pathogenesis of the inflammatory disorders. The transcription factors NF-κB and PPARγ represent two key regulators during IBD that are differentially regulated. Interestingly, a bioactive lipid metabolite of PGD$_2$ that activates PPARγ also inactivates NF-κB, in the presence of all selenoprotein expression. This review highlights areas that exploit such a unique relationship between NF-κB and PPARγ pathways, which could potentially present as an approach to mitigate inflammation while promoting sustained resolution and remission. Emerging studies point to resolution of IBD through inhibition of NF-κB and the activation of PPARγ in a number of immune cell types including macrophages, Th1, Th17 and ILC3s, where Se could play an important role (Figure 1). As discussed, it is probable that Se, through its effect on the activation of NF-κB and PPARγ, could impact the immune mechanisms to "fine tune" for effective remission. Interestingly, commensal microbiota, which can lead to IBD when the epithelial barrier is breached, can also regulate the activation of both NF-κB and PPARγ [76,77]. Studies have shown that the butyrate producing commensal *Clostridia* can activate PPARγ, while the commensal *Streptococcus salivarius* can prevent the activation of NF-κB [76,77]. It has also been reported that Se can alter the composition of the gut microbiota, which in turn can also impact the Se status of the host and consequently, the selenoproteome of the host [78]. Therefore, it appears that Se could impact commensal bacteria that regulate NF-κB and PPARγ. Furthermore, the effect of Se during an infection brought about by pathogenic bacteria could result in different immune responses when compared to the action of Se as it pertains to commensal bacteria. This review provides insights into the role of Se as a potential dietary factor that could be used as an adjunct therapy in IBD; however, further studies are needed to completely understand the intricate mechanisms the underlie the disease pathogenesis as well as the ones that follow remission.

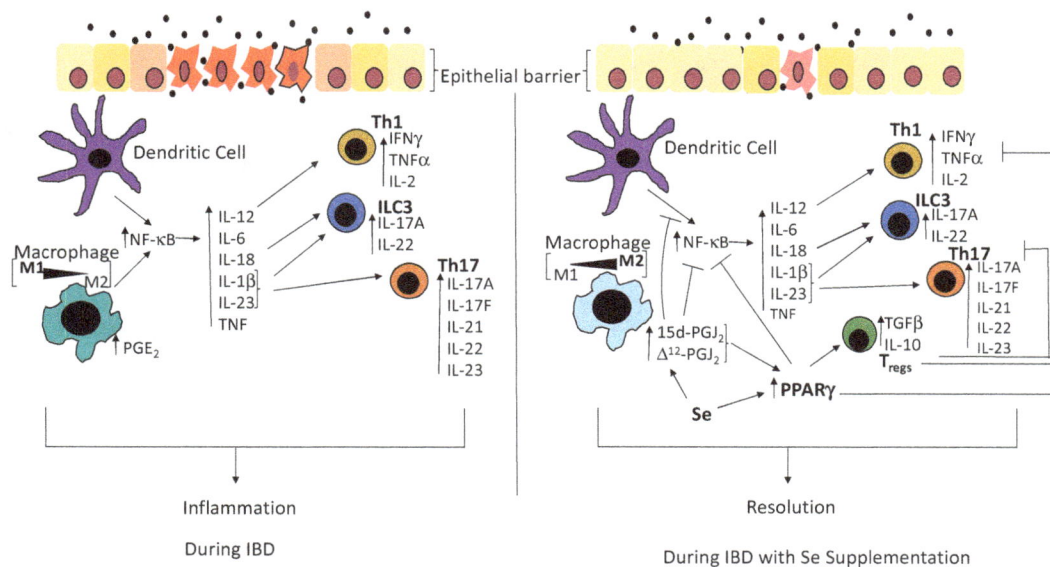

Figure 1. Schematic showing disruption of the epithelial barrier results in activation of immune networks that are regulated by Se. Consequently, innate immune cells such as macrophages and dendritic cells sense the presence of the bacteria and mount an immune response through the upregulation of the transcription factor, nuclear factor-kappa B (NF-κB), leading to the production of pro-inflammatory cytokines such as interleukin (IL)-18 and interleukin (IL)-12, as well as IL-1β and IL-23, which are involved in the differentiation of innate lymphoid cells (ILC3s), Th1 and Th17 cells respectively [36]. In the presence of Se, macrophages produce 15d-prostaglandin J_2 (15d-PGJ$_2$) and Δ^{12}-prostaglandin J_2 (Δ^{12}-PGJ$_2$). The nuclear hormone receptor, peroxisome proliferator-activated receptor gamma (PPARγ), is upregulated and inhibits Th1, Th17 as well as the action of NF-κB, thus inhibiting the production of the pro-inflammatory cytokines that are required for the differentiation of T helper cells and ILC3s. Simultaneously, PPARγ leads to the differentiation of T_{regs}, which inhibit the function of T helper cells. As 15d-PGJ$_2$ and Δ^{12}-PGJ$_2$ are ligands of PPARγ, they bind to PPARγ and potentiates its action on NF-κB and T_{regs}, as well as directly inhibit the activation of NF-κB. Commensal bacteria are represented by filled black circles. IFNγ: interferon gamma; TNFα: tumor necrosis factor alpha; PGE$_2$: prostaglandin E$_2$; IBD: Inflammatory bowel disease; IL-2: interleukin-2; IL-17A: interleukin-17A; IL-22: interleukin-22; IL-6: interleukin-6; IL-1β: interleukin-1β; IL23: interleukin-23; IL-17F: interleukin-17F; IL-21: interleukin-21; TGF-β: transforming growth factor beta; IL-10: interleukin-10.

Acknowledgments: We thank all present and past members of the Prabhu laboratory for their help and advice. K. Sandeep Prabhu thanks the National Institutes of Health (DK077152 and Office of Dietary Supplements; CA 162665) and United States Department of Agriculture (Hatch Fund #4605).

Conflicts of Interest: The authors declare no conflict of interest.

References

1. De Lange, K.M.; Barrett, J.C. Understanding inflammatory bowel disease via immunogenetics. *J. Autoimmun.* **2015**, *64*, 91–100. [CrossRef] [PubMed]

2. Abraham, C.; Cho, J.H. Inflammatory bowel disease. *N. Engl. J. Med.* **2009**, *361*, 2066–2078. [CrossRef] [PubMed]

3. Zhang, Y.Z.; Li, Y.Y. Inflammatory bowel disease: Pathogenesis. *World J. Gastroenterol.* **2014**, *20*, 91–99. [CrossRef] [PubMed]

4. Han, Y.M.; Koh, J.; Kim, J.W.; Lee, C.; Koh, S.J.; Kim, B.G.; Lee, K.L.; Im, J.P.; Kim, J.S. NF-kappa B activation correlates with disease phenotype in Crohn's disease. *PLoS ONE* **2017**, *12*, 1–13. [CrossRef] [PubMed]

5. Dubuquoy, L.; Rousseaux, C.; Thuru, X.; Peyrin-Biroulet, L.; Romano, O.; Chavatte, P.; Chamaillard, M.; Desreumaux, P. PPARγ as a new therapeutic target in inflammatory bowel diseases. *Gut* **2006**, *55*, 1341–1349. [CrossRef] [PubMed]

6. Sang, L.; Chang, B.; Zhu, J.; Yang, F.; Li, Y.; Jiang, X.; Sun, X.; Lu, C.; Wang, D. Dextran sulfate sodium-induced acute experimental colitis in C57BL/6 mice is mitigated by selenium. *Int. Immunopharmacol.* **2016**, *39*, 359–368. [CrossRef] [PubMed]

7. Han, E.S.; Oh, J.Y.; Park, H.J. Cordyceps militaris extract suppresses dextran sodium sulfate-induced acute colitis in mice and production of inflammatory mediators from macrophages and mast cells. *J. Ethnopharmacol.* **2011**, *134*, 703–710. [CrossRef] [PubMed]

8. Papp, L.V.; Lu, J.; Holmgren, A.; Khanna, K.K. From selenium to selenoproteins: Synthesis, identity, and their role in human health. *Antioxid. Redox Signal.* **2007**, *9*, 775–806. [CrossRef] [PubMed]

9. Andoh, A.; Hirashima, M.; Maeda, H.; Hata, K.; Inatomi, O.; Tsujikawa, T.; Sasaki, M.; Takahashi, K.; Fujiyama, Y. Serum selenoprotein-P levels in patients with inflammatory bowel disease. *Nutrition* **2005**, *21*, 574–579. [CrossRef] [PubMed]

10. Geerling, B.J.; Badart-Smook, A.; Stockbrugger, R.W.; Brummer, R.J.M. Comprehensive nutritional status in recently diagnosed patients with inflammatory bowel disease compared with population controls. *Eur. J. Clin. Nutr.* **2000**, *54*, 514–521. [CrossRef] [PubMed]

11. Reimund, J.M.; Hirth, C.; Koehl, C.; Baumann, R.; Duclos, B. Antioxidant and immune status in active Crohn's disease. A possible relationship. *Clin. Nutr.* **2000**, *19*, 43–48. [CrossRef] [PubMed]

12. Seiderer, J.; Dambacher, J.; Kühnlein, B.; Pfennig, S.; Konrad, A.; Török, H.P.; Haller, D.; Göke, B.; Ochsenkühn, T.; Lohse, P.; et al. The role of the selenoprotein S (*SELS*) gene -105G>A promoter polymorphism in inflammatory bowel disease and regulation of *SELS* gene expression in intestinal inflammation. *Tissue Antigens* **2007**, *70*, 238–246. [CrossRef] [PubMed]

13. Hoffmann, P.R. An emerging picture of the biological roles of selenoprotein K. In *Selenium: Its Molecular Biology and Role in Human Health*; Springer Science & Business Media: New York, NY, USA, 2012; pp. 335–344. ISBN 978-1-4614-1024-9.

14. Liu, J.; Rozovsky, S. Membrane-bound selenoproteins. *Antioxid. Redox Signal.* **2015**, *23*, 795–813. [CrossRef] [PubMed]

15. Wiercinska-Drapalo, A.; Jaroszewicz, J.; Tarasow, E.; Flisiak, R.; Prokopowicz, D. Transforming growth factor beta(1) and prostaglandin E2 concentrations are associated with bone formation markers in ulcerative colitis patients. *Prostaglandins Other Lipid Mediat.* **2005**, *78*, 160–168. [CrossRef] [PubMed]

16. Barrett, C.W.; Reddy, V.K.; Short, S.P.; Motley, A.K.; Lintel, M.K.; Bradley, A.M.; Freeman, T.; Vallance, J.; Ning, W.; Parang, B.; et al. Selenoprotein P influences colitis-induced tumorigenesis by mediating stemness and oxidative damage. *J. Clin. Investig.* **2015**, *125*, 2646–2660. [CrossRef] [PubMed]

17. Barrett, C.W.; Singh, K.; Motley, A.K.; Lintel, M.K.; Matafonova, E.; Bradley, A.M.; Ning, W.; Poindexter, S.V.; Parang, B.; Reddy, V.K.; et al. Dietary selenium deficiency exacerbates DSS-induced epithelial injury and AOM/DSS-induced tumorigenesis. *PLoS ONE* **2013**, *8*, 1–11. [CrossRef] [PubMed]

18. Gandhi, U.H.; Kaushal, N.; Ravindra, K.C.; Hegde, S.; Nelson, S.M.; Narayan, V.; Vunta, H.; Paulson, R.F.; Prabhu, K.S. Selenoprotein-dependent up-regulation of hematopoietic prostaglandin D_2 synthase in macrophages is mediated through the activation of Peroxisome Proliferator-activated Receptor (PPAR)g. *J. Biol. Chem.* **2011**, *286*, 27471–27482. [CrossRef] [PubMed]

19. Kaushal, N.; Kudva, A.K.; Patterson, A.D.; Chiaro, C.; Kennett, M.J.; Desai, D.; Amin, S.; Carlson, B.A.; Cantorna, M.T.; Prabhu, K.S. Crucial role of macrophage selenoproteins in experimental colitis. *J. Immunol.* **2014**, *193*, 3683–3692. [CrossRef] [PubMed]

20. Hayden, M.S.; Ghosh, S. NF-κB in immunobiology. *Cell Res.* **2011**, *21*, 223–244. [CrossRef] [PubMed]

21. Ahmed, S.; Dewan, M.Z.; Xu, R. Nuclear factor-kappaB in inflammatory bowel disease and colorectal cancer. *Am. J. Digest. Dis.* **2014**, *1*, 84–96.

22. Baeuerle, P.A.; Baltimore, D. IκB: A specific inhibitor of the NFκB transcription factor. *Science* **1988**, *242*, 540–546. [CrossRef] [PubMed]

23. Oh, H.; Ghosh, S. NF-κB: Roles and regulation in different CD4$^+$ T cell subsets. *Immunol. Rev.* **2013**, *252*, 41–51. [CrossRef] [PubMed]

24. Nenci, A.; Becker, C.; Wullaert, A.; Gareus, R.; Van Loo, G.; Danese, S.; Huth, M.; Nikolaev, A.; Neufert, C.; Madison, B.; et al. Epithelial NEMO links innate immunity to chronic intestinal inflammation. *Nature* **2007**, *446*, 557–561. [CrossRef] [PubMed]

25. Pasparakis, M. IKK/NF-κB signaling in intestinal epithelial cells controls immune homeostasis in the gut. *Mucosal Immunol.* **2008**, *1*, 54–57. [CrossRef] [PubMed]

26. Pasparakis, M. Role of NF-κB in epithelial biology. *Immunol. Rev.* **2012**, *246*, 346–358. [CrossRef] [PubMed]

27. Kang, J.-H.; Choi, S.; Jang, J.-E.; Ramalingam, P.; Ko, Y.T.; Kim, S.Y.; Oh, S.H. Wasabia japonica is a potential functional food to prevent colitis via inhibiting the NF-κB signaling pathway. *Food Funct.* **2017**, *8*, 2865–2874. [CrossRef] [PubMed]

28. Seo, J.; Lee, C.; Hwang, S.; Chun, J. Nimbolide inhibits nuclear factor-κB pathway in intestinal epithelial cells and macrophages and alleviates experimental colitis in mice. *Phytother. Res.* **2016**, *30*, 1605–1614. [CrossRef] [PubMed]

29. Vunta, H.; Davis, F.; Palempalli, U.D.; Bhat, D.; Arner, R.J.; Thompson, J.T.; Peterson, D.G.; Reddy, C.C.; Prabhu, K.S. The anti-inflammatory effects of selenium are mediated through 15-deoxy-$\Delta^{12,14}$-prostaglandin J_2 in macrophages. *J. Biol. Chem.* **2007**, *282*, 17964–17973. [CrossRef] [PubMed]

30. Rossi, A.; Kapahi, P.; Natoli, G.; Takahashi, T.; Chen, Y.; Karin, M.; Santoro, M.G. Anti-inflammatory cyclopentenone prostaglandins are direct inhibitors of IκB kinase. *Nature* **2000**, *403*, 103–108. [CrossRef] [PubMed]

31. Pande, V.; Ramos, M.J. Molecular recognition of 15-deoxy-$\Delta^{12,14}$-prostaglandin J_2 by nuclear factor-kappa B and other cellular proteins. *Bioorg. Med. Chem. Lett.* **2005**, *15*, 4057–4063. [CrossRef] [PubMed]

32. Christensen, M.J.; Nartey, E.T.; Hada, A.L.; Legg, R.L.; Barzee, B.R. High selenium reduces NF-κB-regulated gene expression in uninduced human prostate cancer cells. *Nutr. Cancer* **2007**, *58*, 197–204. [CrossRef] [PubMed]

33. Zhu, C.; Zhang, S.; Song, C.; Zhang, Y.; Ling, Q.; Hoffmann, P.R.; Li, J.; Chen, T.; Zheng, W.; Huang, Z. Selenium nanoparticles decorated with Ulva lactuca polysaccharide potentially attenuate colitis by inhibiting NF-κB mediated hyper inflammation. *J. Nanobiotechnol.* **2017**, *15*, 1–15. [CrossRef] [PubMed]

34. Atreya, I.; Atreya, R.; Neurath, M.F. NF-κB in inflammatory bowel disease. *J. Intern. Med.* **2008**, *263*, 591–596. [CrossRef] [PubMed]

35. Neurath, M.; Finotto, S.; Glimcher, L. The role of Th1/Th2 polarization in mucosal immunity. *Nat. Med.* **2002**, *8*, 567–573. [CrossRef] [PubMed]

36. Giuffrida, P.; Corazza, G.R.; Di Sabatino, A. Old and new lymphocyte players in inflammatory bowel disease. *Dig. Dis. Sci.* **2018**. [CrossRef] [PubMed]

37. Maloy, K.J.; Kullberg, M.C. IL-23 and Th17 cytokines in intestinal homeostasis. *Mucosal Immunol.* **2008**, *1*, 339–349. [CrossRef] [PubMed]

38. Cortés, A.; Muñoz-Antoli, C.; Esteban, J.G.; Toledo, R. Th2 and Th1 responses: Clear and hidden sides of immunity against intestinal helminths. *Trends Parasitol.* **2017**, *33*, 678–693. [CrossRef] [PubMed]

39. Victor, A.R.; Nalin, A.P.; Dong, W.; McClory, S.; Wei, M.; Mao, C.; Kladney, R.D.; Youssef, Y.; Chan, W.K.; Briercheck, E.L.; et al. IL-18 drives ILC3 proliferation and promotes IL-22 production via NF-κB. *J. Immunol.* **2017**, 1601554. [CrossRef] [PubMed]

40. Monteleone, G.; Biancone, L.; Marasco, R.; Morrone, G.; Marasco, O.; Luzza, F.; Pallone, F. Interleukin 12 is expressed and actively released by Crohn's disease intestinal lamina propria mononuclear cells. *Gastroenterology* **1997**, 1169–1178. [CrossRef]

41. Sugihara, T.; Kobori, A.; Imaeda, H.; Tsujikawa, T.; Amagase, K.; Takeuchi, K.; Fujiyama, Y.; Andoh, A. The increased mucosal mRNA expressions of complement C3 and interleukin-17 in inflammatory bowel disease. *Clin. Exp. Immunol.* **2010**, *160*, 386–393. [CrossRef] [PubMed]

42. Fujino, S. Increased expression of interleukin 17 in inflammatory bowel disease. *Gut* **2003**, *52*, 65–70. [CrossRef] [PubMed]

43. Geremia, A.; Arancibia-Cárcamo, C.V.; Fleming, M.P.P.; Rust, N.; Singh, B.; Mortensen, N.J.; Travis, S.P.L.; Powrie, F. IL-23–Responsive innate lymphoid cells are increased in inflammatory bowel disease. *J. Exp. Med.* **2011**, *208*, 1127–1133. [CrossRef] [PubMed]

44. Michel, M.-L.; Keller, A.C.; Paget, C.; Fujio, M.; Trottein, F.; Savage, P.B.; Wong, C.-H.; Schneider, E.; Dy, M.; Leite-de-Moraes, M.C. Identification of an IL-17-producing NK1.1^{neg} iNKT cell population involved in airway neutrophilia. *J. Exp. Med.* **2007**, *204*, 995–1001. [CrossRef] [PubMed]

45. Sutton, C.E.; Lalor, S.J.; Sweeney, C.M.; Brereton, C.F.; Lavelle, E.C.; Mills, K.H.G. Interleukin-1 and IL-23 induce innate IL-17 production from $\gamma\delta$ T cells, amplifying Th17 responses and autoimmunity. *Immunity* **2009**, *31*, 331–341. [CrossRef] [PubMed]

46. Venken, K.; Elewaut, D. IL-23 responsive innate-like T cells in spondyloarthritis: The less frequent they are, the more vital they appear. *Curr. Rheumatol. Rep.* **2015**, *17*, 30. [CrossRef] [PubMed]

47. Freudlsperger, C.; Bian, Y.; Contag Wise, S.; Burnett, J.; Coupar, J.; Yang, X.; Chen, Z.; Van Waes, C. TGF-β and NF-κB signal pathway cross-talk is mediated through TAK1 and SMAD7 in a subset of head and neck cancers. *Oncogene* **2013**, *32*, 1549–1559. [CrossRef] [PubMed]

48. MohanKumar, K.; Namachivayam, K.; Chapalamadugu, K.; Garzon, S.A.; Premkumar, M.; Tipparaju, S.; Maheshwari, A. Smad7 interrupts TGF-β signaling in intestinal macrophages and promotes inflammatory activation of these cells during necrotizing enterocolitis. *Pediatr. Res.* **2016**, *79*, 951–961. [CrossRef] [PubMed]

49. Nakao, S.; Ogtata, Y.; Shimizu, E.; Yamazaki, M.; Furuyama, S.; Sugiya, H. Tumor necrosis factor a (TNF-a)-induced prostaglandin E_2 release is mediated by the activation of cyclooxygenase-2 (COX-2) transcription via NFκB in human gingival fibroblasts. *Mol. Cell. Biochem.* **2002**, *238*, 11–18. [CrossRef] [PubMed]

50. Vong, L.; Ferraz, J.G.P.; Panaccione, R.; Beck, P.L.; Wallace, J.L. A pro-resolution mediator, prostaglandin D_2, is specifically up-regulated in individuals in long-term remission from ulcerative colitis. *Proc. Natl. Acad. Sci. USA* **2010**, *107*, 12023–12027. [CrossRef] [PubMed]

51. Tian, T.; Wang, Z.; Zhang, J. Pathomechanisms of oxidative stress in inflammatory bowel disease and potential antioxidant therapies. *Oxid. Med. Cell. Longev.* **2017**, *2017*. [CrossRef] [PubMed]

52. Chu, F.F.; Esworthy, R.S.; Doroshow, J.H. Role of Se-dependent glutathione peroxidases in gastrointestinal inflammation and cancer. *Free Radic. Biol. Med.* **2004**, *36*, 1481–1495. [CrossRef] [PubMed]

53. Te Velde, A.A.; Pronk, I.; de Kort, F.; Stokkers, P.C.F. Glutathione peroxidase 2 and aquaporin 8 as new markers for colonic inflammation in experimental colitis and inflammatory bowel diseases: An important role for H_2O_2? *Eur. J. Gastroenterol. Hepatol.* **2008**, *20*, 555–560. [CrossRef] [PubMed]

54. Kudva, A.K.; Shay, A.E.; Prabhu, K.S. Selenium and inflammatory bowel disease. *Am. J. Physiol. Gastrointest. Liver Physiol.* **2015**, *309*, G71–G77. [CrossRef] [PubMed]

55. Narayan, V.; Kudva, A.K.; Prabhu, K.S. Reduction of tetrathionate by mammalian thioredoxin reductase. *Biochemistry* **2015**, *54*, 5121–5124. [CrossRef] [PubMed]

56. Kliewer, S.A.; Lenhard, J.M.; Willson, T.M.; Patel, I.; Morris, D.C.; Lehmann, J.M. A prostaglandin J_2 metabolite binds peroxisome proliferator-activated receptor γ and promotes adipocyte differentiation. *Cell* **1995**, *83*, 813–819. [CrossRef]

57. Forman, B.M.; Tontonoz, P.; Chen, J.; Brun, R.P.; Spiegelman, B.M.; Evans, R.M. 15-Deoxy-$\Delta^{12,14}$-Prostaglandin J_2 is a ligand for the adipocyte determination factor PPARγ. *Cell* **1995**, *83*, 803–812. [CrossRef]

58. Schupp, M.; Lazar, M.A. Endogenous ligands for nuclear receptors: Digging deeper. *J. Biol. Chem.* **2010**, *285*, 40409–40415. [CrossRef] [PubMed]

59. Kliewer, S.A.; Umesono, K.; Noonan, D.J.; Heyman, R.A.; Evans, R.M. Convergence of 9-*cis* retinoic acid and peroxisome proliferator signalling pathways through heterodimer formation of their receptors. *Nature* **1992**, *358*, 771–774. [CrossRef] [PubMed]

60. Yamamoto-Furusho, J.K.; Jacintez-Cazares, M.; Furuzawa-Carballeda, J.; Fonseca-Camarillo, G. Peroxisome proliferator-activated receptors family is involved in the response to treatment and mild clinical course in patients with ulcerative colitis. *Dis. Markers* **2014**, *2014*. [CrossRef] [PubMed]

61. Ricote, M.; Glass, C.K. PPARs and molecular mechanisms of transrepression. *Biochim. Biophys. Acta* **2009**, *1771*, 926–935. [CrossRef] [PubMed]

62. Auboeuf, D.; Rieusset, J.; Fajas, L.; Vallier, P.; Frering, V.; Riou, J.; Staels, B.; Auwerx, J.; Laville, M.; Vidal, H. Tissue distribution and quantification of the expression of mRNAs of peroxisome proliferator-activated receptors and liver X receptor-alpha in humans: No alteration in adipose tissue of obese and NIDDM patients. *Diabtetes* **1997**, *46*, 1319–1327. [CrossRef]

63. Choi, J.M.; Bothwell, A.L.M. The nuclear receptor PPARs as important regulators of T-cell functions and autoimmune diseases. *Mol. Cells* **2012**, *33*, 217–222. [CrossRef] [PubMed]

64. Yang, X.Y.; Wang, L.H.; Chen, T.; Hodge, D.R.; Resau, J.H.; DaSilva, L.; Farrar, W.L. Activation of human T lymphocytes is inhibited by peroxisome proliferator-activated receptor γ (PPARγ) agonists. *J. Biol. Chem.* **2000**, *275*, 4541–4544. [CrossRef] [PubMed]

65. Dubuquoy, L.; Å Jansson, E.; Deeb, S.; Rakotobe, S.; Karoui, M.; Colombel, J.F.; Auwerx, J.; Pettersson, S.; Desreumaux, P. Impaired expression of peroxisome proliferator-activated receptor γ in ulcerative colitis. *Gastroenterology* **2003**, *124*, 1265–1276. [CrossRef]

66. Desreumaux, P.; Dubuquoy, L.; Nutten, S.; Peuchmaur, M.; Englaro, W.; Schoonjans, K.; Derijard, B.; Desvergne, B.; Wahli, W.; Chambon, P.; et al. Attenuation of colon inflammation through activators of the retinoid X receptor (RXR)/peroxisome proliferator-activated receptor g (PPARg) heterodimer. A basis for new therapeutic strategies. *J. Exp. Med.* **2001**, *193*, 827–838. [CrossRef] [PubMed]

67. Choo, J.; Lee, Y.; Yan, X.; Noh, T.H.; Kim, S.J.; Son, S.; Pothoulakis, C.; Moon, H.R.; Jung, J.H.; Im, E. A novel peroxisome proliferator-activated receptor (PPAR)γ agonist 2-hydroxyethyl 5-chloro-4,5-didehydrojasmonate exerts anti-inflammatory effects in colitis. *J. Biol. Chem.* **2015**, *290*, 25609–25619. [CrossRef] [PubMed]

68. Bassaganya-Riera, J.; Reynolds, K.; Martino-Catt, S.; Cui, Y.; Hennighausen, L.; Gonzalez, F.; Rohrer, J.; Benninghoff, A.U.; Hontecillas, R. Activation of PPAR γ and δ by conjugated linoleic acid mediates protection from experimental inflammatory bowel disease. *Gastroenterology* **2004**, *127*, 777–791. [CrossRef] [PubMed]

69. Clark, R.B.; Bishop-Bailey, D.; Estrada-Hernandez, T.; Hla, T.; Puddington, L.; Padula, S.J. The nuclear receptor PPARg and immunoregulation: PPARg mediates inhibition of helper T cell responses. *J. Immunol.* **2000**, *164*, 1364–1371. [CrossRef] [PubMed]

70. Maul, J.; Loddenkemper, C.; Mundt, P.; Berg, E.; Giese, T.; Stallmach, A.; Zeitz, M.; Duchmann, R. Peripheral and intestinal regulatory $CD_4+CD_{25}^{high}$ T cells in inflammatory bowel disease. *Gastroenterology* **2005**, *128*, 1868–1878. [CrossRef] [PubMed]

71. Roncarolo, M.-G.; Gregori, S. Is FOXP3 a bona fide marker for human regulatory T cells? *Eur. J. Immunol.* **2008**, *38*, 925–927. [CrossRef] [PubMed]

72. Speca, S.; Giusti, I.; Rieder, F.; Latella, G. Cellular and molecular mechanisms of intestinal fibrosis. *World J. Gastroenterol.* **2012**, *18*, 3635–3661. [CrossRef] [PubMed]

73. Zhao, C.; Chen, W.; Yang, L.; Chen, L.; Stimpson, S.A.; Diehl, A.M. PPARγ agonists prevent TGFbeta1/Smad3-signaling in human hepatic stellate cells. *Biochem. Biophys. Res. Commun.* **2006**, *350*, 385–391. [CrossRef] [PubMed]

74. Kulkarni, A.A.; Thatcher, T.H.; Olsen, K.C.; Maggirwar, S.B.; Phipps, R.P.; Sime, P.J. PPAR-γ ligands repress TGFβ-induced myofibroblast differentiation by targeting the PI3K/Akt pathway: Implications for therapy of fibrosis. *PLoS ONE* **2011**, *6*. [CrossRef] [PubMed]

75. Peters, U.; Takata, Y. Selenium and the prevention of prostate and colorectal cancer. *Mol. Nutr. Food Res.* **2008**, *52*, 1261–1272. [CrossRef] [PubMed]

76. Kaci, G.; Lakhdari, O.; Dore, J.; Ehrlich, S.D.; Renault, P.; Blottiere, H.M.; Delorme, C. Inhibition of the NF-κB pathway in human intestinal epithelial cells by commensal *Streptococcus salivarius*. *Appl. Environ. Microbiol.* **2011**, *77*, 4681–4684. [CrossRef] [PubMed]

77. Byndloss, M.X.; Olsan, E.E.; Rivera-Chávez, F.; Tiffany, C.R.; Cevallos, S.A.; Lokken, K.L.; Torres, T.P.; Byndloss, A.J.; Faber, F.; Gao, Y.; et al. Microbiota-activated PPAR-γ signaling inhibits dysbiotic *Enterobacteriaceae* expansion. *Science* **2017**, *357*, 570–575. [CrossRef] [PubMed]

78. Kasaikina, M.V.; Kravtsova, M.A.; Lee, B.C.; Seravalli, J.; Peterson, D.A.; Walter, J.; Legge, R.; Benson, A.K.; Hatfield, D.L.; Gladyshev, V.N. Dietary selenium affects host selenoproteome expression by influencing the gut microbiota. *FASEB J.* **2011**, *25*, 2492–2499. [CrossRef] [PubMed]

4

High Glucose-Mediated Tyrosine Nitration of PI3-Kinase: A Molecular Switch of Survival and Apoptosis in Endothelial Cells

Sally L. Elshaer [†], Tahira Lemtalsi and Azza B. El-Remessy * [iD]

Retinopathy Research, Augusta Biomedical Research Corporation Charlie Norwood VA Medical Center, Augusta, GA 30912, USA; dr_s_elshaer@mans.edu.eg or slelshaer@gmail.com (S.L.E.); tlemtalsi@augusta.edu (T.L.)

* Correspondence: Azza.El-Remessy@va.gov or aelremessy@outlook.com

† Currently at Determent of Pharmacology& Toxicology, Faculty of Pharmacy, Mansoura University, Mansoura, Dakahlia Governorate 35516, Egypt.

Abstract: Diabetes and hyperglycemia are associated with increased retinal oxidative and nitrative stress and vascular cell death. Paradoxically, high glucose stimulates expression of survival and angiogenic growth factors. Therefore, we examined the hypothesis that high glucose-mediated tyrosine nitration causes inhibition of the survival protein PI3-kinase, and in particular, its regulatory p85 subunit in retinal endothelial cell (EC) cultures. Retinal EC were cultured in high glucose (HG, 25 mM) for 3 days or peroxynitrite (PN, 100 µM) overnight in the presence or absence of a peroxynitrite decomposition catalyst (FeTPPs, 2.5 µM), or the selective nitration inhibitor epicatechin (100 µM). Apoptosis of ECs was assessed using TUNEL assay and caspase-3 activity. Immunoprecipitation and Western blot were used to assess protein expression and tyrosine nitration of p85 subunit and its interaction with the p110 subunit. HG or PN accelerated apoptosis of retinal ECs compared to normal glucose (NG, 5 mM) controls. HG- or PN-treated cells also showed significant increases in tyrosine nitration on the p85 subunit of PI3-kinase that inhibited its association with the catalytic p110 subunit and impaired PI3-kinase/Akt kinase activity. Decomposing peroxynitrite or blocking tyrosine nitration of p85 restored the activity of PI3-kinase, and prevented apoptosis and activation of p38 MAPK. Inhibiting p38 MAPK or overexpression of the constitutively activated Myr-Akt construct prevented HG- or peroxynitrite-mediated apoptosis. In conclusion, HG impairs pro-survival signals and causes accelerated EC apoptosis, at least in part via tyrosine nitration and inhibition of PI3-kinase. Inhibitors of nitration can be used in adjuvant therapy to delay diabetic retinopathy and microvascular complication.

Keywords: peroxynitrite; tyrosine nitration; high glucose; PI3-kinase; apoptosis; endothelial cells; p38 MAPK; survival; Akt

1. Introduction

Exposure to hyperglycemia contributes to diabetes-associated microvascular and macrovascular complications. The Diabetic Complication Clinical Trial (DCCT) and the United Kingdom Prospective Diabetes Study (UKPDS) epidemiological studies correlated poor glycemic control with the development of vascular complications in patients with type 1 or type 2 diabetes mellitus [1,2]. These studies indicated that early exposure to hyperglycemia predisposes individuals to the development of diabetic complications, a phenomenon referred to as metabolic memory or the legacy effect [3]. It has been well-documented that high glucose-mediated oxidative and nitrative stress are integral to the development of diabetes-induced microvascular injury (reviewed in [4]). Microvascular endothelial cells (ECs) are sensitive targets of diabetic and hyperglycemia resulting in vascular injury [5]. Our previous work demonstrated that high glucose triggered formation of peroxynitrite in retinal EC cultures [6]. Diabetic retinopathy is broadly classified into two stages; a non-proliferative background stage, and the blinding proliferative retinopathy stage. By the end of the early non-proliferative stage, clinically significant ischemia takes place when a critical number of retinal capillaries become occluded and non-perfused [7]. Therefore, treatments that prevent or slow down retinal capillary cell death and consequent ischemia are critical for slowing progression of diabetic retinopathy into late sight-threatening proliferative stage.

Peroxynitrite, a highly reactive oxidant, can cause reduction of cellular antioxidant defenses, lipid peroxidation, and inhibition of key metabolic enzymes via nitration of the protein tyrosine residues or by oxidation of thiol pools [8]. Growing evidence supports the concept that covalent modification of various proteins by tyrosine nitration is associated with modification of biological functions (reviewed in [9]). Moreover, we have shown that increased formation of peroxynitrite mediates apoptosis in endothelial cells cultured in high oxygen [10], and in a model for oxygen-induced retinopathy [11] and in the diabetic retina [12].

It has been reported that retinal endothelial cells in diabetic patients and animals undergo accelerated death by a process consistent with apoptosis [13–15]. Paradoxically, high glucose stimulates expression of survival and angiogenic growth factors within retinal capillaries, suggesting uncoupling of survival signaling. Tyrosine nitration is a post-translational protein modification that has been postulated to alter protein function and contribute to metabolic memory and legacy effect [16]. Together, the pivotal role of tyrosine nitration in altering survival signal under diabetic conditions has prompted us to study the effects of high glucose-induced peroxynitrite on cell death in retinal EC cultures. The study attempted also to define the molecular mechanism by which peroxynitrite-mediated tyrosine nitration inhibits the survival signaling pathway.

2. Materials and Methods

2.1. Cell Culture

Retinal endothelial cells were isolated from bovine retinas as described previously [6]. The cells (passages 6–8) were grown to confluence and switched to serum free media, then treated in conditions of normal glucose (NG, 5 mM glucose) or high glucose (HG, 25 mM glucose) for 3 days, as described before [17]. Additional group of cells were treated with peroxynitrite 0.5 mM (Cayman, Ann Arbor, MI, USA) overnight (16 h), as described before [10]. Serum starvation is known to induce apoptosis in endothelial cells [18]. Stock concentrations of peroxynitrite were provided in 0.1 N NaOH. Inhibitors for peroxynitrite (FeTPPs) and epicatechin were obtained from Millipore-Sigma, (Saint Louis, MO, USA), and inhibitor for p38 MAPK (SB203580) was obtained from Calbiochem (La Jolla, CA, USA).

2.2. Caspase-3 Activity

The activity of caspase-3 enzyme was determined using a kit from R&D systems (Cat. #: K105-25, Minneapolis, MN, USA) according to the manufacturer's instruction, as described earlier by our group [19]. Briefly, cells were lysed on ice for 10 min with lysis buffer provided with the kit. To 50 µL of cell lysate, 50 µL of 2X reaction buffer was added, followed by 5µL of caspase-3 fluorogenic substrate (DEVD-AFC). The mixture was incubated for 2 h at 37 °C, and fluorescence was measured with a fluorescent plate reader (BioTek Synergy2, Winooski, VT, USA) with an excitation of 400 nm and an emission of 505 nm. Results were normalized to non-starved EC cultures.

2.3. TUNEL Assay

ApopTag® Fluorescein In Situ Apoptosis Detection Kit was used to determine cell death in EC cultures according to the manufacturer's instructions (S7110, Millipore, Darmstadt, Germany).

Cells were grown on coverslips and treated with high glucose or peroxynitrite as described previously [12]. EC cultures were counterstained with propidium iodide (PI) and cover-slipped with Vectashield (Vector Laboratories, Burlingame, CA, USA). Micrographs were captured at 20X by fluorescent microscope (AxioObserver.Z1; Zeiss, Jena, Germany).

2.4. Western Blotting Analysis

EC cultures were harvested after various treatments and lysed in modified radioimmunoprecipitation assay (RIPA) buffer (Cat# 20-188, Millipore-Sigma, Burlington, MA, USA) and 50 μg of total protein was separated on a 10–12% SDS-polyacrylamide gel by electrophoresis, transferred to nitrocellulose, and incubated with specific antibody. Antibodies for phospho-p38 MAPK, p38 MAPK, Akt, and Akt kinase were purchased from Cell Signaling Technology, Inc. (Beverly, MA, USA). The primary antibody was detected using a horseradish peroxidase-conjugated goat anti-mouse or anti-rabbit antibody (EMD, La Jolla, CA, USA) and enhanced chemiluminescence. The films were scanned, and the band intensity was quantified using ImageJ densitometry software version, and expressed as optical density (OD).

2.5. Immunoprecipitation

EC cultures were incubated in high glucose or peroxynitrite for the desired time in the presence or absence of peroxynitrite decomposition catalyst FeTPPs or nitration inhibitor, epicatechin. EC lysates were prepared, as described above, for immunoblotting. For PI3-kinase tyrosine nitration, 100 μg protein was incubated with p85. The precipitated proteins were analyzed by SDS-PAGE, and blotted with nitrotyrosine antibody or p85 for equal loading. To study the effects on the interaction of the regulatory subunit with the catalytic subunit of PI3-kinase, 100 μg protein was incubated with p110. Antibodies for nitrotyrosine, p85, and p110 subunits of PI3-kinase were purchased from Millipore (Millipore-Sigma, Burlington, MA, USA). For immunoprecipitation, signals were captured, and band intensities were measured using alphaEaseFC (Santa Clara, CA, USA)

2.6. Akt Kinase Assay

Lysates from HG- or PN-treated culture (100 μg) protein were incubated with immobilized Akt (Cell Signaling Technology, Danvers, MA, USA) monoclonal antibody-containing beads with gentle rocking at 4 °C overnight. The beads were washed then incubated in 40 μL kinase buffer supplemented with 200 μM ATP and 1 μg GSK-3 fusion protein for 30 min at 30 °C. The reaction was terminated with sample buffer. The supernatant was separated on a 12% SDS-PAGE gel, transferred to nitrocellulose membrane. Western immunoblotting was performed with anti-phopho-GSK-3α/β (Ser21/9) antibody, and total loading with anti-Akt antibody. Horseradish peroxidase-conjugated goat anti-rabbit antibody and enhanced chemiluminescence were used to detect the primary antibody. The films were scanned, and the band intensity was quantified using the National Institute of Health densitometry ImageJ software version.1 and expressed as optical density (OD).

2.7. Adenoviral Constructs

β-Galactosidase and C-terminal HA-tagged constitutively active Akt (Myr-Akt) were provided as a kind gift from Dr. David Fulton (Augusta University, Augusta, GA, USA) and generated as described previously [20]. EC cultures were infected with adenovirus containing the β-galactosidase and Myr-Akt. The virus was removed, and EC were left to recover for 12 h in complete medium. Western blot analysis using antibodies against total Akt (Cell Signaling Technology, Inc. Beverly, MA, USA) confirmed the overexpression in EC cultures transfected with Myr-Akt, but not in cells transfected with β-galactosidase.

2.8. Statistical Analysis

Results are expressed as mean ± SE, and the data was processed for statistical analysis. For experiments that examined apoptotic insult against control, one-way ANOVA was used.

For experiments that examined effects of apoptotic insults (HG, PN) and treatments (Fe, Epi) against controls, two-way ANOVA was used, followed by Bonferroni post hoc multiple comparisons to assess significant differences among individual groups by GraphPad Software Version.6 (San Diego, CA, USA). Significance was defined at probability $p < 0.05$.

3. Results

3.1. High Glucose-Induced Peroxynitrite Induces Apoptosis in Retinal Endothelial Cells

Our previous studies showed that high glucose (HG) triggered significant increases in peroxynitrite formation in retinal EC at 3 and 5 days [6]. In the present study, we examined the effects of HG-induced nitrative stress (3-days) on EC survival in comparison to normal glucose (NG). Due to powerful apoptotic effects of exogenous peroxynitrite (PN), treatment was limited to overnight (16 h), as described previously [10]. As shown in Figure 1A,B, high glucose and peroxynitrite treatment accelerated EC death as indicated by significant increases in the number of TUNEL-positive cells compared to NG-controls. Caspase-3 is an intracellular cysteine protease that exists as a pro-enzyme, becoming activated during the cascade of intracellular signaling events that culminates in apoptosis. HG and PN significantly increased caspase-3 activity compared to NG controls (Figure 1C). Co-treatment with the specific peroxynitrite decomposition catalyst FeTPPs (Fe, 2.5 μM) or the epicatechin (Epi, 100 μM) significantly reduced cell death in high glucose and peroxynitrite-treated cells. Epicatechin, a dietary flavenol, has been shown to selectively blunt the nitrating effect of peroxynitrite on tyrosine residues [21,22]. These findings suggest that the effect of HG in accelerating apoptosis in retinal EC cultures likely involves PN-mediated alteration of cell survival pathways.

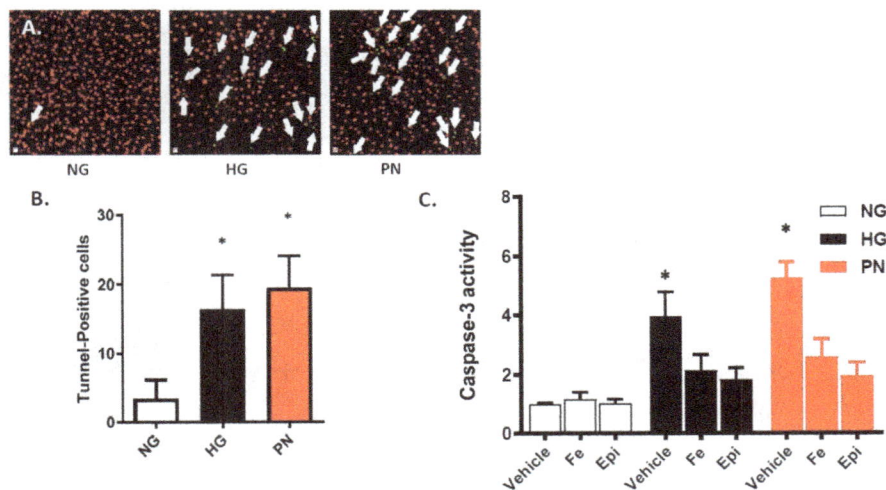

Figure 1. High glucose and peroxynitrite accelerated apoptosis in epithelial cell (EC) cultures. (**A**) Representative micrographs of TUNEL-positive nuclei (green, indicated by white arrows) in EC cultures counterstained with propidium iodide (red), and images were taken at 20× magnification. (**B**) Statistical analysis using one-way ANOVA showing significant increase in the number of TUNEL-positive cells in ECs treated with high glucose (HG, 25 mM) for 3 days or peroxynitrite (PN, 0.5 mM) for overnight, compared with normal glucose (NG) controls. (* $p < 0.05$, $n = 6$). (**C**) Statistical analysis of caspase-3 enzyme activity using two-way ANOVA showed significant interaction among examined groups. Treatment of EC cultures with HG (25 mM) for 3 days or PN (0.5 mM) overnight significantly increased activity of caspase-3 compared to NG. Co-treatment with the specific peroxynitrite decomposition catalyst FeTTPs (Fe, 2.5 μM) or the nitration inhibitor epicatechin (Epi, 100 μM) significantly reduced the increase in caspase-3 activity. (* $p < 0.05$, significant using Bonferroni test compared to the rest of the groups, $n = 5$–6).

3.2. High Glucose and Peroxynitrite-Mediated Tyrosine Nitration of p85 Subunits Causes PI3-Kinase Dysfunction

Previous studies have shown that the p85 regulatory subunit of PI3-kinase is a sensitive target for peroxynitrite-induced tyrosine nitration [11,23,24]. Our immunoprecipitation assay showed that EC cultured in HG or treated with PN showed a significant increase in tyrosine nitration of p85 compared to EC cultured in normal glucose (Figure 2A, B). The increase in tyrosine nitration was markedly attenuated by the specific peroxynitrite decomposition catalyst FeTTPs (Fe, 2.5 μM) and by the specific nitration inhibitor epicatechin (Epi, 100 μM) (Figure 2B,C). In order to confirm the inhibitory effect of tyrosine nitration on PI3-kinase function, we determined the effects of HG and exogenous PN on the association between the regulatory p85 subunit and the catalytic p110 subunit in response to peroxynitrite, and in the presence or absence of nitration inhibitors. Treatment with HG or PN caused dissociation of p85 from p110 as the band for p85 could no longer be detected in the immune-precipitates (Figure 3A). Meanwhile, re-probing the blots with antibody against p110 subunit revealed the presence of p110 protein band. Treatments with FeTPPs or epicatechin restored the association between p85 and p110 in HG- or PN-treated EC cultures, and did not affect normal glucose controls. These results suggest that PN-mediated tyrosine nitration of p85 could alter the cell survival responses mediated normally by PI3-kinase activation.

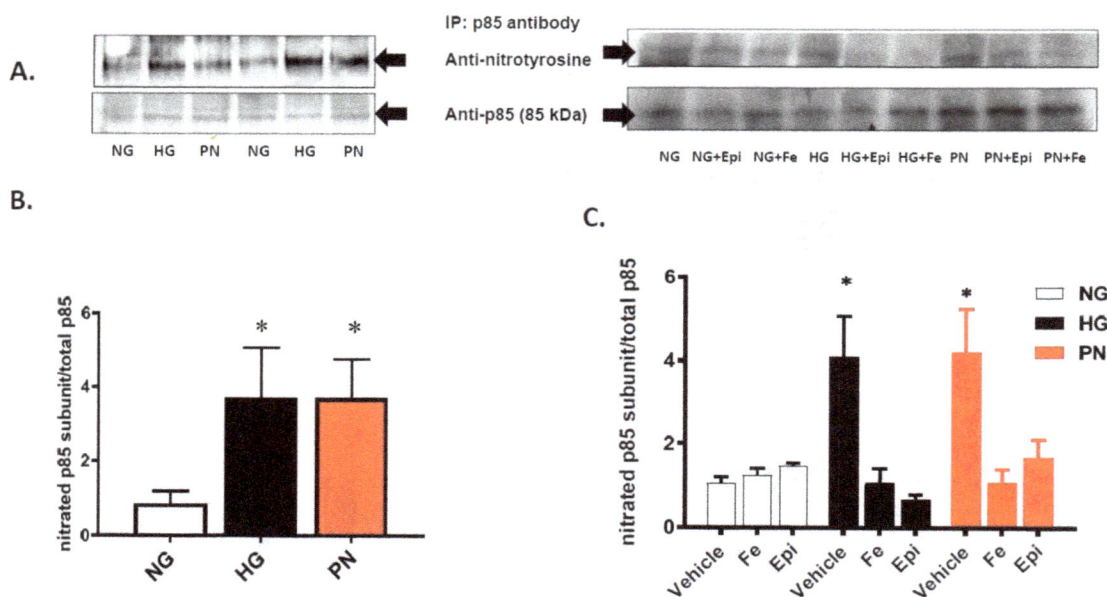

Figure 2. High glucose and peroxynitrite cause tyrosine nitration of the p85 subunit in ECs. (**A**) Representative blots of EC cultured in normal glucose (NG, 5 mM), high glucose (HG, 25 mM) for 3 days, or peroxynitrite (PN, 0.5 mM) overnight (left panel), alone or in the presence or absence of the specific peroxynitrite decomposition catalyst FeTTPs (Fe, 2.5 μM) or the nitration inhibitor epicatechin (Epi, 100 μM) (right panel). EC lysates were immune-precipitated with antibody against p85 subunit, and immunoblotted with antibodies that detect nitrotyrosine (NY) or anti-p85 s-subunit as loading control. (**B**) Statistical analysis of densitometry ratio of tyrosine-nitrated (NY) p85 subunit to total p85 using one-way ANOVA showed significant tyrosine nitration of p85 subunit in HG- and PN-treated cultures compared to normal glucose (* $p < 0.05$ vs. NG, $n = 4$). (**C**) Statistical analysis of densitometric ratio of tyrosine-nitrated (NY) p85 subunit to total p85 using two-way ANOVA showed significant interaction among examined groups. There was significant increase of tyrosine nitration of p85 subunit in HG- or PN-treated EC lysates compared to NG controls. Inhibiting tyrosine nitration using FeTTPs or epicatechin significantly reduced tyrosine nitration in HG- or PN-treated cells (* $p < 0.05$ versus rest of the groups, significant using Bonferroni test compared to the rest of the groups, $n = 4$–5).

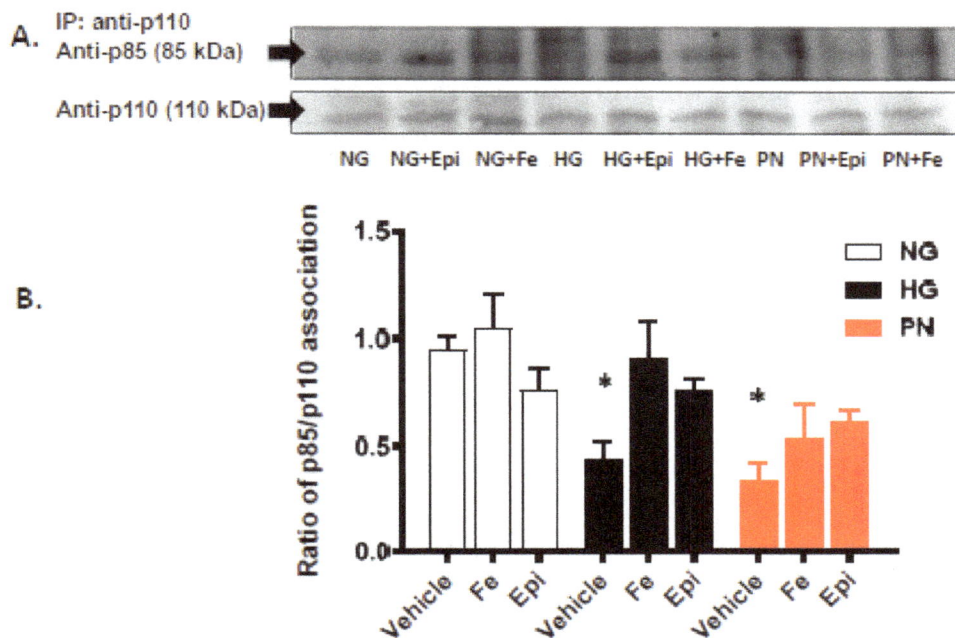

Figure 3. High glucose and peroxynitrite inhibit association between p85 and p110 subunits of PI3- kinase. (**A**) Representative blot of the catalytic subunit (p110) immunoprecipitation showing protein–protein interaction between p110 and the regulatory subunit (p85) that was decreased under high glucose (HG, 25 mM) for 3 days, or peroxynitrite (PN, 0.5 mM) overnight, as compared to normal glucose (NG, 5 mM) but restored back in the presence of FeTTPs (Fe, 2.5 μM) or epicatechin (Epi, 100 μM). (**B**) Statistical analysis of the ratio of p85 subunit and p110 subunit using two-way ANOVA showed significant impact of apoptotic insult and also for treatment compared to insult. EC cultures treated with HG or PN showed significant decrease in association of p85 subunit and p110 subunit compared to NG. The association between p85 and p110 was restored in cultures co-treated with the specific peroxynitrite decomposition catalyst FeTTPs (Fe, 2.5 μM) or the nitration inhibitor epicatechin (Epi, 100 μM) (* $p < 0.05$ versus vehicle, significant using Bonferroni test compared to the rest of the groups, $n = 4$–5).

3.3. High Glucose-Induced Peroxynitrite Inhibits Akt and Activates P38 MAPK in ECs

In response to survival factors, activation of PI3-kinase/Akt pathway is essential for EC survival, whereas dysfunction of PI3-kinase can result in activation of p38 MAPK and EC death. Next, we examined whether HG and PN-mediated nitration and dysfunction of PI3 kinase can result in alterations of the pro-survival Akt pathway or activation of the proapoptotic p38 MAPK pathway. As shown in Figure 4A, HG and PN significantly reduced the activity of Akt kinase activity evident by significant decreases in phosphorylation of its downstream target GSK-3. Meanwhile, re-probing the blots with Akt showed comparable levels of Akt protein. Moreover, treatment with HG or PN was associated with significant increases in phosphorylation of p38 MAPK (representative (Figure 5A) and bar graph (Figure 5B)). Co-treatment of EC maintained in HG or PN with the specific peroxynitrite decomposition catalyst FeTPPs attenuated the increases in p38 MAPK phosphorylation (Figure 5A,B). These findings suggest that nitration-mediated dysfunction of PI-3kinase is associated with activation of proapoptotic p38 MAPK signal and inhibition of the survival Akt signal in EC.

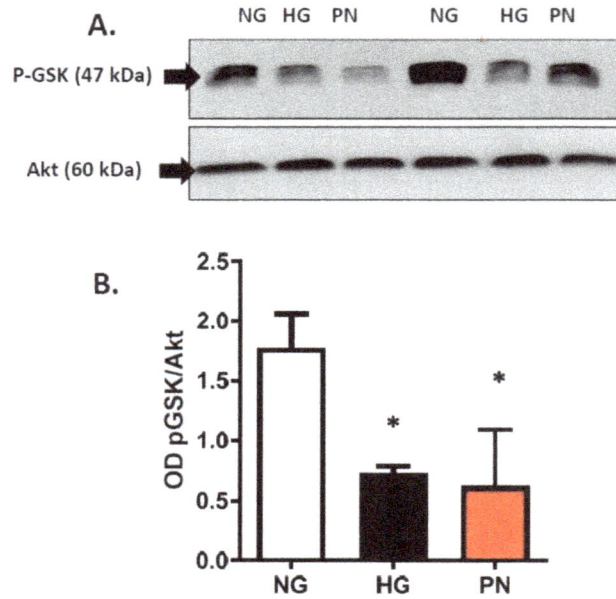

Figure 4. High glucose and peroxynitrite impaired Akt kinase activity. (**A**) Representative Western blot images of p-GSK-3α/β (Ser21/9) associated with total Akt that were immune-precipitated from EC cultures treated with normal glucose (NG, 5 mM), high glucose (HG, 25 mM) for 3 days, or peroxynitrite (PN, 0.5 mM) for overnight. (**B**) Statistical analysis using one-way ANOVA showed that HG or PN significantly inhibited survival signal evident by significant decrease in GSK-3α/β phosphorylation compared with NG. (* $p < 0.05$ versus NG, $n = 3$–4).

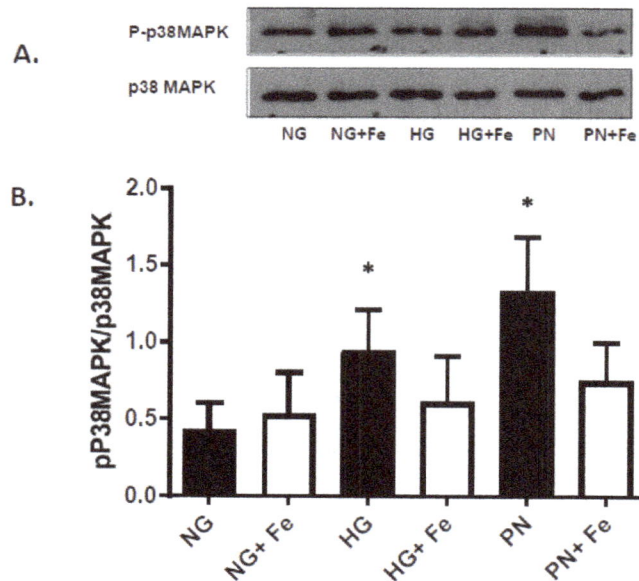

Figure 5. High glucose and peroxynitrite increased p38 MAPK activation that was reversed by FeTTPs. (**A**) Representative Western blot of total and phosphorylated p38 MAPK in lysates of retinal EC cultures treated with normal glucose (NG), high glucose (HG, 25 mM) for 3 days, or peroxynitrite (PN, 0.5 mM) overnight. **B.** Statistical analysis using two-way ANOVA showed significant impact of apoptotic insult and treatment effect. EC treated with HG or PN caused significant increase in p38 MAPK activation compared to NG. This effect was significantly reduced by co-treatment with FeTTPs (Fe, 2.5 μM) in HG- or PN-treated cultures. (* $p < 0.05$, significant using Bonferroni test compared to the rest of the groups, $n = 5$–6).

3.4. Overexpression of Active Akt Restores EC Cultures' Survival

To confirm the inhibitory role of PI3-kinase dysfunction in inhibiting pro-survival effects of Akt under HG or PN, we used adenoviral-mediated gene transfer of constitutively active Akt (Myr-Akt) into retinal EC cultures. A representative image of Western blot confirmed the selective overexpression of Akt in EC cultures transfected with Myr-Akt, but not in cells transfected with β-galactosidase (Figure 6A). Interestingly, the anti-apoptotic effect of Myr-Akt was associated with significant decreases in p38 MAPK expression in HG- or PN-treated EC compared to cultures infected with β-galactosidase constructs. Figure 6B shows that overexpression of the constituently activated Akt (Myr-Akt) significantly mitigated HG- or PN-induced increase in caspase-3 activity, as compared to EC transfected with β-galactosidase constructs. The above data imply that when the Akt pro-survival pathway is activated, the proapoptotic of p38 MAPK-driven pathway is downplayed.

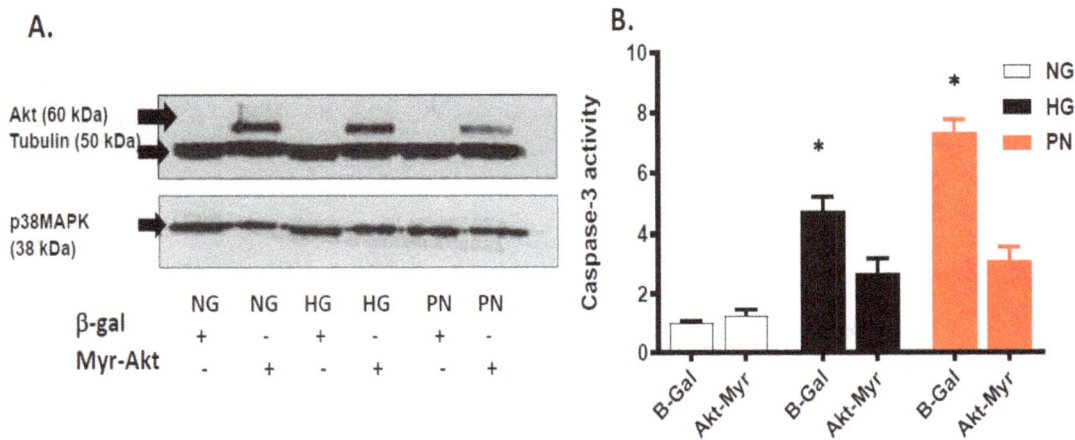

Figure 6. Overexpression of Myr-Akt attenuates proapoptotic effect of high glucose and peroxynitrite. (**A**) Representative Western blot showing selective expression of Akt in retinal EC cultures transfected with constitutively active Akt (Myr-Akt), but not in cultures transfected with adenovirus construct of β-galactosidase (β-Gal). Overexpression of Myr-Akt decreased expression of p38 MAPK. These observations were consistent in ECs cultured in normal glucose (NG, 5 mM), high glucose (HG, 25 mM) for 3 days, or peroxynitrite (PN, 0.5 mM) for overnight. (**B**) Statistical analysis of caspase-3 activity using two-way ANOVA showed significant effect of apoptotic insult and for treatment. Overexpression of Myr-Akt significantly reduced HG- or PN-induced increase in caspase-3 activity compared to EC cultures transfected with β-Gal (* $p < 0.05$, significant using Bonferroni test compared to the rest of the groups, $n = 5$).

3.5. Inhibition of p38 MAPK Restores Cell Survival in Retinal EC Cultures

To confirm the role of p38 MAPK activation in the proapoptotic effects of HG or PN, we treated the cells with the specific p38 MAPK inhibitor; SB203580 (25 μM). As shown in Figure 7, treatment of HG or PN induced apoptosis evidenced by significant increases in caspase-3 activity. Co-treatment with the p38 MAPK inhibitor significantly reduced the apoptosis induced in HG-maintained or PN-treated cultures. Treatment with SB203580 did not affect cell death in the normal glucose control. It is interesting that protective effect of SB203580 was more prominent in HG-treated cultures than in PN-treated cultures.

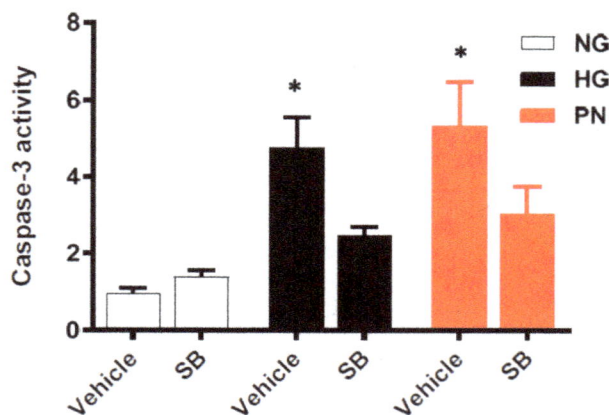

Figure 7. Inhibition of p38 MAPK using SB203580 attenuated high glucose and peroxynitrite-induced apoptosis in retinal EC cultures. Retinal EC cultures were co-treated with normal glucose (NG), high glucose (HG, 25 mM) for 3 days, or peroxynitrite (PN, 0.5 mM) for overnight in the presence or absence of the p38 MAPK inhibitor; SB203580 (25 μM). Statistical analysis using two-way ANOVA showed significant impact of both apoptotic insult and treatment. Inhibiting p38 MAPK significantly attenuated caspase-3 activity in HG- or PN-treated EC cultures compared with controls. (* $p < 0.05$ versus vehicle, significant using Bonferroni test compared to the rest of the groups, $n = 5$).

4. Discussion

Tyrosine nitration is a post-translational protein modification that can result in dramatic changes in protein structure and can modulate protein function (reviewed in [8]). In this study, we demonstrate that tyrosine nitration of the PI3-kinase p85 subunit inactivates the survival signaling pathway in ECs cultured in HG or PN (Figures 1–3). These effects are blocked by the specific peroxynitrite decomposition catalyst FeTPPs, and by the specific nitration inhibitor epicatechin. We show also that the proapoptotic effect of HG or PN is associated with an imbalance between Akt and p38 MAPK activation (Figures 4 and 5). Inhibiting p38 MAPK or overexpression of the constitutively active Akt masks the proapoptotic effect of HG or PN, and restores survival function in retinal EC cultures (Figures 6 and 7). The present study examined the impact of tyrosine nitration to confer inhibition of PI-3kinase/Akt, and activation of p38 MAPK pathway, resulting in apoptosis. Here, we provide evidence that inhibition of PI3-kinase by peroxynitrite-mediated tyrosine nitration triggers a molecular switch, resulting in reducing Akt activation, activating the proapoptotic p38 MAPK pathway, and eventually, cell death. A schematic presentation of these findings and the proposed mechanism by which tyrosine nitration of p85 subunit is serving as molecular switch between survival and apoptosis are illustrated in Figure 8.

Peroxynitrite, the combination product of nitric oxide and superoxide anion, is a powerful and short-lived free radical formed in vivo, that can directly react with different biomolecules by nitration and thiol oxidation (reviewed in [8]). When one molecule of superoxide-anion is formed, it may undergo the superoxide anion dismutase (SOD)-catalyzed dismutation reaction to hydrogen peroxide or interact with nitric oxide in a much faster reaction [25]. While superoxide anion and hydrogen peroxide-mediated oxidative effects are widely studied and well-documented [26,27], peroxynitrite remains a more relevant biological mediator of oxidative effects of both superoxide anion and nitric oxide in biological systems. Diabetes-mediated vascular dysfunction is highly linked to oxidative and nitrative stress [6,28]. Significant increases in tyrosine nitration have been demonstrated in plasma from diabetic patients [29], retinas from diabetic patients [12], and in experimental diabetes [30–33]. Previous in vitro work demonstrated that the p85 regulatory subunit of PI3-kinase is a susceptible target for peroxynitrite-induced tyrosine nitration [23]. Thus, we tested the hypothesis that HG-mediated apoptosis in EC cultures involves the action of peroxynitrite-mediated nitration and inhibition of the survival signal pathway. Indeed, EC cultures treated with HG or PN showed significant increases in tyrosine nitration of the regulatory p85 subunit and dysfunction of PI3-kinase (Figures 2 and 3). The inhibitory effect of nitration of p85 is evident by dramatic decreases in the association of the p85 subunit with the catalytic p110 subunit, as well as by significant decreases in Akt kinase activity.

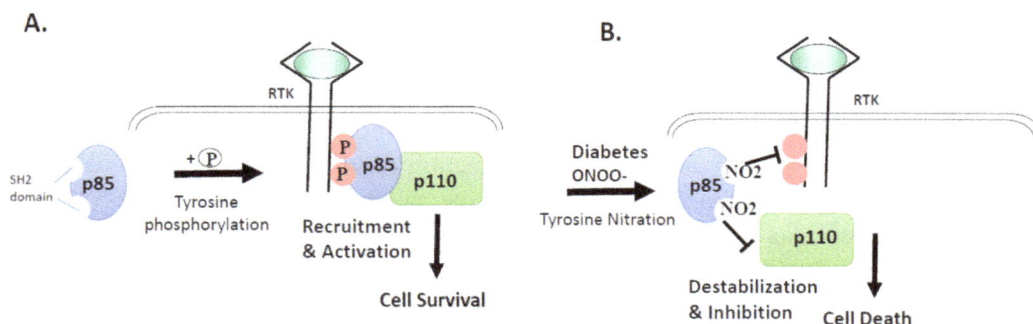

Figure 8. Conceptual frame of the study results. (**A**) Under normal physiological conditions, proper phosphorylation of regulatory subunit of PI3-kinase: p85 by receptor tyrosine kinases (RTK) takes place, resulting in strong association with the catalytic subunit p110, and initiation of cell survival signal. (**B**) Under diabetic or nitrative stress conditions, nitration of p85 subunit—instead of phosphorylation—occurs, resulting in its dissociation from p110 subunit and dysfunction of PI3-kinase and initiation of cell death signal.

Moreover, decomposing peroxynitrite (FeTPPs) and inhibiting tyrosine nitration (epicatechin) attenuated tyrosine nitration of p85 subunit and restored the interaction between the regulatory p85 subunit and the catalytic p110 subunit of PI3-kinase and survival promoting activity. FeTPPs, a selective peroxynitrite scavenger, is an iron porphyrin complex that catalytically isomerizes peroxynitrite into nitrate, while epicatechin is a natural flavonoid that selectively blocks nitration reactions, which does not affect the antioxidant defense [11,34]. Of note, our prior in vivo work demonstrated protective effects of FeTPPs and epicatechin in experimental diabetes and ischemic retinopathy [11,12,34]. Our findings showing the inhibitory effect of tyrosine nitration of p85 subunit resulting in vascular cell death lend further support to prior reports that showed the inhibitory effect of tyrosine nitration of p85 subunit and vascular cell death in oxygen-induced retinopathy [11] and nitration of p85 in brain of diabetic animals [24]. Additional targets were identified, including tyrosine nitration and inhibition of the nerve growth factor (NGF) survival receptor, TrkA, resulting in neurodegeneration in experimental diabetes [12,34] and nitration of actin, resulting in loss of vascular tone in smooth muscles [35]. These results confirm the relationship between nitration of p85, the decreases in Akt activity, and the proapoptotic effects of high glucose and peroxynitrite.

HG- and PN-induced apoptosis was evident by TUNEL and caspase-3 enzyme activity. The proapoptotic effects of HG and PN were associated with activation of p38 MAPK and decreases in Akt kinase activity. It is interesting that expression of constitutively active Akt (Myr-Akt) masked the proapoptotic effects of high glucose and exogenous peroxynitrite in treated EC cultures (Figure 6). In addition, inhibition of p38 MAPK also rescued retinal EC cultures from accelerated cell death (Figure 7). The protective effects of SB203580 were more prominent in high glucose cultures than in peroxynitrite-treated cells, probably because of the magnitude of peroxynitrite-induced cell death. Our results are in agreement with previous reports in other vascular cells [11,36,37]. Furthermore, the anti-apoptotic effect of Myr-Akt was associated with significant inhibition of p38 MAPK. These findings lend further support to a prior study that demonstrated that inhibition of p38 activation is mediated through phosphorylation and inhibition of MEKK3 by Akt in aortic EC cultures [18]. Similar results were reported [36] in HUVEC in response to angiopoietin-1 and in cardiac microvascular EC cultures in response to IL-18 [38], suggesting that the inhibitory influence of Akt on p38 MAPK is a general phenomenon in EC cultures. Moreover, similar findings of the mutual regulatory effects of Akt and p38 MAPK were observed in breast cancer cells [39].

Uncontrolled diabetes is characterized by hyperglycemia that has been shown to drive oxidative and nitrative stress [6,28] and to trigger EC death [14,28]. Paradoxically, HG also stimulates expression of multiple survival factors, including vascular endothelial growth factor (VEGF), NGF, and fibroblast growth factor (FGF) [12,40–43]. Under physiological conditions, survival factors normally mediate its signal via activation of ligand-mediated receptor tyrosine kinase (RTK). As illustrated in Figure 8, activation of regulatory subunit of PI3-kinase, p85, results in strong association with the catalytic subunit, p110, and initiation of cell survival signal under physiological conditions. By contrast, under diabetic and/or pro-oxidative conditions, tyrosine nitration of the regulatory p85 subunit will prevent its subsequent activation, and lead to dysfunction of PI3-kinase. The inhibitory effect of nitration of p85 is evident by dramatic decreases in the association of the regulatory p85 subunit with the catalytic p110 subunit, as well as by significant decreases in Akt kinase activity. In conclusion, our report is the first to elucidate the causal and inhibitory effects of tyrosine nitration of regulatory p85 subunit leading to inactivation of the pro-survival effects of Akt, and activation of the proapoptotic effect of p38MAPK in retinal EC cultures. This proposed pathway may provide a conceptual frame to explain the paradox of increased production of growth factors and uncoupling of its survival effects under diabetic conditions. Thus, therapeutic strategies to restore survival signals, rather than to target growth factors, should be considered to combat diabetic complications.

5. Conclusions

While tight glycemic control can delay microvascular complications, most diabetic patients experience uncontrolled hyperglycemia that predisposes them to the development of diabetic complications. Exposure to HG promotes expression of survival and angiogenic factors, such as VEGF and FGF, however, HG-induced PN inactivates pro-survival function in retinal EC cultures and triggers apoptosis. A schematic representation of the proposed mechanism is shown in Figure 8. The findings that decomposing peroxynitrite and inhibiting tyrosine nitration restored survival function open the door for new therapeutic strategies. Preventing tyrosine nitration and restoring protein function in response to high glucose and diabetes will be essential to interrupt the metabolic memory and legacy effect. Nitration inhibitors, including epicatechin, can be attractive in adjuvant therapy, in addition to anti-hyperglycemic drugs, in controlling early diabetic microvascular complication.

Acknowledgments: This work is supported by pre-doctoral fellowship from American Heart Association (15PRE22830019) to Sally Elshaer. This material is the result of work supported with resources and the use of facilities at the Charlie Norwood VA medical center, Augusta, GA. We would like to thank David Fulton (Vascular Biology Center, Augusta University) for providing Myr-Akt constructs.

Author Contributions: Sally L. Elshaer and Tahira Lemtalsi performed the experiments, analyzed the data and drafted the manuscript. This study was designed, coordinated by Azza B. El-Remessy as the principal investigator, providing conceptual and technical guidance for all aspects of the project in addition to editing the manuscript.

Conflicts of Interest: The authors declare no conflict of interest. The contents do not represent the views of the U.S. Department of Veterans Affairs or American Heart Association funding.

References

1. The Diabetes Control and Complications Trial Research Group. The effect of intensive treatment of diabetes on the development and progression of long-term complications in insulin-dependent diabetes mellitus. *N. Engl. J. Med.* **1993**, *329*, 977–986.

2. United Kingdom Prospective Diabetes Study Group. United Kingdom prospective diabetes study 24: A 6-year, randomized, controlled trial comparing sulfonylurea, insulin, and metformin therapy in patients with newly diagnosed type 2 diabetes that could not be controlled with diet therapy. *Ann. Int. Med.* **1998**, *128*, 165–175.

3. Pirola, L.; Balcerczyk, A.; Okabe, J.; El-Osta, A. Epigenetic phenomena linked to diabetic complications. *Nat. Rev. Endocrinol.* **2010**, *6*, 665–675. [CrossRef] [PubMed]

4. Testa, R.; Bonfigli, A.R.; Prattichizzo, F.; La Sala, L.; De Nigris, V.; Ceriello, A. The "metabolic memory" theory and the early treatment of hyperglycemia in prevention of diabetic complications. *Nutrients* **2017**, *9*, 437. [CrossRef] [PubMed]

5. Keating, S.T.; El-Osta, A. Glycemic memories and the epigenetic component of diabetic nephropathy. *Curr. Diab. Rep.* **2013**, *13*, 574–581. [CrossRef] [PubMed]

6. El-Remessy, A.B.; Abou-Mohamed, G.; Caldwell, R.W.; Caldwell, R.B. High glucose-induced tyrosine nitration in endothelial cells: Role of eNOS uncoupling and aldose reductase activation. *Investig. Ophthalmol. Vis. Sci.* **2003**, *44*, 3135–3143. [CrossRef]

7. Fouda, A.Y.; Artham, S.; El-Remessy, A.B.; Fagan, S.C. Renin-angiotensin system as a potential therapeutic target in stroke and retinopathy: Experimental and clinical evidence. *Clin. Sci. (Lond.)* **2016**, *130*, 221–238. [CrossRef] [PubMed]

8. Bartesaghi, S.; Radi, R. Fundamentals on the biochemistry of peroxynitrite and protein tyrosine nitration. *Redox Biol.* **2018**, *14*, 618–625. [CrossRef] [PubMed]

9. Chakravarti, B.; Chakravarti, D.N. Protein tyrosine nitration: Role in aging. *Curr. Aging Sci.* **2017**, *10*, 246–262. [CrossRef] [PubMed]

10. Gu, X.; El-Remessy, A.B.; Brooks, S.E.; Al-Shabrawey, M.; Tsai, N.T.; Caldwell, R.B. Hyperoxia induces retinal vascular endothelial cell apoptosis through formation of peroxynitrite. *Am. J. Physiol. Cell Physiol.* **2003**, *285*, C546–C554. [CrossRef] [PubMed]

11. Abdelsaid, M.A.; Pillai, B.A.; Matragoon, S.; Prakash, R.; Al-Shabrawey, M.; El-Remessy, A.B. Early intervention of tyrosine nitration prevents vaso-obliteration and neovascularization in ischemic retinopathy. *J. Pharmacol. Exp. Ther.* **2010**, *332*, 125–134. [CrossRef] [PubMed]

12. Ali, T.K.; Matragoon, S.; Pillai, B.A.; Liou, G.I.; El-Remessy, A.B. Peroxynitrite mediates retinal neurodegeneration by inhibiting nerve growth factor survival signaling in experimental and human diabetes. *Diabetes* **2008**, *57*, 889–898. [CrossRef] [PubMed]

13. Mizutani, M.; Kern, T.S.; Lorenzi, M. Accelerated death of retinal microvascular cells in human and experimental diabetic retinopathy. *J. Clin. Investig.* **1996**, *97*, 2883–2890. [CrossRef] [PubMed]

14. Mohr, S.; Xi, X.; Tang, J.; Kern, T.S. Caspase activation in retinas of diabetic and galactosemic mice and diabetic patients. *Diabetes* **2002**, *51*, 1172–1179. [CrossRef] [PubMed]

15. Kim, D.; Mecham, R.P.; Trackman, P.C.; Roy, S. Downregulation of lysyl oxidase protects retinal endothelial cells from high glucose-induced apoptosis. *Investig. Ophthalmol. Vis. Sci.* **2017**, *58*, 2725–2731. [CrossRef] [PubMed]

16. Kowluru, R.A. Effect of reinstitution of good glycemic control on retinal oxidative stress and nitrative stress in diabetic rats. *Diabetes* **2003**, *52*, 818–823. [CrossRef] [PubMed]

17. Wu, H.; Xia, X.; Jiang, C.; Wu, J.; Zhang, S.; Zheng, Z.; Liu, W.; Zhang, Y.; Ren, H.; Wei, C.; et al. High glucose attenuates insulin-induced VEGF expression in bovine retinal microvascular endothelial cells. *Eye (Lond.)* **2010**, *24*, 145–151. [CrossRef] [PubMed]

18. Gratton, J.P.; Morales-Ruiz, M.; Kureishi, Y.; Fulton, D.; Walsh, K.; Sessa, W.C. Akt down-regulation of p38 signaling provides a novel mechanism of vascular endothelial growth factor-mediated cytoprotection in endothelial cells. *J. Biol. Chem.* **2001**, *276*, 30359–30365. [CrossRef] [PubMed]

19. Shanab, A.Y.; Mysona, B.A.; Matragoon, S.; El-Remessy, A.B. Silencing p75(NTR) prevents proNGF-induced endothelial cell death and development of acellular capillaries in rat retina. *Mol. Ther. Methods Clin. Dev.* **2015**, *2*, 15013. [CrossRef] [PubMed]

20. Fulton, D.; Gratton, J.P.; McCabe, T.J.; Fontana, J.; Fujio, Y.; Walsh, K.; Franke, T.F.; Papapetropoulos, A.; Sessa, W.C. Regulation of endothelium-derived nitric oxide production by the protein kinase Akt. *Nature* **1999**, *399*, 597–601. [CrossRef] [PubMed]

21. Pannala, A.S.; Rice-Evans, C.A.; Halliwell, B.; Singh, S. Inhibition of peroxynitrite-mediated tyrosine nitration by catechin polyphenols. *Biochem. Biophys. Res. Commun.* **1997**, *232*, 164–168. [CrossRef] [PubMed]

22. Schroeder, P.; Klotz, L.O.; Sies, H. Amphiphilic properties of (−)-epicatechin and their significance for protection of cells against peroxynitrite. *Biochem. Biophys. Res. Commun.* **2003**, *307*, 69–73. [CrossRef]

23. Hellberg, C.B.; Boggs, S.E.; Lapetina, E.G. Phosphatidylinositol 3-kinase is a target for protein tyrosine nitration. *Biochem. Biophys. Res. Commun.* **1998**, *252*, 313–317. [CrossRef] [PubMed]

24. Abdelsaid, M.; Prakash, R.; Li, W.; Coucha, M.; Hafez, S.; Johnson, M.H.; Fagan, S.C.; Ergul, A. Metformin treatment in the period after stroke prevents nitrative stress and restores angiogenic signaling in the brain in diabetes. *Diabetes* **2015**, *64*, 1804–1817. [CrossRef] [PubMed]

25. Ferrer-Sueta, G.; Radi, R. Chemical biology of peroxynitrite: Kinetics, diffusion, and radicals. *ACS Chem. Biol.* **2009**, *4*, 161–177. [CrossRef] [PubMed]

26. Munzel, T.; Sorensen, M.; Schmidt, F.; Schmidt, E.; Steven, S.; Kroller-Schon, S.; Daiber, A. The adverse effects of environmental noise exposure on oxidative stress and cardiovascular risk. *Antioxid. Redox Signal.* **2018**, *28*, 873–908. [CrossRef] [PubMed]

27. Lassegue, B.; San Martin, A.; Griendling, K.K. Biochemistry, physiology, and pathophysiology of NADPH oxidases in the cardiovascular system. *Circ. Res.* **2012**, *110*, 1364–1390. [CrossRef] [PubMed]

28. Zou, M.H.; Shi, C.; Cohen, R.A. High glucose via peroxynitrite causes tyrosine nitration and inactivation of prostacyclin synthase that is associated with thromboxane/prostaglandin H(2) receptor-mediated apoptosis and adhesion molecule expression in cultured human aortic endothelial cells. *Diabetes* **2002**, *51*, 198–203. [PubMed]

29. Ceriello, A.; Mercuri, F.; Quagliaro, L.; Assaloni, R.; Motz, E.; Tonutti, L.; Taboga, C. Detection of nitrotyrosine in the diabetic plasma: Evidence of oxidative stress. *Diabetologia* **2001**, *44*, 834–838. [PubMed]

30. El-Remessy, A.B.; Behzadian, M.A.; Abou-Mohamed, G.; Franklin, T.; Caldwell, R.W.; Caldwell, R.B. Experimental diabetes causes breakdown of the blood-retina barrier by a mechanism involving tyrosine nitration and increases in expression of vascular endothelial growth factor and urokinase plasminogen activator receptor. *Am. J. Pathol.* **2003**, *162*, 1995–2004. [CrossRef]

31. El-Remessy, A.B.; Al-Shabrawey, M.; Khalifa, Y.; Tsai, N.T.; Caldwell, R.B.; Liou, G.I. Neuroprotective and blood-retinal barrier-preserving effects of cannabidiol in experimental diabetes. *Am. J. Pathol.* **2006**, *168*, 235–244. [CrossRef] [PubMed]

32. Zou, M.H.; Li, H.; He, C.; Lin, M.; Lyons, T.J.; Xie, Z. Tyrosine nitration of prostacyclin synthase is associated with enhanced retinal cell apoptosis in diabetes. *Am. J. Pathol.* **2011**, *179*, 2835–2844. [CrossRef] [PubMed]

33. Nie, H.; Wu, J.L.; Zhang, M.; Xu, J.; Zou, M.H. Endothelial nitric oxide synthase-dependent tyrosine nitration of prostacyclin synthase in diabetes in vivo. *Diabetes* **2006**, *55*, 3133–3141. [CrossRef] [PubMed]

34. Al-Gayyar, M.M.; Matragoon, S.; Pillai, B.A.; Ali, T.K.; Abdelsaid, M.A.; El-Remessy, A.B. Epicatechin blocks pro-nerve growth factor (proNGF)-mediated retinal neurodegeneration via inhibition of p75 neurotrophin receptor expression in a rat model of diabetes [corrected]. *Diabetologia* **2011**, *54*, 669–680. [CrossRef] [PubMed]

35. Coucha, M.; Abdelsaid, M.; Li, W.; Johnson, M.H.; Orfi, L.; El-Remessy, A.B.; Fagan, S.C.; Ergul, A. Nox4 contributes to the hypoxia-mediated regulation of actin cytoskeleton in cerebrovascular smooth muscle. *Life Sci.* **2016**, *163*, 46–54. [CrossRef] [PubMed]

36. Harfouche, R.; Gratton, J.P.; Yancopoulos, G.D.; Noseda, M.; Karsan, A.; Hussain, S.N. Angiopoietin-1 activates both anti- and proapoptotic mitogen-activated protein kinases. *FASEB J.* **2003**, *17*, 1523–1525. [CrossRef] [PubMed]

37. Huang, W.Y.; Wu, H.; Li, D.J.; Song, J.F.; Xiao, Y.D.; Liu, C.Q.; Zhou, J.Z.; Sui, Z.Q. Protective effects of blueberry anthocyanins against H_2O_2-induced oxidative injuries in human retinal pigment epithelial cells. *J. Agric. Food Chem.* **2018**, *66*, 1638–1648. [CrossRef] [PubMed]

38. Chandrasekar, B.; Valente, A.J.; Freeman, G.L.; Mahimainathan, L.; Mummidi, S. Interleukin-18 induces human cardiac endothelial cell death via a novel signaling pathway involving NF-kappaB-dependent PTEN activation. *Biochem. Biophys. Res. Commun.* **2006**, *339*, 956–963. [CrossRef] [PubMed]

39. Kello, M.; Kulikova, L.; Vaskova, J.; Nagyova, A.; Mojzis, J. Fruit peel polyphenolic extract-induced apoptosis in human breast cancer cells is associated with ROS production and modulation of p38MAPK/ERK1/2 and the Akt signaling pathway. *Nutr. Cancer* **2017**, *69*, 920–931. [CrossRef] [PubMed]

40. El-Remessy, A.B.; Franklin, T.; Ghaley, N.; Yang, J.; Brands, M.W.; Caldwell, R.B.; Behzadian, M.A. Diabetes-induced superoxide anion and breakdown of the blood-retinal barrier: Role of the VEGF/uPAR pathway. *PLoS ONE* **2013**, *8*, e71868. [CrossRef] [PubMed]

41. Park, K.S.; Kim, S.S.; Kim, J.C.; Kim, H.C.; Im, Y.S.; Ahn, C.W.; Lee, H.K. Serum and tear levels of nerve growth factor in diabetic retinopathy patients. *Am. J. Ophthalmol.* **2008**, *145*, 432–437. [CrossRef] [PubMed]

42. Wu, Y.; Zhang, Q.; Zhang, R. Kaempferol targets estrogen-related receptor alpha and suppresses the angiogenesis of human retinal endothelial cells under high glucose conditions. *Exp. Ther. Med.* **2017**, *14*, 5576–5582. [PubMed]

43. Clyne, A.M.; Zhu, H.; Edelman, E.R. Elevated fibroblast growth factor-2 increases tumor necrosis factor-alpha induced endothelial cell death in high glucose. *J. Cell. Physiol.* **2008**, *217*, 86–92. [CrossRef] [PubMed]

5

Effects of Mulberry Fruit (*Morus alba* L.) Consumption on Health Outcomes

Hongxia Zhang [1,†], Zheng Feei Ma [2,3,*,†] (iD), Xiaoqin Luo [4] and Xinli Li [5]

[1] Department of Food Science, University of Otago, Dunedin 9016, New Zealand; zhanghongxia326@hotmail.com
[2] Department of Public Health, Xi'an Jiaotong-Liverpool University, Suzhou 215123, China
[3] School of Medical Sciences, Universiti Sains Malaysia, Kota Bharu 15200, Malaysia
[4] Department of Nutrition and Food Safety, School of Public Health, Xi'an Jiaotong University Health Science Center, Xi'an 710061, China; luoxiaoqin2012@mail.xjtu.edu.cn
[5] Department of Nutrition and Food Hygiene, School of Public Health, Medical College of Soochow University, Suzhou 215123, China; lixinli@suda.edu.cn
* Correspondence: Zhengfeei.Ma@xjtlu.edu.cn
† These authors contributed equally to this work.

Abstract: Mulberry (*Morus alba* L.) belongs to the Moraceae family and is widely planted in Asia. Mulberry fruits are generally consumed as fresh fruits, jams and juices. They contain considerable amounts of biologically active ingredients that might be associated with some potential pharmacological activities that are beneficial for health. Therefore, they have been traditionally used in traditional medicine. Studies have reported that the presence of bioactive components in mulberry fruits, including alkaloids and flavonoid, are associated with bioactivities such as antioxidant. One of the most important compounds in mulberry fruits is anthocyanins which are water-soluble bioactive ingredients of the polyphenol class. Studies have shown that mulberry fruits possess several potential pharmacological health benefits including anti-cholesterol, anti-obesity and hepatoprotective effects which might be associated with the presence of some of these bioactive compounds. However, human intervention studies on the pharmacological activities of mulberry fruits are limited. Therefore, future studies should explore the effect of mulberry fruit consumption on human health and elucidate the detailed compounds. This paper provides an overview of the pharmacological activities of mulberry fruits.

Keywords: mulberry; polyphenols; anthocyanins; health; nutrition

1. Introduction

Natural products have always been a rich source of biologically active compounds [1–3]. These substances present in fruits and vegetables have received increasing attention because of their antioxidant properties and potential strategy in reducing the risk of certain types of diseases such as metabolic syndrome [1,4,5]. About 50% of the drugs approved are natural products [5]. About 80% of the populations living in many countries rely on the phytomedicines and the plant-derived drug market is estimated to reach approximately $35 billion in 2020 [5,6].

Mulberry (*Morus alba* L.) belongs to the Morus genus of the Moraceae family [7]. Mulberry is also known as *Ramulus Mori* or Sangzhi [8]. To date, this genus has 24 species and 100 varieties that have been known [7]. Mulberry is a species native to China and has been widely cultivated in many regions including Asia, Africa, America, Europe and India [9]. China has planted mulberry for more than 5000 years and mulberry is a traditional Chinese edible fruit that can be eaten fresh [10]. According to traditional Chinese Medicine, mulberry fruits are used to improve eyesight and protect against liver damage [11]. They are grown to feed silkworms [12,13] The season of fresh mulberry fruit in China is usually less than 1 month. Mulberry fruits are difficult to preserve because they have high water content (i.e., ~80%) [11]. Mulberry has been used in traditional Oriental medicine to treat diabetes and premature white hair [14].

Mulberry fruits are appetising and low in calories [15]. Mulberry fruits have a sour taste with a pH < 3.5, providing a more concentrated flavour for fruit production and fresh-eating [16]. Mulberry fruits possess several potential pharmacological properties including anti-cholesterol, anti-diabetic, antioxidative and anti-obesity effects [8,17–19]. These pharmacological properties are due to the presence of polyphenol compounds including anthocyanins, however, different colours of mulberry fruits even from the same species may have different amounts of anthocyanins [20]. Cyanidin-3-rutinoside and cyanidin-3-glucoside are the major anthocyanins isolated from mulberry fruits [21,22].

Although different mulberry varieties with the same genotype are likely to have differences in nutritional values and pharmacological properties [23], the aim of this work was to review some potential roles of mulberry fruits (*Morus alba* L.) and their bioactive compounds in health. Also, some of the potential mechanisms of their actions will be discussed briefly. We hope that this work would provide a valuable reference resource for future studies in this area.

Search Strategy

An electronic literature search was conducted using Google Scholar, Medline (OvidSP) and PubMed until February 2018. Additional articles were identified and obtained from references in the retrieved articles. Search terms included combinations of the following: mulberry, fruits, hypertension, diabetes, anti-tumour, hepatoprotective, anti-obesity, anti-oxidative stress and phytochemicals. For the purpose of this mini-review, the search was restricted to experimental, epidemiological and clinical studies published in English that address the phytochemical constituents and pharmacological properties of mulberry fruits (*Morus alba* L.).

2. Phytochemical Compounds

Compared with mulberry leaves and barks, mulberry fruits are less commonly used in traditional Chinese Medicine. The possible reasons might be due to the lack of awareness of their health benefits and limited production [24]. However, there is increasing interest in isolating and quantifying the phytochemical compounds from mulberry fruits. This is because mulberry fruits can be also consumed as foods [24]. Mulberry fruits have strong antioxidant property which is due primarily to the presence of polyphenols [25]. Figure 1 shows the major polyphenol composition found in mulberry fruits.

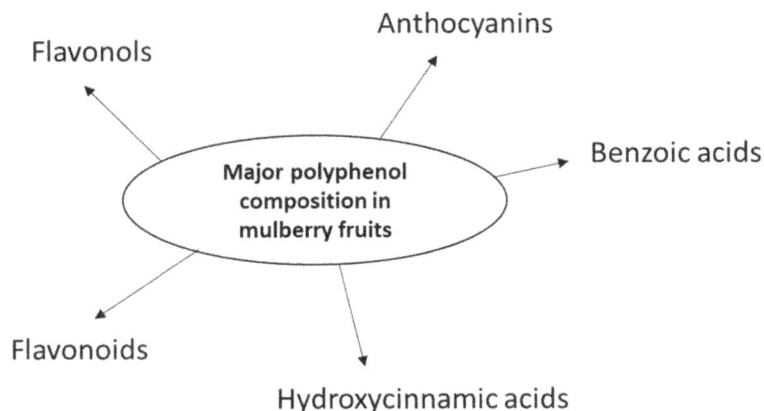

Figure 1. Major polyphenol composition in mulberry fruits.

Phytochemical compounds of mulberry fruits (*Morus nigra*, *Morus indica* and *Morus rubra*) have been reported in several studies [26–28]. Kang, Hur, Kim, Ryu and Kim [17] isolated cyanidin-3-*O*-β-D-glucopyranoside (C3G) from 1% HCl-MeOH mulberry fruit extracts using Amberlite IRC-50 ion exchange chromatography. C3G was identified and quantified by liquid chromatography-mass spectroscopy (LC-MS) and High-Performance Liquid Chromatography (HPLC) [17]. C3G is an aglycon of anthocyanin that has inflammation-suppressing and free radical scavenging activity, which might protect against endothelial dysfunction [17].

In a study assessing the polyphenolic composition of five major mulberry fruit varieties (i.e., Pachungsipyung, Whazosipmunja, Suwonnosang, Jasan and Mocksang) cultivated in Korea using spectrophotometric methods, Bae and Suh [29] reported that the total phenols, total anthocyanins, coloured (ionised) anthocyanins and total flavanols ranged from 960 to 2570 µg/g gallic acid equivalents, 137 to 2057 µg/g malvidin-3-glucoside equivalents, 10 to 190 µg/g malvidin-3-glucoside equivalents and 6 to 65 µg/g catechin equivalents.

Kusano, Orihara, Tsukamoto, Shibano, Coskun, Guvenc and Erdurak [24] isolated five new nortropane alkaloids (i.e., 2α,3β-dihydroxynortropane, 2β,3β-dihydroxynortropane, 2α,3β-6exo-trihydroxynortropane, 2α,3β,4α-trihydroxynortropane, 3β,6exo-dihydroxynortropane) along with nor-ψ-tropine from ripened mulberry fruits grown in Turkey. In addition, Kusano, Orihara, Tsukamoto, Shibano, Coskun, Guvenc and Erdurak [24] also isolated and determined the new structures of six amino acids, which were morusimic acid A, morusimic acid B, morusimic acid C, morusimic acid D, morusimic acid E and morusimic acid F using spectroscopic data.

Kim, et al. [30] identified five pyrrole alkaloids in mulberry fruits, which were morrole B, morrole C, morrole D, morrole E and morrole F based on spectroscopic data. In addition, the authors [30] also isolated 11 pyrrole alkaloids, which were 4-[formyl-5-(hydroxymethyl)-1H-pyrrol-1-yl]butanoate, 2-(5-hydroxymethyl-2′,5′-dioxo-2′,3′,4′,5′-tetrahydro-1′H-1,3′-bipyrrole)carbaldehyde, 4-[formyl-5-(hydroxymethyl)-1H-pyrrol-1-yl]butanoate, 4-[formyl-5-(methoxymethyl)-1H-pyrrol-1-yl]butanoic acid, methyl 2-[2-formyl-5-(methoxymethyl)-1H-pyrrole-1-yl]propanoate, 2-(5′-hydroxymethyl-2′-formylpyrrol-1′-yl)-3-phenyl-propionic acid lactone, methyl 2-[2-formyl-5-(methoxymethyl)-1H-pyrrol-1-yl]-3-(4-hydroxyphenyl)propanoate, 2-(5′- hydroxymethyl-2′-formylpyrrol-1′-yl)-3-(4-hydroxyphenyl)-propionic acid lactone, 2-(5-hydroxymethyl- 2-formylpyrrole-1-yl)propionic acid lactone, 2-(5-hydroxymethyl-2-formylpyrrol-1-yl)isovaleric acid lactone, 2-(5-hydroxymethyl-2-formylpyrrole-1-yl)isocaproic acid lactone and 2-[2-formyl-5-(hydroxymethyl)-1-pyrrolyl-]3-methylpentanoic acid lactone.

Natić, et al. [31] isolated epigallocatechin, epigallocatechin gallate, gallocatechin, gallocatechin gallate, isorhamnetin glucuronide, isorhamnetin hexoside, isorhamnetin hexosylhexoside, kaempferol glucuronide, kaempferol hexoside, kaempferol hexosylhexoside, kaempferol rhamnosylhexoside, morin and naringin from mulberry fruits grown in Vojvodina, North Serbia. Quercetin glucoronide, quercetin hexoside, quercetin hexosylhexoside, quercetrin from mulberry fruits were also isolated using ultra HPLC (UHPLC) system coupled to a high resolution mass spectrophotometer [31]. In addition, the authors [31] also reported the presence of cyanidin galloylhexoside, cyanidin hexoside, cyanidin hexosylhexoside, cyanidin pentoside, cyanidin rhamnosylhexoside, delphinidin acetylhexoside, delphinidin hexoside, delphinidin rhamnosylhexoside, pelargonidin hexoside, pelargonidin rhamnosylhexoside and petunidin rhamnosylhexoside from mulberry fruits.

Qin, et al. [32] isolated cyanidin 3-*O*-glucoside, cyanidin 3-*O*-rutinoside, pelargonidin 3-*O*-glucoside and pelargonidin 3-*O*-rutinoside ultraviolet-visible from mulberry fruits grown in Shaanxi, China using UV-Visible spectroscopy, HPLC-pulsed amperometric detector (PAD), LC-MS and proton nuclear magnetic resonance (1HNMR). Du, et al. [33] isolated cyanidin 3-*O*-β-D-galactopyranoside, cyanidin 3-*O*-β-D-glucopyranoside and cyanidin 7-*O*-β-D-glucopyranoside from mulberry fruits bought from local stores in Hangzhou, China. In addition, the authors [33] also isolated cyanidin 3-*O*-(6″-*O*-α-rhamnopyranosyl-β-D-galactopyranoside) and cyanidin

3-O-(6''-O-α-rhamnopyranosyl-β-D-glucopyranoside) from mulberry fruits. While Memon, et al. [34] isolated gallic acid, protocatechuic acid, protocatechuic aldehyde, p-hydroxybenzoic acid, vanillic acid, chlorogenic acid, syringic acid, syringealdehyde and m-coumaric acid from mulberry fruits grown in Pakistan. A study by Peng, et al. [35] identified eight major compounds which were gallic acid, chlorogenic acid, protocatechuic acid, rutin, caffeic acid, 3-caffeoyl quinic acid, 4-caffeoyl quinic acid and quercetin-3-O-glucoside in mulberry fruit water extract.

Another study by Kim, et al. [36] identified four pyrrole alkaloids from mulberry fruits planted in Chonbuk, Korea which were 2-formyl-5-(hydroxymethyl)-1H-pyrrole-1-butanoic acid, 5-(hydroxymethyl)-1H-pyrrole-2-carboxaldehyde, 2-formyl-1H-pyrrole-1-butanoic acid and 2-formyl-5-(methoxymethyl)-1H-pyrrole-1-butanoic acid. In addition, the authors [36] also isolated a new pyrrole alkaloid, which was morrole A. All the structures of isolated pyrrole alkaloids were determined using 1D and 2D nuclear magnetic resonance (NMR) analyses [36].

Isabelle, et al. [37] reported the presence of 3-caffeoyl quinic acid, 5-caffeoyl quinic acid, cyanidin-3-glucoside, 4-caffeoyl quinic acid, cyanidin-3-rutinoside, pelargonidin-3-glucoside, rutin, quercetin and kaempferol-3-rutinoside in the Chinese mulberry fruit cultivar Guo-2. In addition, the authors [37] also found the presence of α-tocopherol, α-tocotrienol, δ-tocopherol, γ-tocopherol, β-carotene, lutein, neoxanthin and violaxanthin in the Chinese mulberry fruit cultivar Bei-2-5, Guiyou-154, Heipisang, Xuan-27 and Tang-10. Rutin, 1-deoxynojirimycin (DJN), cyanidin-3-O-β-glucoside, cyanidin-3-O-β-rutinoside, resveratrol and oxyresveratrol were also present in the Chinese mulberry fruits [38,39].

Wang, Xiang, Wang, Tang and He [15] isolated quercetin-3-O-β-D-glucopyranoside, quercetin 3-O-(6''-O-acetyl)-β-D-glucopyranoside, quercetin 3-O-β-D-rutinoside, quercetin 7-O-β-D-glucopyranoside, quercetin 3,7-di-O-β-D-glucopyranoside, kaempferol 3-O-β-D-glucopyranoside, kaempferol 3-O-β-D-rutinoside, isobavachalcone, 2,4,2',4',-tetrahydroxy-3'-(3-methyl-2-butenyl)-chalcone (morachalcone), (2E)-1-[2,3-dihydro-4-hydroxy-2-(1-methylethenyl)-5-benzofuranyl]-3-(4-hydroxyphenyl)-1-propanone, 5,7,3'-trihydroxy-flavanone-49-O-β-D-glucopyranoside, 5,7,4'-trihydroxy-flavanone-3'-O-β-D-glucopyranoside, dihydrokaempferol 7-O-ß-D-glucopyranoside, 2-O-(3,4-dihydroxybenzoyl)-2,4,6-trihydroxyphenylacetic acid, 2-O-(3,4-dihydroxybenzoyl)-2,4,6-trihydroxyphenylmethylacetate (jaboticabin), p-hydroxybenzoic acid, protocatechuic acid, 3-methoxy-4-hydroxybenzoic acid (vanillic acid), protocatechuic acid methyl ester, protocatechuic acid ethyl ester, 4-hydroxyphenylacetic acid methyl ester, 5,7-dihydroxychromone, 2-(4-hydroxyphenyl)ethanol (tyrosol) and pyrocatecholin in ethyl acetate-soluble extract of mulberry fruits. The authors [15] determined the structures of isolated compounds based on MS and NMR analysis.

Jiang and Nie [40] reported that mulberry fruit cultivar Hetianbaisang contains many types of essential amino acids (i.e., isoleucine, leucine, threonine, lysine, valine, phenylalanine, tyrosine, tryptophan, histidine, methionine and cysteine) and seven non-essential amino acids (i.e., arginine, alanine, proline, glutamic acid, glycine, serine and aspartic acid). In addition, the authors [40] also found the presence of minerals including potassium, calcium, magnesium, iron, sodium, zinc, copper, selenium and manganese in mulberry fruit cultivar Hetianbaisang. Mulberry fruit cultivar Hetianbaisang also contains organic acids including malic acid, succinic acid, citric acid, tartaric acid, acetic acid [40]. In addition, linoleic acid, myristic acid, stearic acid, palmitic acid and α-linoleic acid were also detected in mulberry fruit cultivar Hetianbaisang [40].

Yang, Yang and Zheng [11] reported that the total phenolics, total flavonoids and anthocyanins in the freeze-dried powder of mulberry fruits were 23.0 mg/g gallic acid equivalents, 3.9 mg/g rutin equivalents, 0.87 mg/g cyanidin-3-glucoside equivalents, respectively. The major flavonol in mulberry fruit powder was rutin (0.43 mg/g), followed by morin (0.16 mg/g), quercetin (0.01 mg/g) and myricetin (0.01 mg/g) [11]. HPLC was used to determine the flavonols in mulberry fruit powder [11]. In addition, the freeze-dried powder of mulberry fruits also contained 1.20 mg/g ascorbic acid, 0.32 mg/g vitamin E and 243.0 mg/g dietary fibre [11].

Fatty acid content and composition of mulberry can vary according to different ecological conditions. For example, Yang, Yang and Zheng [11] found that Chinese mulberry fruits had 7.55% total lipids, with 87.5% of unsaturated fatty acids. The highest fatty acid content in Chinese mulberry fruits was linoleic acid C18:2 (79.4%), followed by palmitic acid C16:2 (8.6%) and oleic acid C18:1 (7.5%) [11]. In addition, Chinese mulberry also contained 0.6% α-linolenic acid C18:3 [11]. Although the highest fatty acid content in Turkish mulberry was linoleic acid C18:2 (57.3%) followed by palmitic acid C16:0 (22.4%); no presence of linolenic acid C18:3 was reported [7].

Different colours of mulberry fruits (*M. alba* L) such as red, purple and purple-red have been reported [41]. Aramwit, Bang and Srichana [41] reported that purple mulberry fruit extract had higher contents of total sugars and anthocyanins than red and purple-red mulberry fruit extracts. This is because sugars are needed as the precursors to synthesis anthocyanins [41]. However, red mulberry fruit had a higher ascorbic acid and ß-carotene than purple and purple-red mulberry fruit extracts [41].

Many volatile compounds have also been found in mulberry fruits [42]. Calin-Sanchez, Martinez-Nicolas, Munera-Picazo, Carbonell-Barrachina, Legua and Hernandez [42] reported that volatile compounds found in mulberry fruits grown in Spain included acetic acid, 3-hydroxyl-2-butanone, ethyl butyrate, ethyl acetate, 3-methylbutanal, 2-methybutanal, heptanal, methional, hexanal, trans-2-hexanal, 2-octenone,hexanoic acid, benzaldehyde, methyl hexanoate, 2-ethylhexanal, octanal, limonene, 6-methyl-5-hepten-2on, ethyl hexanoate, 2,4-nonanadienal, phenylacetaldehyde, trans-2-octenal, cis-α-ocimene, terpinonene, 2-nonanone, nonanal, octanoic acid, cis-2-nonenal, dodecanoic acid, terpinen-4-ol, ethyl octanoate, ethyl dodecanoate, decanal, decanoic acid and ethyl decanoate. The authors [42] suggested that these volatile compounds in mulberry fruits might present better sensory profiles for the market demands from consumers.

Chen, et al. [43] reported that the levels of phenolic compounds in mulberry fruits are higher than blackberry, blueberry, raspberry and strawberry, suggesting that mulberry fruits can be used as good sources of phenolic compounds. Therefore, mulberry fruits are rich in diverse phenolic compounds including polyhenols, anthocyanins and flavonoids.

3. Pharmacological Properties

As mentioned previously, mulberry fruits are rich in anthocyanins [44], which have attracted attention of researchers and consumers because of their potential pharmacological activities on health [45–49]. Anthocyanins from mulberry fruits can inhibit the oxidation of low-density lipoprotein (LDL) and scavenge free radicals [33,50]. Many studies have showed that mulberry leaves exhibit a wide range of pharmacological activities [51–57]. However, there are limited studies that have been conducted on the pharmacological properties of mulberry fruits [15,58,59]. Also, most studies have been conducted in animal models using mulberry fruits as a dietary supplement [15,58,59]. Although existing literature shows that there is relationship between mulberry fruit consumption and improved health outcomes, these studies often infer a causal correlation between a bioactive substance of mulberry fruits and the observed health outcomes. This approach is more likely to oversimplify the complicated body mechanisms that will eventually lead to the observed health outcomes. Therefore, the conclusions based on such studies should always be interpreted with caution [60] because the observed health outcomes may not be attributed to the action of a single bioactive compound of mulberry fruits.

3.1. Hypolipidemic

Cardiovascular disease (CVD) is one of the most common causes of deaths, with about 17 million people die of CVD (including stroke and coronary heart disease) every year worldwide [61,62]. It is estimated that CVD will continue to be the largest contributor to global mortality in the future [63] Hyperlipidemia is one of the major risk factors for CVD [64]. Therefore, an increasing focus has been reported in research studies that determine the effectiveness of natural alternative medicine in reducing blood lipid levels [11]. This is because majority of the hypolipidemic drugs can potentially cause side effects and they are expensive [11].

Yang, Yang and Zheng [11] reported that rat fed with high fat diet supplemented with 5% or 10% mulberry fruit powder had a significant decrease in the concentration of serum and liver triglyceride, total cholesterol and serum LDL cholesterol. An increase in the serum high-density lipoprotein (HDL) cholesterol was reported in rat fed with high fat diet supplemented with 5% or 10% mulberry fruit powder [11]. It is suggested that the presence of dietary fiber in mulberry fruits inhibits the hepatic lipogenesis and increases LDL-receptor activity [65]. In addition, the authors suggested that mulberry fruits might have a hypolipidemic effect because mulberry fruits have high content of dietary fiber and linoleic acid [11].

Chen, Liu, Hsu, Huang, Yang and Wang [50] reported that New Zealand white rabbits fed with high cholesterol diet (HCD) (containing 95.7% standard Purina chow, 3% lard oil and 1.3% cholesterol) plus 0.5% or 1.0% water extract of mulberry fruits for 10 weeks had lower levels of total cholesterol, LDL cholesterol, and triglycerides than those fed with only lard oil diet. The authors [50] also showed that rabbits fed with HCD plus 0.5% or 1.0% water extract of mulberry fruits had significantly reduced severe atherosclerosis in the aorta by 42–63% and these findings were supported by histopathological examination of blood vessel of rabbits. The effect of water extract of mulberry fruits on the levels of total cholesterol and LDL cholesterol was reported to be dose-dependent [50]. No adverse effects on the changes of liver or renal functions in rabbits fed with HCD plus 0.5% or 1.0% water extract of mulberry fruits were reported [50].

In a randomised controlled study of 58 hypercholesterolemic adults aged 30–60 years, Sirikanchanarod, et al. [66] reported that after 6 weeks of 45 g freeze-dried mulberry fruit consumption (325 mg anthocyanins), the intervention group had a significantly lower level of total cholesterol and LDL (both p-values < 0.001) than the control group. The authors [66] suggested that mulberry fruits might be used as an alternative treatment for hypercholesterolemic patients. Therefore, the consumption of mulberry fruits might reduce the risk of atherosclerosis because mulberry fruits possess anti-hyperlipidemic and anti-oxidative abilities to prevent the oxidation of LDL [50].

3.2. Anti-Diabetic

Diabetes is characterised by hyperglycemia which results from the defects of secretion of insulin [67]. It is associated with a series of health complications including CVD and failure of various organs [67]. Jiao, Wang, Jiang, Kong, Wang and Yan [59] reported that diabetic rats fed with two different fractions of mulberry fruit polysaccharides (MFP50 and MFP90) for seven weeks had a significant decrease in the levels of fasting glucose, fasting serum insulin, homeostasis model of assessment-insulin resistance, triglyceride and oral glucose tolerance test-area under the curve. The MFP50 and MFP90 had a final ethanol concentration of 50% and 90%, respectively [59]. When compared with diabetic rats fed with pure water, diabetic rats fed with MFP50 and MFP90 had a lower serum insulin level at a rate of 26.5% and 32.5%, respectively [59]. The MFP50 group had a significant increase in the level of HDL cholesterol and the proportion of HDL cholesterol to total cholesterol [59]. The authors [59] also found that both MFP50 and MFP90 reduced the levels of serum alanine transaminase (ALT), suggesting that they have potential hepatoprotective effects. Although MFP50 had a more stable hypoglycemic effect than MFP90, MFP90 had a better hypolipidemic effect than MFP50 [59].

Similar findings were also reported by Guo, Li, Zheng, Xu, Liang and He [58] who found that diabetic rats fed with mulberry fruit polysaccharides for 2 weeks had a decrease in fasting blood glucose. Another study by Wang, Xiang, Wang, Tang and He [15] reported that diabetic rats fed with ethyl acetate-soluble extract of mulberry fruits for 2 weeks had a significant decrease in the levels of fasting blood glucose and glycosylated serum protein. The authors [15] also found that ethyl acetate-soluble extract of mulberry fruits had significantly increased the antioxidant activities of catalase (CAT), glutathione peroxidase (GSH-Px) and superoxide dismutase (SOD) in diabetic rats. Ethyl acetate-soluble extract of mulberry fruits also possesses strong α-glucoside inhibitory activity and radical-scavenging activities against 2,2-diphenyl-1-picrylhdrazyl (DPPH) and superoxide anion radicals [15]. A study by Xu, et al. [68] reported that diabetic mice fed with mulberry fruit polysaccharides had a lower level of haemoglobin A1c (HbA1c) and a reduction in streptozotocin (STZ)-lesioned pancreatic cells. In addition, diabetic mice fed with mulberry fruit polysaccharides also had an increase in insulin level and B-cell lymphoma 2 (bcl-2) expression [68].

Yan, et al. [69] reported that male C57BL6/J genetic background (db/db) mice fed with anthocyanin extract of mulberry fruit in the doses of 50 and 125 mg/kg body weight per day for 8 weeks had a significant decrease in the levels of cholesterol, fasting blood glucose, leptin, serum insulin and triglyceride as well as an increase in adiponectin level. Therefore, the authors [69] suggested that anthocyanin extract of mulberry fruit can be used to improve the resistance of insulin and leptin. Taken together, these results [15,58,59] suggest that mulberry fruits might play an important role in the treatment of diabetes because of their anti-hyperglycemic and anti-hyperlipidemic effects.

3.3. Anti-Obesity

Several studies have shown that obesity plays a major role in contributing to dyslipidemia [70–73]. Lim, et al. [74] reported that high fat diet-induced obese mice fed with a combination of mulberry leaf extract and mulberry fruit extract at low and high doses had a significant decrease in body weight gain, fasting plasma glucose, insulin and homeostasis model assessment of insulin resistance. The low dose of combination of mulberry leaf extract and mulberry fruit extract was 133 mg mulberry leaf extract and 67 mg mulberry fruit extract/kg/day, while the high dose of combination of mulberry leaf extract and mulberry fruit extract was 333 mg mulberry leaf extract and 167 mg mulberry fruit extract/kg/day [74]. The high dose of combination of mulberry leaf extract and mulberry fruit extract had significantly improved the glucose control [74]. In addition, the high dose of combination of mulberry leaf extract and mulberry fruit extract also decreased the protein levels of manganese superoxide dismutase, inducible nitric oxide synthase, monocyte chemoattractant protein-1, C-reactive protein (CRP), tumour necrosis factor-α and interleukin-1 [74]. Therefore, it is suggested that the combination of mulberry leaf extract and mulberry fruit extract possess the anti-obesity and anti-diabetic properties by modulating oxidative stress and inflammation induced by obesity [74].

Peng, Liu, Chuang, Chyau, Huang and Wang [35] reported that male hamsters fed with mulberry fruit water extract for 12 weeks had a lower high fat diet-induced body weight and visceral fat, accompanied with a decrease in serum triacylglycerol, cholesterol, LDL/HDL ratio and free fatty acid. In addition, mulberry fruit water extract also reduced fatty acid synthase and 3-hydroxy-3-methylglutaryl-coenzyme A (HMG-CoA) reductase and elevated hepatic peroxisome proliferator-activated receptor α and carnitine palmitoyltransferase-1 [35]. No physiological burdens in terms of levels of serum blood urea nitrogen, creatinine, potassium and sodium ions were exerted by the administration of mulberry fruit extract [35]. The authors [35] suggested that mulberry fruit water extracts regulate lipolysis and lipogenesis, which can be used to reduce the body weight.

3.4. Anti-Tumour

Gastrointestinal tract cancers are also one of the most common types of cancers in the world [75,76] and *Helicobacter pylori* is one of the common suspects in triggering the gastric carcinogenesis [77,78]. Huang, et al. [79] reported that after male balb/c nude mice were fed with anthocyanin-rich mulberry fruit extract for 7 weeks, atypical glandular cells (AGS) tumour xenograft growth in mice was inhibited, suggesting that anthocyanins from mulberry fruits might be used to prevent gastric carcinoma formation.

3.5. Hepatoprotective

In a study investigating the protective effect of mulberry fruit marc (the solid component after juicing) anthocyanins on carbon tetrachloride (CC14)-induced liver fibrosis in male Sprague Dawley rats, Li, et al. [80] reported that rats fed with mulberry fruit marc anthocyanins had a decrease in the levels of ALT, aspartate amino transferase, collagen type-III hyaluronidase acid and hydroxyproline. Another study by Chang, et al. [81] reported that mulberry fruit extracts suppressed the synthesis and enhanced the oxidation of fatty acids. Therefore, the mulberry fruits might prevent the non-alcoholic fatty liver disease.

3.6. Protective against Cytotoxicity and Oxidative Stress

In a study investigating the protective effect of mulberry fruit extract against ethyl carbamate (EC)-induced cytotoxicity in human liver HepG2 cells, Chen, Li, Bao and Gowd [43] reported no decrease in cell viability with the treatments of mulberry fruit extract (0.5 mg/mL, 1.0 mg/mL and 2.0 mg/mL). Therefore, the authors [43] suggested that mulberry fruits can be used to protect against EC-induced cytotoxicity and oxidative stress. Also, in a study investigating the effect of mulberry fruit consumption on the anti-fatigue activity in mice using a weight-loaded swimming test, Jiang, Guo, Xu, Huang, Yuan and Lv [44] reported that mice fed with mulberry juice purification and mulberry marc purification had an increase endurance capacity than the control group. The authors [44] suggested that the presence of anthocyanins in mulberry fruits might act as an antioxidant to reduce exercise-induced oxidative stress and physical fatigue.

3.7. Protective against Brain Damage

Kang, Hur, Kim, Ryu and Kim [17] reported that that C3G isolated from mulberry fruit extracts had shown a cytoprotective effect on PC12 cells exposed to hydrogen peroxide in vitro and a neuroprotective effect on cerebral ischemic damage caused by oxygen glucose deprivation (OGD) in vivo. Therefore, it is suggested that mulberry fruits possess neuroprotective effects in vivo and vitro ischemic oxidative stress [17]. Table 1 shows an overview of animal studies investigating the pharmacological properties of mulberry fruits.

Table 1. An overview of animal studies investigating the pharmacological properties of mulberry fruits.

Pharmacological Properties	References
Hypolipidemic	Yang et al. [11]; Chen et al. [50]; Sirikanchanarod et al. [66]
Anti-diabetic	Wang et al. [15]; Jiao et al. [59]; Guo et al. [58]; Xu et al. [68]; Yan et al. [69]
Anti-obesity	Peng et al. [35]; Lim et al. [74]
Anti-tumour	Huang et al. [79]
Hepatoprotective	Li et al. [80]; Chang et al. [81]
Protective against cytotoxicity and oxidative stress	Jiang et al. [44]; Chang et al. [81]
Protective against brain damage	Kang et al.[17]

3.8. Adverse Effects

Due to a limited number of human studies, it is difficult to assess the safety of mulberry fruit consumption. Moreover, there is insufficient evidence regarding the recommended consumption of mulberry fruits (i.e., dosage) and its treatment duration. It is necessary that all future clinical studies that investigate the effects of mulberry fruit consumption on health should follow the Consolidated Standards of Reporting Trials (CONSORT) guidelines for generating scientifically rigorous evidence [82–84].

4. Conclusions and Future Research

Literature reviews have highlighted that mulberry fruits contain high content of polyphenolic compounds and antioxidants [85]. This suggests that there are many opportunities for the food and healthcare industry to explore the health benefits of mulberry fruits because there is a potential growing market for mulberry fruits. However, the contents of bioactive compounds such as anthocyanins, alkaloids, flavonoids and polyphenols are dependent on the cultivars. Although the bioactive compounds may work synergistically to promote health, such claims still require further investigation in order to establish the causative relationship between mulberry fruit consumption and health.

There are limited studies with sufficient data to support whether mulberry fruits are beneficial to human health especially in terms of the management and prevention of chronic diseases such as diabetes and CVD. The majority of the studies that reported beneficial effects of mulberry fruits on health are animal-based studies. Moreover, these studies used different varieties of mulberry fruits, types of solvents and methods of preparation, which cause the evaluation of activity of mulberry fruits to be difficult and these studies involve quite heterogeneous data. Therefore, larger well-designed, randomised controlled trials are needed to examine the effects of mulberry fruit consumption on human health. Similar to other plants and food products [1,86], the fate of polyphenol compounds in the body, especially after undergoing intestinal transformations by enzymes produced by gut microbiota should also be addressed. The elucidation of some active ingredient structures in mulberry fruits and their mechanisms in promoting pharmacological properties are also worthy of further research.

Author Contributions: The project idea was developed by Z.F.M. Z.F.M. wrote the first draft of the manuscript. Z.F.M., H.X., X.L. and X.L. conducted the literature search and revised the manuscript.

Acknowledgments: The authors received no specific funding for this work.

Conflicts of Interest: The authors declare no conflict of interest.

References

1. Ma, Z.F.; Zhang, H. Phytochemical constituents, health benefits, and industrial applications of grape seeds: A mini-review. *Antioxidants* **2017**, *6*, 71. [CrossRef] [PubMed]

2. Ji, H.-F.; Li, X.-J.; Zhang, H.-Y. Natural products and drug discovery. Can thousands of years of ancient medical knowledge lead us to new and powerful drug combinations in the fight against cancer and dementia? *EMBO Rep.* **2009**, *10*, 194–200. [CrossRef] [PubMed]

3. Zhang, H.; Ma, Z.F. Phytochemical and pharmacological properties of *Capparis spinosa* as a medicinal plant. *Nutrients* **2018**, *10*, 116. [CrossRef] [PubMed]

4. Cao, Y.; Ma, Z.F.; Zhang, H.; Jin, Y.; Zhang, Y.; Hayford, F. Phytochemical properties and nutrigenomic implications of yacon as a potential source of prebiotic: Current evidence and future directions. *Foods* **2018**, *7*, 59. [CrossRef] [PubMed]

5. Veeresham, C. Natural products derived from plants as a source of drugs. *J. Adv. Pharm. Technol. Res.* **2012**, *3*, 200–201. [CrossRef] [PubMed]

6. Gryn-Rynko, A.; Bazylak, G.; Olszewska-Slonina, D. New potential phytotherapeutics obtained from white mulberry (*Morus alba* L.) leaves. *Biomed. Pharmacother.* **2016**, *84*, 628–636. [CrossRef] [PubMed]

7. Ercisli, S.; Orhan, E. Chemical composition of white (*Morus alba*), red (*Morus rubra*) and black (*Morus nigra*) mulberry fruits. *Food Chem.* **2007**, *103*, 1380–1384. [CrossRef]

8. Ye, F.; Shen, Z.; Xie, M. Alpha-glucosidase inhibition from a Chinese medical herb (*Ramulus mori*) in normal and diabetic rats and mice. *Phytomedicine* **2002**, *9*, 161–166. [CrossRef] [PubMed]

9. Khan, M.A.; Rahman, A.A.; Islam, S.; Khandokhar, P.; Parvin, S.; Islam, M.B.; Hossain, M.; Rashid, M.; Sadik, G.; Nasrin, S.; et al. A comparative study on the antioxidant activity of methanolic extracts from different parts of *Morus alba* L. (moraceae). *BMC Res. Notes* **2013**, *6*, 24. [CrossRef] [PubMed]

10. Ning, D.; Lu, B.; Zhang, Y. The processing technology of mulberry series product. *China Fruit Veg. Proc.* **2005**, *5*, 38–40.

11. Yang, X.; Yang, L.; Zheng, H. Hypolipidemic and antioxidant effects of mulberry (*Morus alba* L.) fruit in hyperlipidaemia rats. *Food Chem. Toxicol.* **2010**, *48*, 2374–2379. [CrossRef] [PubMed]

12. Arabshahi-Delouee, S.; Urooj, A. Antioxidant properties of various solvent extracts of mulberry (*Morus Indica* L.) leaves. *Food Chem.* **2007**, *102*, 1233–1240. [CrossRef]

13. Sohn, B.-H.; Park, J.-H.; Lee, D.-Y.; Cho, J.-G.; Kim, Y.-S.; Jung, I.-S.; Kang, P.-D.; Baek, N.-I. Isolation and identification of lipids from the silkworm (*Bombyx mori*) droppings. *J. Korean Soc. Appl. Biol. Chem.* **2009**, *52*, 336–341. [CrossRef]

14. Liu, H.; Qiu, N.; Ding, H.; Yao, R. Polyphenols contents and antioxidant capacity of 68 Chinese herbals suitable for medical or food uses. *Food Res. Int.* **2008**, *41*, 363–370. [CrossRef]

15. Wang, Y.; Xiang, L.; Wang, C.; Tang, C.; He, X. Antidiabetic and antioxidant effects and phytochemicals of mulberry fruit (*Morus alba* L.) polyphenol enhanced extract. *PLoS ONE* **2013**, *8*, e71144. [CrossRef] [PubMed]

16. Yang, Y.; Zhang, T.; Xiao, L.; Yang, L.; Chen, R. Two new chalcones from leaves of *Morus alba* L. *Fitoterapia* **2010**, *81*, 614–616. [CrossRef] [PubMed]

17. Kang, T.H.; Hur, J.Y.; Kim, H.B.; Ryu, J.H.; Kim, S.Y. Neuroprotective effects of the cyanidin-3-*O*-beta-D-glucopyranoside isolated from mulberry fruit against cerebral ischemia. *Neurosci. Lett.* **2006**, *391*, 122–126. [CrossRef] [PubMed]

18. Kim, A.J.; Park, S. Mulberry extract supplements ameliorate the inflammation-related hematological parameters in carrageenan-induced arthritic rats. *J. Med. Food* **2006**, *9*, 431–435. [CrossRef] [PubMed]

19. Zhang, Z.; Shi, L. Anti-inflammatory and analgesic properties of *cis*-mulberroside a from *Ramulus mori*. *Fitoterapia* **2010**, *81*, 214–218. [CrossRef] [PubMed]

20. Gerasopoulos, D.; Stavroulakis, G. Quality characteristics of four mulberry (*Morus* sp) cultivars in the area of Chania, Greece. *J. Sci. Food Agric.* **1997**, *73*, 261–264. [CrossRef]

21. Suhl, H.J.; Noh, D.O.; Kang, C.S.; Kim, J.M.; Lee, S.W. Thermal kinetics of color degradation of mulberry fruit extract. *Die Nahr.* **2003**, *47*, 132–135.

22. Liu, X.; Xiao, G.; Chen, W.; Xu, Y.; Wu, J. Quantification and purification of mulberry anthocyanins with macroporous resins. *J. Biomed. Biotechnol.* **2004**, 326–331. [CrossRef] [PubMed]

23. Bao, T.; Xu, Y.; Gowd, V.; Zhao, J.; Xie, J.; Liang, W.; Chen, W. Systematic study on phytochemicals and antioxidant activity of some new and common mulberry cultivars in China. *J. Funct. Foods* **2016**, *25*, 537–547. [CrossRef]

24. Kusano, G.; Orihara, S.; Tsukamoto, D.; Shibano, M.; Coskun, M.; Guvenc, A.; Erdurak, C.S. Five new nortropane alkaloids and six new amino acids from the fruit of *Morus alba* Linne growing in Turkey. *Chem. Pharm. Bull.* **2002**, *50*, 185–192. [CrossRef] [PubMed]

25. Yang, J.; Liu, X.; Zhang, X.; Jin, Q.; Li, J. Phenolic profiles, antioxidant activities, and neuroprotective properties of mulberry (*Morus atropurpurea* Roxb.) fruit extracts from different ripening stages. *J. Food Sci.* **2016**, *81*, C2439–C2446. [CrossRef] [PubMed]

26. Chan, E.W.; Lye, P.Y.; Wong, S.K. Phytochemistry, pharmacology, and clinical trials of *Morus alba*. *Chin. J. Nat. Med.* **2016**, *14*, 17–30. [PubMed]

27. Arfan, M.; Khan, R.; Rybarczyk, A.; Amarowicz, R. Antioxidant activity of mulberry fruit extracts. *Int. J. Mol. Sci.* **2012**, *13*, 2472–2480. [CrossRef] [PubMed]

28. Imran, M.; Khan, H.; Shah, M.; Khan, R.; Khan, F. Chemical composition and antioxidant activity of certain *Morus* species. *J. Zhejiang Univ. Sci. B* **2010**, *11*, 973–980. [CrossRef] [PubMed]

29. Bae, S.-H.; Suh, H.-J. Antioxidant activities of five different mulberry cultivars in Korea. *Food Sci. Technol.* **2007**, *40*, 955–962. [CrossRef]

30. Kim, S.B.; Chang, B.Y.; Hwang, B.Y.; Kim, S.Y.; Lee, M.K. Pyrrole alkaloids from the fruits of *Morus alba*. *Bioorgan. Med. Chem. Lett.* **2014**, *24*, 5656–5659. [CrossRef] [PubMed]

31. Natić, M.M.; Dabić, D.Č.; Papetti, A.; Fotirić Akšić, M.M.; Ognjanov, V.; Ljubojević, M.; Tešić, Ž.L. Analysis and characterisation of phytochemicals in mulberry (*Morus alba* L.) fruits grown in Vojvodina, North Serbia. *Food Chem.* **2015**, *171*, 128–136. [CrossRef] [PubMed]

32. Qin, C.; Li, Y.; Niu, W.; Ding, Y.; Zhang, R.; Shang, X. Analysis and characterisation of anthocyanins in mulberry fruit. *Czech J. Food Sci.* **2010**, *28*, 117–126. [CrossRef]

33. Du, Q.; Zheng, J.; Xu, Y. Composition of anthocyanins in mulberry and their antioxidant activity. *J. Food Comp. Anal.* **2008**, *21*, 390–395. [CrossRef]

34. Memon, A.A.; Memon, N.; Luthria, D.L.; Bhanger, M.I.; Pitafi, A.A. Phenolic acids profiling and antioxidant potential of mulberry (*Morus laevigata* W., *Morus nigra* L., *Morus alba* L.) leaves and fruits grown in Pakistan. *Pol. J. Food Nutr. Sci.* **2010**, *60*, 25–32.

35. Peng, C.-H.; Liu, L.-K.; Chuang, C.-M.; Chyau, C.-C.; Huang, C.-N.; Wang, C.-J. Mulberry water extracts possess an anti-obesity effect and ability to inhibit hepatic lipogenesis and promote lipolysis. *J. Agric. Food Chem.* **2011**, *59*, 2663–2671. [CrossRef] [PubMed]

36. Kim, S.B.; Chang, B.Y.; Jo, Y.H.; Lee, S.H.; Han, S.-B.; Hwang, B.Y.; Kim, S.Y.; Lee, M.K. Macrophage activating activity of pyrrole alkaloids from *Morus alba* fruits. *J. Ethnopharmacol.* **2013**, *145*, 393–396. [CrossRef] [PubMed]

37. Isabelle, M.; Lee, B.L.; Ong, C.N.; Liu, X.; Huang, D. Peroxyl radical scavenging capacity, polyphenolics, and lipophilic antioxidant profiles of mulberry fruits cultivated in southern China. *J. Agric. Food Chem.* **2008**, *56*, 9410–9416. [CrossRef] [PubMed]

38. Liu, C.; Xiang, W.; Yu, Y.; Shi, Z.-Q.; Huang, X.-Z.; Xu, L. Comparative analysis of 1-deoxynojirimycin contribution degree to α-glucosidase inhibitory activity and physiological distribution in *Morus alba* L. *Ind. Crops Prod.* **2015**, *70*, 309–315. [CrossRef]

39. Song, W.; Wang, H.J.; Bucheli, P.; Zhang, P.F.; Wei, D.Z.; Lu, Y.H. Phytochemical profiles of different mulberry (*Morus* sp.) species from China. *J. Agric. Food Chem.* **2009**, *57*, 9133–9140. [CrossRef] [PubMed]

40. Jiang, Y.; Nie, W.-J. Chemical properties in fruits of mulberry species from the Xinjiang province of China. *Food Chem.* **2015**, *174*, 460–466. [CrossRef] [PubMed]

41. Aramwit, P.; Bang, N.; Srichana, T. The properties and stability of anthocyanins in mulberry fruits. *Food Res. Int.* **2010**, *43*, 1093–1097. [CrossRef]

42. Calin-Sanchez, A.; Martinez-Nicolas, J.J.; Munera-Picazo, S.; Carbonell-Barrachina, A.A.; Legua, P.; Hernandez, F. Bioactive compounds and sensory quality of black and white mulberries grown in Spain. *Plant Foods Hum. Nutr.* **2013**, *68*, 370–377. [CrossRef] [PubMed]

43. Chen, W.; Li, Y.; Bao, T.; Gowd, V. Mulberry fruit extract affords protection against ethyl carbamate-induced cytotoxicity and oxidative stress. *Oxid. Med. Cell. Longev.* **2017**, *2017*, 1594963. [CrossRef] [PubMed]

44. Jiang, D.Q.; Guo, Y.; Xu, D.H.; Huang, Y.S.; Yuan, K.; Lv, Z.Q. Antioxidant and anti-fatigue effects of anthocyanins of mulberry juice purification (MJP) and mulberry marc purification (MMP) from different varieties mulberry fruit in China. *Food Chem. Toxicol.* **2013**, *59*, 1–7. [CrossRef] [PubMed]

45. Carvalho, J.C.T.; Perazzo, F.F.; Machado, L.; Bereau, D. Biologic activity and biotechnological development of natural products. *Biomed. Res. Int.* **2013**, 971745. [CrossRef] [PubMed]

46. Lila, M.A. Anthocyanins and human health: An in vitro investigative approach. *J. Biomed. Biotechnol.* **2004**, *2004*, 306–313. [CrossRef] [PubMed]

47. Lee, Y.M.; Yoon, Y.; Yoon, H.; Park, H.M.; Song, S.; Yeum, K.J. Dietary anthocyanins against obesity and inflammation. *Nutrients* **2017**, *9*. [CrossRef] [PubMed]

48. Yang, S.; Wang, B.L.; Li, Y. Advances in the pharmacological study of *Morus alba* L. *Acta Pharm. Sin.* **2014**, *49*, 824–831.

49. Huang, H.P.; Ou, T.T.; Wang, C.J. Mulberry (sang shen zi) and its bioactive compounds, the chemoprevention effects and molecular mechanisms in vitro and in vivo. *J. Tradit. Complement. Med.* **2013**, *3*, 7–15. [CrossRef] [PubMed]

50. Chen, C.-C.; Liu, L.-K.; Hsu, J.-D.; Huang, H.-P.; Yang, M.-Y.; Wang, C.-J. Mulberry extract inhibits the development of atherosclerosis in cholesterol-fed rabbits. *Food Chem.* **2005**, *91*, 601–607. [CrossRef]

51. Adisakwattana, S.; Ruengsamran, T.; Kampa, P.; Sompong, W. In vitro inhibitory effects of plant-based foods and their combinations on intestinal α-glucosidase and pancreatic α-amylase. *BMC Complement. Altern. Med.* **2012**, *12*, 110. [CrossRef] [PubMed]

52. Chang, Y.-C.; Yang, M.-Y.; Chen, S.-C.; Wang, C.-J. Mulberry leaf polyphenol extract improves obesity by inducing adipocyte apoptosis and inhibiting preadipocyte differentiation and hepatic lipogenesis. *J. Funct. Foods* **2016**, *21*, 249–262. [CrossRef]

53. Kwon, H.J.; Chung, J.Y.; Kim, J.Y.; Kwon, O. Comparison of 1-deoxynojirimycin and aqueous mulberry leaf extract with emphasis on postprandial hypoglycemic effects: In vivo and in vitro studies. *J. Agric. Food. Chem.* **2011**, *59*, 3014–3019. [CrossRef] [PubMed]

54. Li, Y.-G.; Ji, D.-F.; Zhong, S.; Lv, Z.-Q.; Lin, T.-B.; Chen, S.; Hu, G.-Y. Hybrid of 1-deoxynojirimycin and polysaccharide from mulberry leaves treat diabetes mellitus by activating PDX-1/insulin-1 signaling pathway and regulating the expression of glucokinase, phosphoenolpyruvate carboxykinase and glucose-6-phosphatase in alloxan-induced diabetic mice. *J. Ethnopharmacol.* **2011**, *134*, 961–970. [PubMed]

55. Naowaratwattana, W.; De-Eknamkul, W.; De Mejia, E.G. Phenolic-containing organic extracts of mulberry (*Morus alba* L.) leaves inhibit HepG2 hepatoma cells through G2/M phase arrest, induction of apoptosis, and inhibition of topoisomerase II alpha activity. *J. Med. Food.* **2010**, *13*, 1045–1056. [CrossRef] [PubMed]

56. Naowaboot, J.; Pannangpetch, P.; Kukongviriyapan, V.; Kukongviriyapan, U.; Nakmareong, S.; Itharat, A. Mulberry leaf extract restores arterial pressure in streptozotocin-induced chronic diabetic rats. *Nutr. Res.* **2009**, *29*, 602–608. [CrossRef] [PubMed]

57. De Oliveira, A.M.; do Nascimento, M.F.; Ferreira, M.R.A.; de Moura, D.F.; dos Santos Souza, T.G.; da Silva, G.C.; da Silva Ramos, E.H.; Paiva, P.M.G.; de Medeiros, P.L.; da Silva, T.G.; et al. Evaluation of acute toxicity, genotoxicity and inhibitory effect on acute inflammation of an ethanol extract of *Morus alba* L. (moraceae) in mice. *J. Ethnopharmacol.* **2016**, *194*, 162–168. [CrossRef] [PubMed]

58. Guo, C.; Li, R.; Zheng, N.; Xu, L.; Liang, T.; He, Q. Anti-diabetic effect of *Ramulus mori* polysaccharides, isolated from *Morus alba* L., on STZ-diabetic mice through blocking inflammatory response and attenuating oxidative stress. *Int. Immunopharmacol.* **2013**, *16*, 93–99. [CrossRef] [PubMed]

59. Jiao, Y.; Wang, X.; Jiang, X.; Kong, F.; Wang, S.; Yan, C. Antidiabetic effects of *Morus alba* fruit polysaccharides on high-fat diet- and streptozotocin-induced type 2 diabetes in rats. *J. Ethnopharmacol.* **2017**, *199*, 119–127. [CrossRef] [PubMed]

60. Willett, W.C. Dietary fats and coronary heart disease. *J. Intern. Med.* **2012**, *272*, 13–24. [CrossRef] [PubMed]

61. Townsend, N.; Wilson, L.; Bhatnagar, P.; Wickramasinghe, K.; Rayner, M.; Nichols, M. Cardiovascular disease in Europe: Epidemiological update 2016. *Eur. Heart J.* **2016**, *37*, 3232–3245. [CrossRef] [PubMed]

62. Ma, Z.F.; Lee, Y.Y. Virgin coconut oil and its cardiovascular health benefits. *Nat. Prod. Commun.* **2016**, *11*, 1151–1152.

63. Lu, H.; Pan, W.-Z.; Wan, Q.; Cheng, L.-L.; Shu, X.-H.; Pan, C.-Z.; Qian, J.-Y.; Ge, J.-B. Trends in the prevalence of heart diseases over a ten-year period from single-center observations based on a large echocardiographic database. *J. Zhejiang Univ. Sci. B* **2016**, *17*, 54–59. [CrossRef] [PubMed]

64. Chobanian, A.V. Single risk factor intervention may be inadequate to inhibit atherosclerosis progression when hypertension and hypercholesterolemia coexist. *Hypertension* **1991**, *18*, 130–131. [CrossRef] [PubMed]

65. Venkatesan, N.; Devaraj, S.N.; Devaraj, H. Increased binding of LDL and VLDL to apo B,E receptors of hepatic plasma membrane of rats treated with Fibernat. *Eur. J. Nutr.* **2003**, *42*, 262–271. [CrossRef] [PubMed]

66. Sirikanchanarod, A.; Bumrungpert, A.; Kaewruang, W.; Senawong, T.; Pavadhgul, P. The effect of mulberry fruits consumption on lipid profiles in hypercholesterolemic subjects: A randomized controlled trial. *J. Pharm. Nutr. Sci.* **2016**, *60*, 7–14.

67. Kalofoutis, C.; Piperi, C.; Kalofoutis, A.; Harris, F.; Phoenix, D.; Singh, J. Type II diabetes mellitus and cardiovascular risk factors: Current therapeutic approaches. *Exp. Clin. Cardiol.* **2007**, *12*, 17–28. [PubMed]

68. Xu, L.; Yang, F.; Wang, J.; Huang, H.; Huang, Y. Anti-diabetic effect mediated by *Ramulus mori* polysaccharides. *Carbohydr. Polym.* **2015**, *117*, 63–69. [CrossRef] [PubMed]

69. Yan, F.; Dai, G.; Zheng, X. Mulberry anthocyanin extract ameliorates insulin resistance by regulating PI3K/AKT pathway in HepG2 cells and db/db mice. *J. Nutr. Biochem.* **2016**, *36*, 68–80. [CrossRef] [PubMed]

70. Ebbert, J.O.; Jensen, M.D. Fat depots, free fatty acids, and dyslipidemia. *Nutrients* **2013**, *5*, 498–508. [CrossRef] [PubMed]

71. Jung, U.J.; Choi, M.-S. Obesity and its metabolic complications: The role of adipokines and the relationship between obesity, inflammation, insulin resistance, dyslipidemia and nonalcoholic fatty liver disease. *Int. J. Mol. Sci.* **2014**, *15*, 6184–6223. [CrossRef] [PubMed]

72. Klop, B.; Elte, J.W.F.; Castro Cabezas, M. Dyslipidemia in obesity: Mechanisms and potential targets. *Nutrients* **2013**, *5*, 1218–1240. [CrossRef] [PubMed]

73. DeFronzo, R.A.; Ferrannini, E. Insulin resistance. A multifaceted syndrome responsible for NIDDM, obesity, hypertension, dyslipidemia, and atherosclerotic cardiovascular disease. *Diabetes Care* **1991**, *14*, 173–194. [CrossRef] [PubMed]

74. Lim, H.H.; Lee, S.O.; Kim, S.Y.; Yang, S.J.; Lim, Y. Anti-inflammatory and antiobesity effects of mulberry leaf and fruit extract on high fat diet-induced obesity. *Exp. Biol. Med.* **2013**, *238*, 1160–1169. [CrossRef] [PubMed]

75. Torre, L.A.; Bray, F.; Siegel, R.L.; Ferlay, J.; Lortet-Tieulent, J.; Jemal, A. Global cancer statistics, 2012. *CA Cancer J.* **2015**, *65*, 87–108. [CrossRef] [PubMed]

76. Pourhoseingholi, M.A.; Vahedi, M.; Baghestani, A.R. Burden of gastrointestinal cancer in Asia: An overview. *Gastroenterol. Hepatol. Bed Bench* **2015**, *8*, 19–27. [PubMed]

77. Ma, Z.F.; Majid, N.A.; Yamaoka, Y.; Lee, Y.Y. Food allergy and helicobacter pylori infection: A systematic review. *Front. Microbiol.* **2016**, *7*, 368. [CrossRef] [PubMed]

78. Nishizawa, T.; Suzuki, H. Gastric carcinogenesis and underlying molecular mechanisms: Helicobacter pylori and novel targeted therapy. *BioMed Res. Int.* **2015**, *2015*, 794378. [CrossRef] [PubMed]

79. Huang, H.-P.; Chang, Y.-C.; Wu, C.-H.; Hung, C.-N.; Wang, C.-J. Anthocyanin-rich *Mulberry* extract inhibit the gastric cancer cell growth in vitro and xenograft mice by inducing signals of p38/p53 and c-jun. *Food Chem.* **2011**, *129*, 1703–1709. [CrossRef]

80. Li, Y.; Yang, Z.; Jia, S.; Yuan, K. Protective effect and mechanism of action of mulberry marc anthocyanins on carbon tetrachloride-induced liver fibrosis in rats. *J. Funct. Foods* **2016**, *24*, 595–601. [CrossRef]

81. Chang, J.-J.; Hsu, M.-J.; Huang, H.-P.; Chung, D.-J.; Chang, Y.-C.; Wang, C.-J. Mulberry anthocyanins inhibit oleic acid induced lipid accumulation by reduction of lipogenesis and promotion of hepatic lipid clearance. *J. Agric. Food Chem.* **2013**, *61*, 6069–6076. [CrossRef] [PubMed]

82. Schulz, K.F.; Altman, D.G.; Moher, D. Consort 2010 statement: Updated guidelines for reporting parallel group randomised trials. *BMJ* **2010**, *340*, c332. [CrossRef] [PubMed]

83. Moher, D.; Hopewell, S.; Schulz, K.F.; Montori, V.; Gøtzsche, P.C.; Devereaux, P.J.; Elbourne, D.; Egger, M.; Altman, D.G. Consort 2010 explanation and elaboration: Updated guidelines for reporting parallel group randomised trials. *BMJ* **2010**, *340*, c869. [CrossRef] [PubMed]

84. Pandis, N.; Fleming, P.S.; Hopewell, S.; Altman, D.G. The consort statement: Application within and adaptations for orthodontic trials. *Am. J. Orthod. Dentofac. Orthop.* **2015**, *147*, 663–679. [CrossRef] [PubMed]

85. Yuan, Q.; Zhao, L. The mulberry (*Morus alba* L.) fruit—A review of characteristic components and health benefits. *J. Agric. Food Chem.* **2017**, *65*, 10383–10394. [CrossRef] [PubMed]

86. Ravichanthiran, K.; Ma, Z.F.; Zhang, H.; Cao, Y.; Wang, C.W.; Muhammad, S.; Aglago, E.K.; Zhang, Y.; Jin, Y.; Pan, B. Phytochemical profile of brown rice and its nutrigenomic implication. *Antioxidants* **2018**, accepted for publication.

6

Resuspendable Powders of Lyophilized Chalcogen Particles with Activity against Microorganisms

Sharoon Griffin [1,2], Muhammad Sarfraz [1], Steffen F. Hartmann [2],
Shashank Reddy Pinnapireddy [2] (iD), Muhammad Jawad Nasim [1], Udo Bakowsky [2],
Cornelia M. Keck [2,*] and Claus Jacob [1,*]

[1] Division of Bioorganic Chemistry, School of Pharmacy, Saarland University, D-66123 Saarbruecken, Germany; sharoon.griffin@uni-saarland.de (S.G.); s8musarf@stud.uni-saarland.de (M.S.); jawad.nasim@uni-saarland.de (M.J.N.)

[2] Department of Pharmaceutics and Biopharmaceutics, University of Marburg, 35037 Marburg, Germany; steffenfhartmann@googlemail.com (S.F.H.); shashank.pinnapireddy@pharmazie.uni-marburg.de (S.R.P.); ubakowsky@aol.com (U.B.)

* Correspondence: cornelia.keck@pharmazie.uni-marburg.de (C.M.K.); c.jacob@mx.uni-saarland.de (C.J.)

Abstract: Many organic sulfur, selenium and tellurium compounds show considerable activity against microorganisms, including bacteria and fungi. This pronounced activity is often due to the specific, oxidizing redox behavior of the chalcogen-chalcogen bond present in such molecules. Interestingly, similar chalcogen-chalcogen motifs are also found in the elemental forms of these elements, and while those materials are insoluble in aqueous media, it has recently been possible to unlock their biological activities using naturally produced or homogenized suspensions of respective chalcogen nanoparticles. Those suspensions can be employed readily and often effectively against common pathogenic microorganisms, still their practical uses are limited as such suspensions are difficult to transport, store and apply. Using mannitol as stabilizer, it is now possible to lyophilize such suspensions to produce solid forms of the nanoparticles, which upon resuspension in water essentially retain their initial size and exhibit considerable biological activity. The sequence of Nanosizing, Lyophilization and Resuspension (NaLyRe) eventually provides access to a range of lyophilized materials which may be considered as easy-to-handle, ready-to-use and at the same time as bioavailable, active forms of otherwise insoluble or sparingly substances. In the case of elemental sulfur, selenium and tellurium, this approach promises wider practical applications, for instance in the medical or agricultural arena.

Keywords: antimicrobial activity; chalcogen nanoparticles; mannitol; resuspended lyophilized nanosuspensions (NaLyRe); sulfur; selenium; tellurium

---

1. Introduction

Organic chalcogen compounds have been investigated for several decades due to their often pronounced biological activities against parasites, microorganisms and cancer cells. Indeed, the field of natural Organic Sulfur Compounds (OSCs) has attracted tremendous attention, as Reactive Sulfur Species (RSS) such as allicin and polysulfanes from garlic or allylisocyanate (mustard oil) from various *Brassica* plants exhibit interesting chemopreventive and possibly even therapeutic properties [1]. Organoselenium compounds, in particular ebselen and its derivatives, pose a similar attraction in the Life Sciences, especially in the context of antioxidants [2,3]. In contrast, organotellurium compounds have long remained marginalized in Biology, yet some of them, such as RT-01 and AS101, have also recently emerged from the chemical closet with some prominence [2,4–6]. Not surprisingly, the field of biologically active organochalcogens has stimulated considerable efforts in chemical synthesis and has produced volumes of more or less exotic molecules [7,8].

One of the predominant modes of action of many of these compounds is due to their ability to oxidize—rather selectively—the thiol groups of cysteine residues in pivotal cellular signalling proteins and enzymes, hence triggering processes which eventually may culminate in an antioxidant response, or the initiation of apoptosis or other forms of cell death. Intriguingly, the chalcogen-chalcogen bond often at the centre of such redox action is also found in the elemental forms of sulfur (S_8, common yellow form), selenium (Se_8, red allotrope) and tellurium (Te_8, dark grey), implying that such elemental modifications, from the perspective of reactivity, may themselves also be biologically active [9]. Indeed, recent studies on inorganic polysulfides, such as the tetrasulfide S_4^{2-}, support this notion of simple, purely inorganic, "carbon free" yet highly active variants of chalcogens [10–12]. Unfortunately, neither of the various elemental forms of any of the three chalcogens in question is soluble in water. Hence traditionally it has mostly been futile to apply elemental sulfur, selenium or tellurium in a biological context, with some notable exceptions, such as colloidal sulfur and its uses as fungicide in vineyards [13,14].

Indeed, the apparent lack of solubility and hence bioavailability can be overcome with suspensions of small particles with diameters in the low or sub-micrometer range. We have recently shown that such particles can be obtained rather easily by physical or chemical methods and, in the case of selenium, even with the assistance of certain bacteria which readily generate natural, protein-coated selenium nanoparticles in adequate quality and yield. Most of these particles show some activity against microorganisms [15]. Nanosized tellurium, in particular, appears to be rather active against organisms such as *Escherichia coli*, *Candida albicans*, *Saccaromyces cerevisiae* and the model nematode *Steinernema feltiae* [16]. While the nanosuspensions employed as part of such studies are rather promising as a first proof-of-concept for production and activity, they also have considerable drawbacks once used in practice. For instance, such liquid suspensions are difficult to maintain and to store for prolonged periods of time, they need to be kept under sterile conditions, are not particularly amenable to transport, and an adjustment of reliable concentrations is generally difficult. We have therefore undertaken a series of studies to produce easier-to-handle solid materials based on elemental chalcogens. Here we report our first results with the underlying NaLyre sequence of processing, which involves nanosizing, then lyophilizing and subsequently resuspending mannitol-stabilized chalcogen nanoparticles, and biological activities associated with them.

2. Materials and Methods

2.1. Production of Chalcogen Nanoparticles

Chalcogens were purchased from the following companies: Sulfur from Carl Roth GmbH + Co. KG (Karlsruhe, Germany), selenium from ThermoFisher Acros Organics (Geel, Belgium) and tellurium from Sigma-Aldrich Chemie GmbH (Taufkirchen, Germany). For every chalcogen, suspensions in distilled water were produced containing 1% of the respective chalcogen as well as 1% of Plantacare® 2000 UP (BASF, Ludwigshafen, Germany) as particle stabilizer. The coarse suspension was produced by dispersing the chalcogen into the surfactant solution under magnetic stirring. These suspensions were stored in the refrigerator at 4 °C until further use. Prior to High Pressure Homogenization (HPH) the coarse suspensions were stirred using a Polytron® PT2100 high-speed stirrer (Kinematica GmbH, Luzern, Switzerland) attached to a Polytron® PT-DA-2112/EC aggregate. Each sample was stirred ten times at 11,000 rpm for 1 min each, a technique known as High Speed Stirring (HSS). Afterwards HPH was performed using an APV Gaulin Lab 40 high pressure homogenizer (APV Deutschland GmbH, Unna, Germany). Initial pre-milling involved 3 cycles each at 250 bar, 500 bar, 750 bar and 1000 bar, respectively. Subsequent main milling consisted of 10 cycles at 1500 bar. Between each cycle the sample was cooled to below 5 °C to guarantee stability and to ensure that the temperature during milling remained below 30 °C. The physical stability of those particles was monitored over time using a combination of analytical techniques routinely employed for size characterization (see Section 2.3). Thereafter, the nanosuspensions were stored at a refrigerator at 4 °C for 30 days and inspected at day 1 (1 day after production) and finally at day 30 after production.

2.2. Lyophilization of Chalcogen Nanoparticles

As part of the lyophilization studies, the appropriate concentration of mannitol (ThermoFisher Acros Organics) was determined first using the selenium nanosuspension. Mannitol, in particular, was selected as it is a popular choice of "cryoprotectant" for freeze-drying of nanoparticles [17–19]. Different concentrations of mannitol (0.01 g, 0.02 g, 0.05 g and 1 g) were added to 5 mL of selenium nanosuspension to yield suspensions with 1%, 2%, 5% and 20% w/v of mannitol. Together with a 5 mL sample without any mannitol (0%), these five samples were lyophilized using an Alpha 1-4 LSC lyophilizer (Martin Christ Gefriertrocknungsanlagen GmbH, Osterode am Harz, Germany). The freeze-drying steps were performed in the following manner: Freezing (−80 °C, overnight), main drying (−50 °C, 0.120 mbar for 48 h) and final drying (25 °C, above 1 mbar pressure for 24 h). The conditions for lyophilization were optimized for mannitol according to the literature with appropriate modifications [17,18,20]. Eventually, the 20% suspension was deemed effective for achieving the respective sizes after freeze-drying. Samples of sulfur and tellurium nanosuspensions were then lyophilized under the same conditions.

2.3. Size Characterization of Chalcogen Nanoparticles

The samples prior to lyophilization (see above) as well as samples of 1.05 g of lyophilized material re-suspended in 5 mL of distilled water were analyzed with regard to their size, size distribution and particle morphology, using Photon Correlation Spectroscopy (PCS, also known as Dynamic Light Scattering), Laser Diffraction (LD, also known as Static Light Scattering) and Light Microscopy (LM). PCS measurements were performed using a Zetasizer Nano ZS (Malvern Instruments, Worcestershire, UK). Prior to the measurements samples were diluted by a factor 1:200. All measurements were performed at 21 °C. LD was performed on a Mastersizer 3000 (Malvern Instruments, UK) attached with a HydroMV dispersion unit. Mie theory was applied by using the optical parameter (real/imaginary refractive index) 1.570/0.010. For the morphological analysis an Olympus BX53 light microscope (Olympus Cooperation, Tokyo, Japan) with an Olympus SC50 CMOS color camera was employed (Olympus soft imaging solutions GmbH, Muenster, Germany).

2.4. Zeta Potential (ZP) Measurements of Chalcogen Nanoparticles

The charge of the chalcogen nanoparticles was assessed via ZP measurements using a Malvern Zetasizer Nano ZS (Malvern Instruments, UK) at 21 °C and a field strength of 20 V/cm. ZP measurements via the laser Doppler anemometry yield the electrophoretic mobility, which was converted to the ZP by using the Helmholtz–Smoluchowski equation. ZP measurements were performed in conductivity-adjusted Milli-Q water (50 S/cm, using 0.9% NaCl solution) and in the original surfactant solution [21]. The measurements in the original solution are important for predicting long term stability, while the measurements in conductivity-adjusted water are indicative of the potential at the Stern layer. Differences in these measurements can be used, among others, to predict the ability of the surfactant to bind to the surface of the particles [22,23].

2.5. Scanning Electron Microscopy (SEM) of Chalcogen Nanoparticles

Scanning electron microscopy (SEM) was performed using a Hitachi S-510 Scanning Electron Microscope (Hitachi-High Technologies Europe GmbH, Krefeld, Germany). The nanoparticle suspensions were pipetted onto SEM pin stubs fixed with conductive carbon tabs and air dried. The samples were then sputtered with gold at 13.3 Pa argon and 30 mA using an Edwards S150 sputter coater (Edwards Vacuum, Crawley, UK) and examined using SEM at an accelerating voltage of 5 kV and 30 μA emission current under 4.6×10^{-4} Pa vacuum [24]. The micrographs were recorded digitally using the DISS 5 digital image acquisition system (Point Electronic GmbH, Halle/Saale, Germany).

2.6. Nematicidal Activity of Chalcogen Nanoparticles

The model nematode *S. feltiae* was purchased from Sautter und Stepper GmbH (Ammerbuch, Germany) in the form of powder and stored at 4 °C in the dark. Fresh samples were used prior to each experiment. A homogeneous mixture was prepared by dissolving 200 mg of nematode powder in 50 mL distilled water. Later on, the nematode suspension was placed for 30 min at room temperature with occasional shaking and in moderate light. Viability was examined under a light microscope at four-fold magnification (TR 200, VWR International, Leuven, Belgium). Viability of nematodes above 80% in each sample was considered as prerequisite for each experiment.

10 μL of nematode suspension were added to each well of a 96-well plate. Suspensions of the nanosized samples (sulfur, selenium and tellurium) were then added into the wells to achieve final concentrations of 25, 50, 100 and 200 μM. Afterwards, the final volume in each well was adjusted to 100 μL by adding Phosphate Buffered Saline (PBS pH = 7.4). PBS and ethanol (10 μL per well) were used as negative and positive control, respectively. Each experiment was performed independently on three different occasions and in triplicate ($n = 9$). Living and dead nematodes were counted under the microscope prior to treatment, and the viability fraction (V_0) was calculated (usually > 0.9). After 24 h, the V_{24} fraction was calculated by once more counting the living and dead nematodes. 50 μL of lukewarm water (50 °C) was added to each well to stimulate the nematodes prior to counting. After 24 h, the viability was calculated and expressed as a percentage of initial viability V_0 according to Equation (1):

$$\text{Viability (\%)} = [V_{24}/V_0] \times 100 \tag{1}$$

Results are represented as mean ± SD and GraphPad Prism (Version 5.03, GraphPad Software, La Jolla, CA, USA) has been used to calculate the statistical significances by one-way ANOVA, with $p < 0.05$ considered to be statistically significant.

2.7. Antimicrobial Activity of Chalcogen Nanoparticles

The activity of nanosized suspensions of sulfur, selenium and tellurium against *E. coli*, *Staphylococcus carnosus*, *C. albicans* and *S. cerevisiae* was investigated in routine microbial growth assays based on optical density and recorded in the form of growth curves [15]. Fresh cultures of *S. carnosus*, *E. coli*, *C. albicans* and *S. cerevisiae* were prepared on bacterial basic media, Luria-Bertani broth (LB) Sabouraud Dextrose Agar (SDA) and Yeast Peptone Dextrose (YPD) agar media, respectively. After 18–24 h of incubation, the microbial colonies from these plates were used to inoculate liquid cultures. Liquid cultures were subsequently incubated at 37 °C until reaching an optical density of 0.8–1.0. These microbial cultures were then exposed to the nanoparticles as described below. Bacterial or yeast culture with growth medium was employed as negative control while the positive control was composed of a mixture of penicillin, streptomycin and amphotericin B (4 U, 0.4 μg/mL and 10 μg/mL, respectively). An additional solvent control—which was required here because of the presence of stabilizers—consisted of a mixture of mannitol (20%) and Plantacare® (1%) whose concentrations were adjusted according to the one present in the sample. Nanosized suspensions were evaluated at various dilutions (formal chalcogen concentrations of 750, 1000, 1500 and 2000 μM) and the plates were incubated at 37 °C for 24 h. It should be mentioned upfront that these are formal concentrations as the particles do not dissolve (see Results). Microbial as well as fungal growth both were monitored by recording the optical density of the samples (A_{540}) at 0, 4, and 24 h (0 h refers to the first measurement immediately after incubation) on a Cary50 Bio UV/VIS spectrophotometer (Varian Australia Pty Ltd., Mulgrave, Australia). These absorbance values were converted to percentage values compared to the negative control whose value was used as a reference at each time interval and set at 100%, respectively.

In essence, growth (%) represents the percentage of UV-Vis spectrophotometric absorbance values compared to the negative control.

As some of the particle suspensions themselves also absorb or scatter light, nanosuspensions without microorganisms were used as additional controls to adjust the readings accordingly. All experiments were carried out in triplicate, at three different occasions ($n = 9$). Results are represented as mean $\pm$ SD and statistical significances have been calculated by two-way ANOVA using GraphPad Prism (Version 5.03, GraphPad Software, La Jolla, CA, USA) with $p < 0.05$ considered to be statistically significant.

3. Results

Overall, the results obtained as part of this study support the idea that suspensions of stabilized chalcogen-nanoparticles can be lyophilized to yield ready-to-use powders which can be resuspended on demand without notable loss of particle quality (i.e., no significant aggregation) and with a range of interesting biological activities against common pathogens such as *E. coli*, *S. carnosus* and *C. albicans*. These results will now be presented and discussed in more detail.

3.1. Nanosizing, Lyophilization and Resuspension (NaLyRe) of Chalcogen Particles

In good agreement with our previous findings, a combination of HSS, pre-milling and HPH resulted in spherical particles of sulfur, selenium and tellurium with diameters in the range of 760 nm for sulfur, 210 nm for selenium and 175 nm for tellurium (Figure 1) [15,25]. Figure 1 confirms that the combination of so-called pre-milling and subsequent cycles of HPH is able to reduce the size of the particles considerably. A lower limit is reached in all cases, implying that the method at hand is able to produce good quality particles with sub-micrometer diameters, yet cannot go much below the 100 nm range.

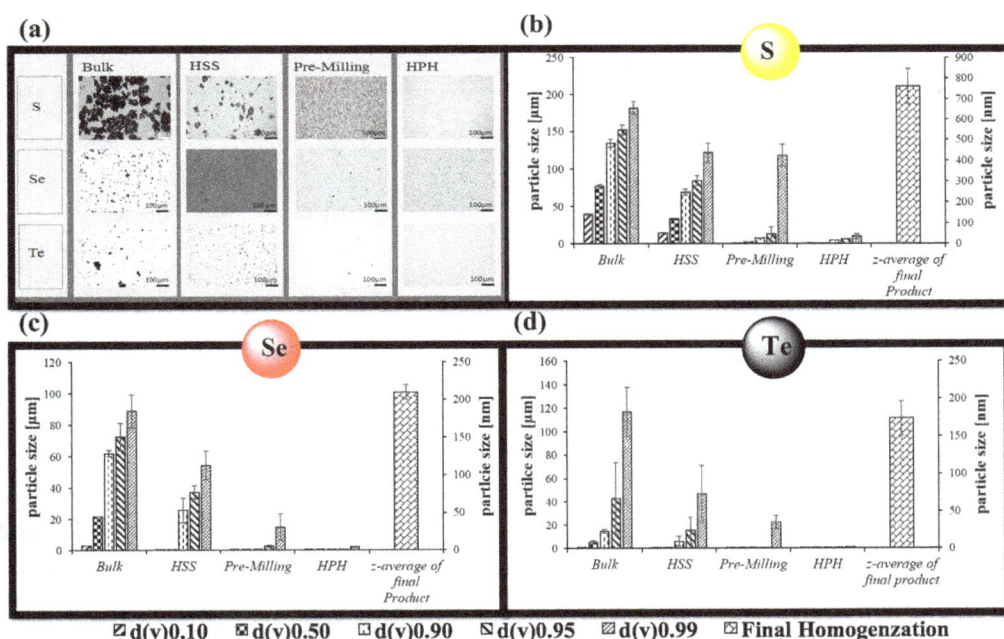

Figure 1. Characterization of nanosized chalcogen particle suspensions. (**a**) 200× magnification of nanoparticles at different generation steps; LD and PCS measurements for (**b**) sulfur; (**c**) selenium and (**d**) tellurium. It should be noted that light microscopy has been used here primarily to monitor the nanosizing process and per se is not an adequate technique to characterize particles in the nanosize range.

The nanosized suspensions shown in Figure 1 are of adequate quality and can be employed for biological studies soon after production. Nonetheless, a prolonged storage may result in aggregation, decomposition or other detrimental events. While the manufacture of such suspensions under high pressure ensures that they are initially sterile, contaminations are common during handling and result in fouling of such samples. Lyophilization in the presence of the well-known cryoprotectant mannitol was therefore seen as a suitable alternative to produce low weight, durable, readily storable and transportable samples. Figure 2 illustrates the ability of mannitol to help prevent possible agglomeration upon freeze-drying, which is clearly concentration depended. In the presence of about 20% w/v of mannitol, the size of particles remains comparably unaffected by a sequence of freeze-drying and subsequent resuspension in distilled water, with an average diameter of 245 nm before and 250 nm afterwards.

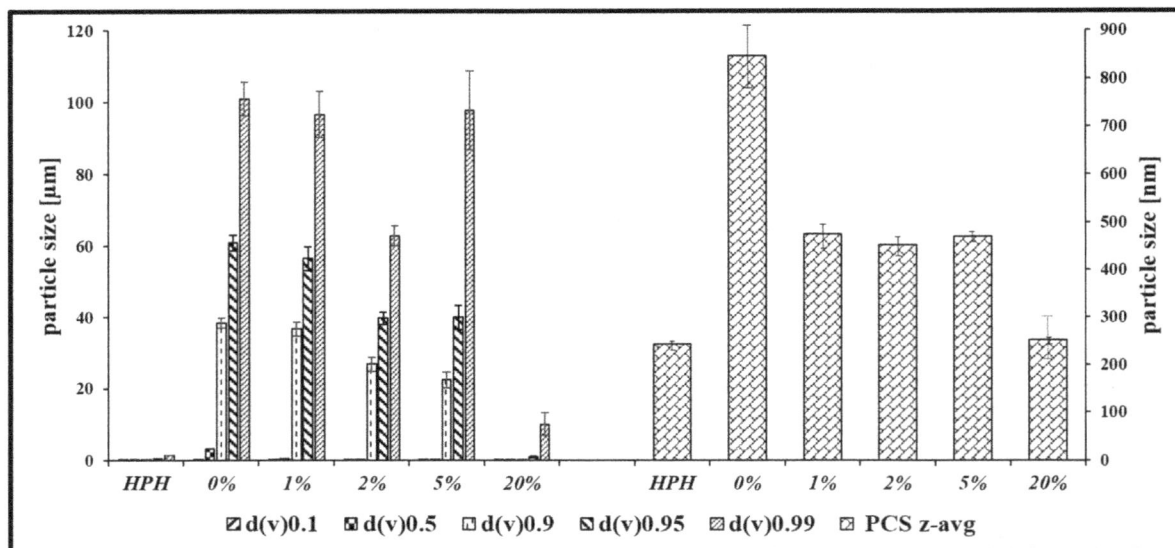

Figure 2. Determination of the effective concentration of mannitol for stabilizing selenium nanoparticles during lyophilization. LD and PCS measurements of selenium nanoparticles at 0%, 1%, 2%, 5% and 20% w/v of mannitol are shown. The HPH sample did not undergo freeze-drying and its quality, which serves as a benchmark, is achieved in the freeze-dried samples in the presence of 20% w/v mannitol.

Once the most appropriate concentration of mannitol as "cryoprotective" was determined, it was applied to the various sulfur, selenium and tellurium suspensions. After freeze-drying, these powder-like samples were stored at 4 °C and then, on demand, resuspended in 5 mL of distilled water by gentle manual shaking for 1 min. The freeze-dried samples could be stored as powders for 30 days in our experiments without notable physical changes.

Figure 3 shows photographic images of the lyophilized samples before and after resuspension in distilled water. In essence, the lyophilized samples shown in Figure 3a are powder-like and show the corresponding colors of the respective nanosized materials somewhat eclipsed by the white color of mannitol, i.e., sulfur (pale yellow), selenium (light pinkish red) and tellurium (grey) (Figure 3a). In some aspects, these materials represent "resuspendable" and biologically available forms of the three elements, which apart from the stabilizers Plantacare® (for particle stability) and mannitol (for freeze-drying) consist *exclusively* of the chalcogen elements. Unlike the elements they are based on, however, these materials can be resuspended readily and easily as shown in Figure 3b.

The native samples before lyophilisation and resuspended samples were then inspected more closely for their stability at storage conditions (at 4 °C and in a dark environment). Here, the average particle size as well as size distribution was monitored employing LD and PCS and with a firm focus on possible aggregation. Figure 4 confirms that the samples stored for 30 days at 4 °C as well as the lyophilized and subsequently resuspended samples both in their liquid forms retained the main physical characteristics of the original, freshly nanosized and pre-lyophilized samples at Day 1, such as average size and size distribution. Indeed, it appears that all native chalcogen suspensions (Figure 4a), re-suspensions (Figure 4a–d) as well as the freeze-dried powders (Figure 3a) were reasonably stable for well over one month at 4 °C, with some possible exceptions, which showed some larger aggregates, as noted with LD. Yet here as well, those larger particles seemed to be the exception as the average diameter did not increase significantly and overall, the suspensions also proved quite stable and without large agglomerates detectable under the light microscope.

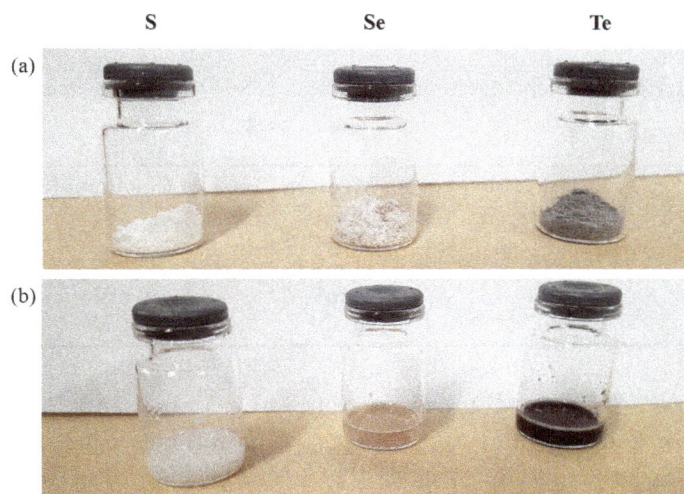

Figure 3. Photographic view of nanosized chalcogens. (**a**) lyophilized powders; (**b**) resuspensions after addition of water and simple manual shaking for 1 min.

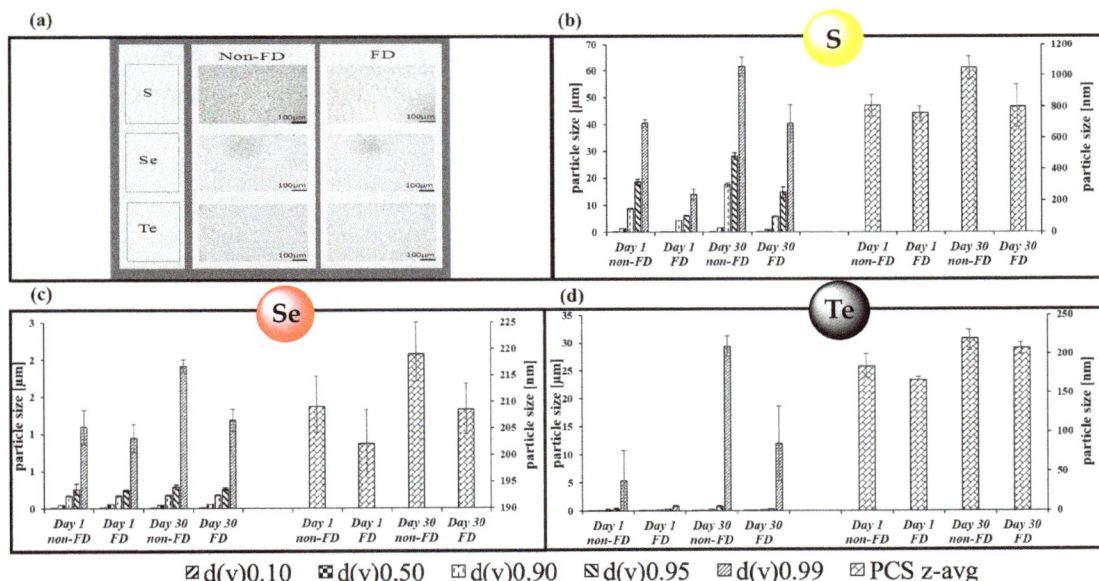

Figure 4. Analysis of the various chalcogen samples. (**a**) Microscopic view of samples after 30 days of storage, with a comparison of samples stored as suspensions at 4 °C in the dark (non-FD or "non-freeze-dried") and resuspended lyophilized samples (FD or "freeze-dried"); LD and PCS measurements of resuspended lyophilized samples of (**b**) sulfur, (**c**) selenium and (**d**) tellurium samples after 1 and 30 days of storage. The values obtained compare well with the results for the native samples provided in Figure 1.

Furthermore, to estimate the long-term stability of the nanosuspensions, measurements of their respective ZPs were performed. The ZP is an indicator of electrokinetic potential and hence can be used to predict the stability of colloidal dispersions. As mentioned already, ZPs were measured in the original suspension medium as well as in conductivity-adjusted Milli-Q water. The measurements in conductivity-adjusted Milli-Q water and in original dispersion medium were important to provide a larger picture of the charges and their effects on stability. The Stern potential, as estimated through measurements in conductivity-adjusted water, corresponds to the potential at the Stern layer and is indicative of possible electrodynamic attractions or repulsions.

The values for the initial nanosuspensions as well as the resuspended lyophilized samples are provided in Table 1.

Table 1. ZP measurements of chalogen nanoparticles. Non-FD or "non-freeze-dried" and FD or "freeze-dried".

Chalogen	In Original Suspension Medium		In Conductivity-Adjusted Water	
	Non-FD	FD	Non-FD	FD
S	−30 mV	−36 mV	−47 mV	−54 mV
Se	−24 mV	−26 mV	−40 mV	−41 mV
Te	−27 mV	−30 mV	−31 mV	−36 mV

The ZPs measured in this medium range between −31 mV and −47 mV in the samples before freeze-drying for tellurium and sulfur, respectively, and between −36 mV and −54 mV for tellurium and sulfur, respectively, in the samples after freeze-drying, with selenium at −40 mV before and −41 mV after freeze-drying. These values correspond to the respective Stern potentials and indicate well-charged particles, whose negative charges in turn prevent aggregation and therefore promote stability. The ZP measurements in original dispersion medium (surfactant and water), provide another perspective on stability. In this instance, the ZPs relate directly to the stabilization efficacy of the particles in the original suspension [22,23]. The chalogen nanosuspensions in the original medium show ZPs between −27 mV to −30 mV for tellurium and sulfur, respectively, before freeze-drying, and between −30 mV to −36 mV for tellurium and sulfur, respectively after freeze-drying, with selenium at −24 mV before and −26 mV after freeze-drying. Overall, ZP values below −30 mV are normally considered adequate for long-term physical stability. Here, one must also take into account that ZPs are not only dependent on the characteristics of the substance but also on the surfactants used. Plantacare® used in the present study is a non-ionic sugar-based surfactant [26]. Future studies should include a variety of surfactants in order to learn more about the surface charges and their impact on the stability of chalcogens. In a nutshell, the particles are charged enough to repel each other and hence do not aggregate and the sequence of lyophilizing and resuspension does not change this aspect dramatically. If at all, these processes may result in a small increase in negative charge by a few millivolts (see Table 1).

Another technique for visualizing the stability of nanoparticles is microscopy of suspensions over time. Since the size of particles was out of the range and reach of light microscopy, SEM imagery was employed [24]. As described earlier (Section 2.5), SEM requires drying of suspensions, which results in extensive agglomeration for the sample before freeze-drying (Figure 5a). This complication was avoided with the freeze-dried samples as these samples were lyophilized in the presence of a cryoprotectant (Figure 5b). Nonetheless, the presence of this cryoprotectant, which is also "dried", complicates the images obtained. The micrographs therefore show the mannitol matrix (Figure 5b (i)) and the selenium particles embedded therein (Figure 5b (ii)). Please note that the samples are dried and hence the presence of slats, composed of mannitol, complicates the images and also results in apparent artefacts.

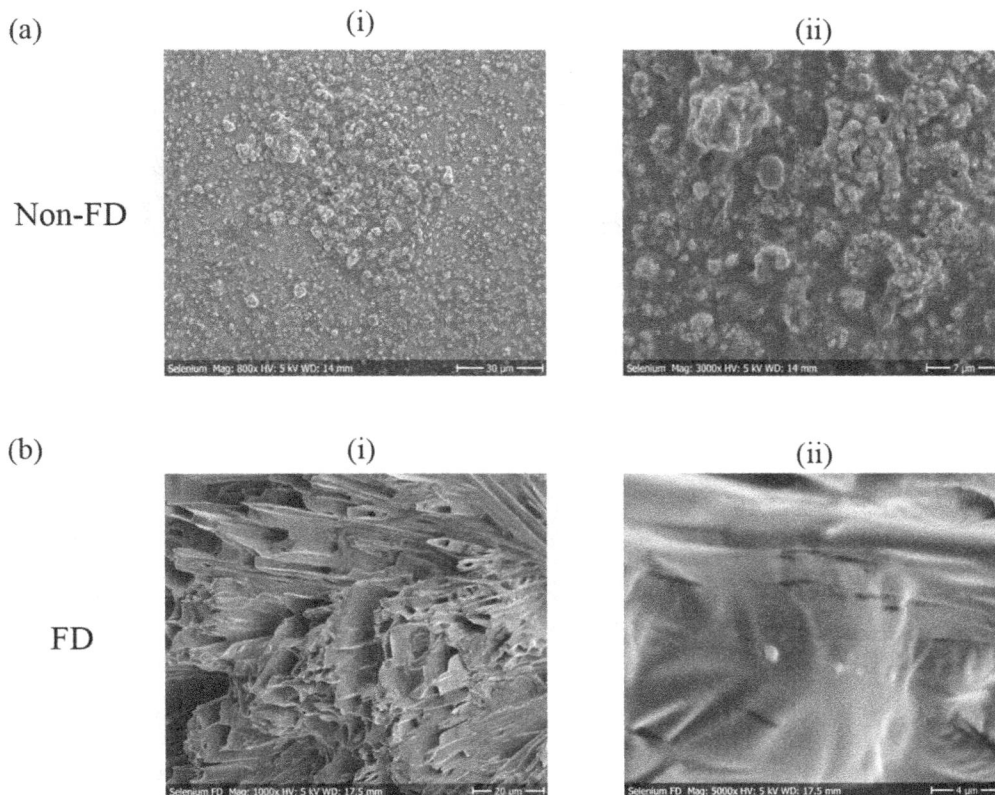

Figure 5. SEM micrographs of selenium particles. (**a**) micrographs of non-FD samples at (i) 800 and (ii) 3000× magnification; (**b**) micrographs of FD samples at (i) 1000× and (ii) 5000× magnification.

3.2. Antimicrobial Activity of Resuspended Samples

The lyophilized samples shown in Figure 3a were resuspended on demand to yield suspensions of defined concentrations. These suspensions were then investigated for their potential antimicrobial and nematicidal activity in assays based on Gram-negative (*E. coli*) and Gram-positive bacteria (*S. carnosus*), yeasts (*S. cerevisiae* and *C. albicans*) and eventually the model nematode *S. feltiae* [15,25]. It must be emphasized from the outset that the concentrations given (in molar units) are for the entire amount of the respective chalcogen in suspension. As the nanoparticles obviously do not dissolve, their chemical action is restricted to the chalcogen atoms exposed to the particle surface, and therefore also critically depends on the shape and size of the particles in question. Hence, as a rough estimate, only between 0.1% and 1% of the total chalcogen atoms are likely to be exposed and able to participate in biological activity, assuming the particles are spherical, smooth and around 100 nm in diameter. This implies, however, that formal "concentrations" shown in the following figures and discussed in the text cannot be compared directly with completely soluble materials as they obviously have to be considerably higher in order to exert the same chemical reactivity and biological activity (see Discussion).

As Figures 6–9 illustrate, overall there is a notable toxicity of the (re-)suspended chalcogen particles against most microorganisms under investigation (*S. cerevisiae, C. albicans, E. coli, S. carnosus* and *C. albicans*). Generally, this toxicity is concentration-dependent and can be noted after 4 h. After 24 h, growth remains reduced in most cases when compared to the control, and in some cases there may even be a slight "recovery" of growth, probably due to the surviving cells which continue or resume their growth.

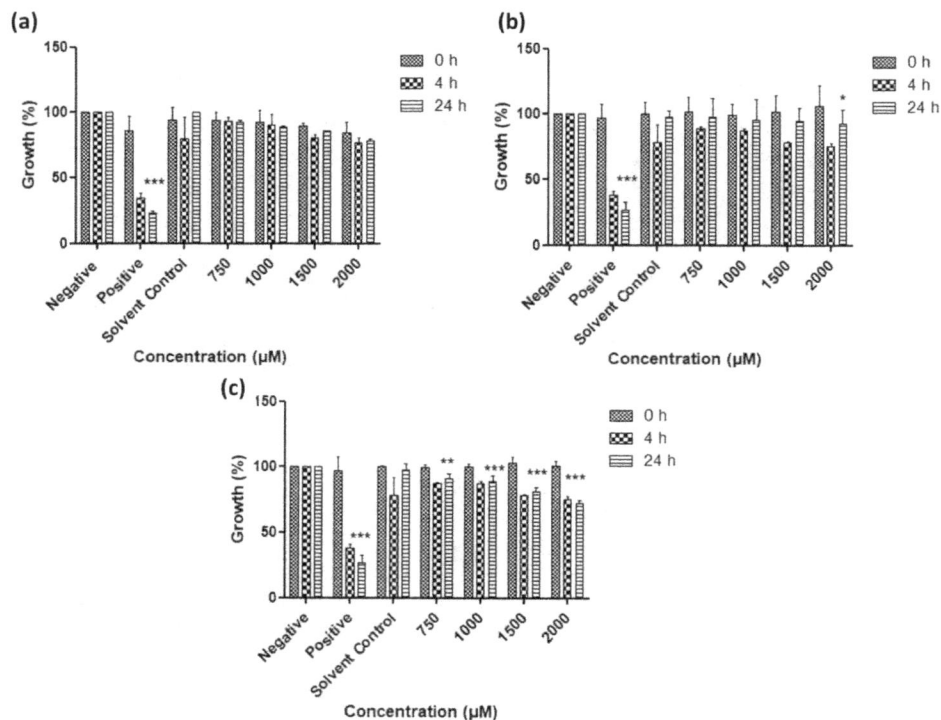

Figure 6. Impact of resuspended nanosized particles of (**a**) sulfur, (**b**) selenium and (**c**) tellurium on the growth of *S. cerevisiae*. Values represent mean ± S.D. * $p < 0.05$, ** $p < 0.01$ and *** $p < 0.001$. See text for further experimental details.

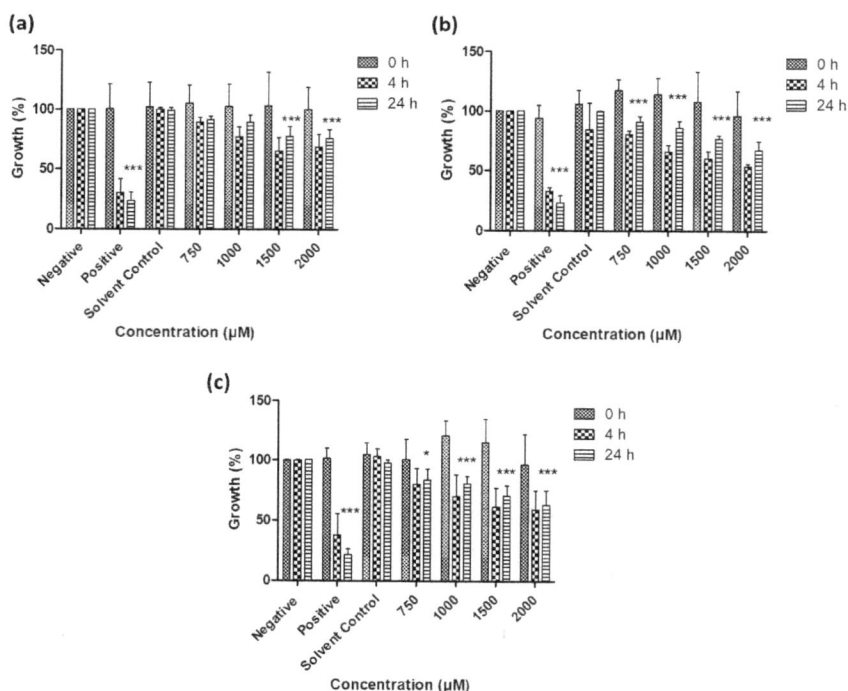

Figure 7. Impact of resuspended nanosized particles of (**a**) sulfur (**b**) selenium and (**c**) tellurium, on the growth of *C. albicans*. Values represent mean ± S.D. * $p < 0.05$ and *** $p < 0.001$. See text for further details.

Baker's yeast exemplifies several aspects of this activity (Figure 6). The growth of *S. cerevisiae* is affected particularly by the tellurium particles, especially at higher concentrations, with some activity also noted for the selenium particles. Still, *S. cerevisiae* is rather resilient towards exposure to these particles, especially in the case of sulfur and selenium.

In contrast, the growth of the pathogenic yeast *C. albicans* is affected significantly by all three types of chalcogen particles. In the case of sulfur particles, a modest reduction in growth by 20% to 30% can be noted after 4 h (Figure 7). The selenium particles are even more active and able to reduce viability by almost 55% at formal concentrations of around 1 mM of total selenium in suspension. The activity of tellurium particles is comparable, possibly slightly lower when compared to selenium.

Gram-negative bacteria currently pose a particular challenge in the development of effective antibiotics, and Figure 8 indicates that resuspended samples of all three chalcogens are active against *E. coli* at formal chalcogen concentrations in the higher micromolar range. Not surprisingly, the rather toxic tellurium is more active when compared to selenium and sulfur, with a reduction in growth to less than 50% (vs. control) after 24 h incubation at 750 μM, while around 75% of growth is retained when the same concentration of selenium is applied. The sulfur nanoparticles are less active and achieve a similar reduction in growth only at higher concentrations of 1000 to 2000 μM.

A similar trend is also observed in the case of the Gram-positive bacterium *S. carnosus* (Figure 9). At a formal tellurium concentration of 750 μM, the tellurium particles reduce growth to less than 40% after just 4 h, while selenium and sulfur both are somewhat less active, with a remaining growth of around 70% in both cases. Indeed, higher formal concentrations of tellurium particles impact dramatically on the growth and survival of *S. carnosus*, with just 20% to 30% growth remaining at formal tellurium concentrations of and above 1000 μM. Once more, it is likely that the active concentration of truly available, surface-exposed tellurium in those samples is considerably lower, probably in the order of 1 to 10 μM at most.

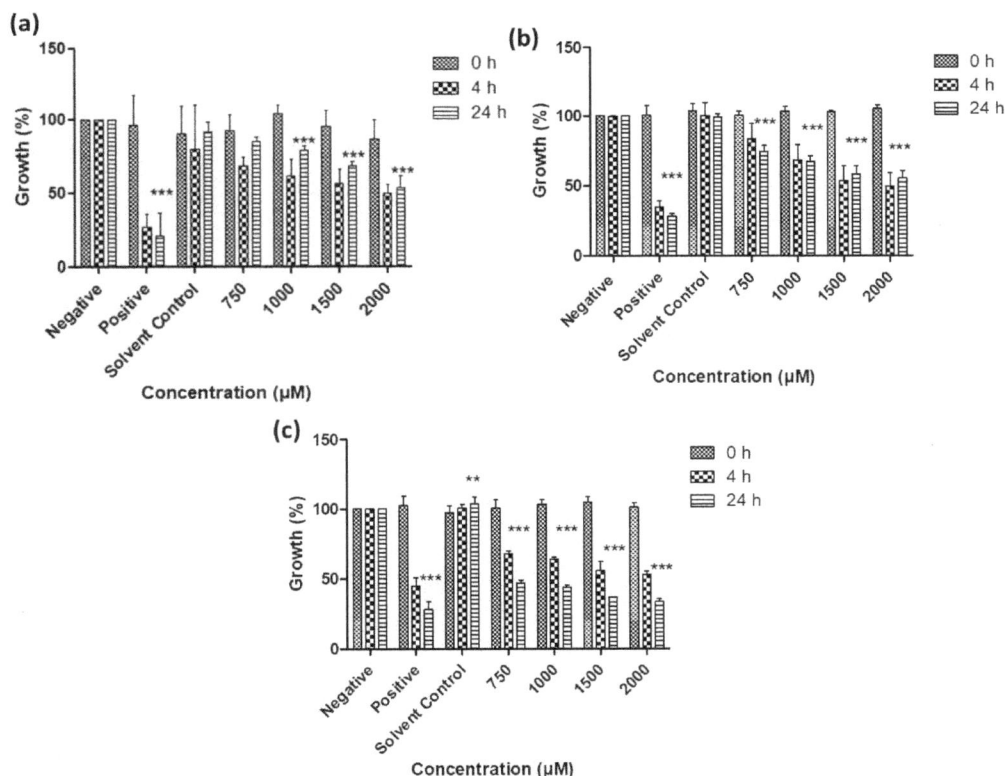

Figure 8. Impact of resuspended nanosized particles of (**a**) sulfur, (**b**) selenium and (**c**) tellurium on the growth of *E. coli*. Values represent mean ± S.D. ** $p < 0.01$ and *** $p < 0.001$. See text for further details.

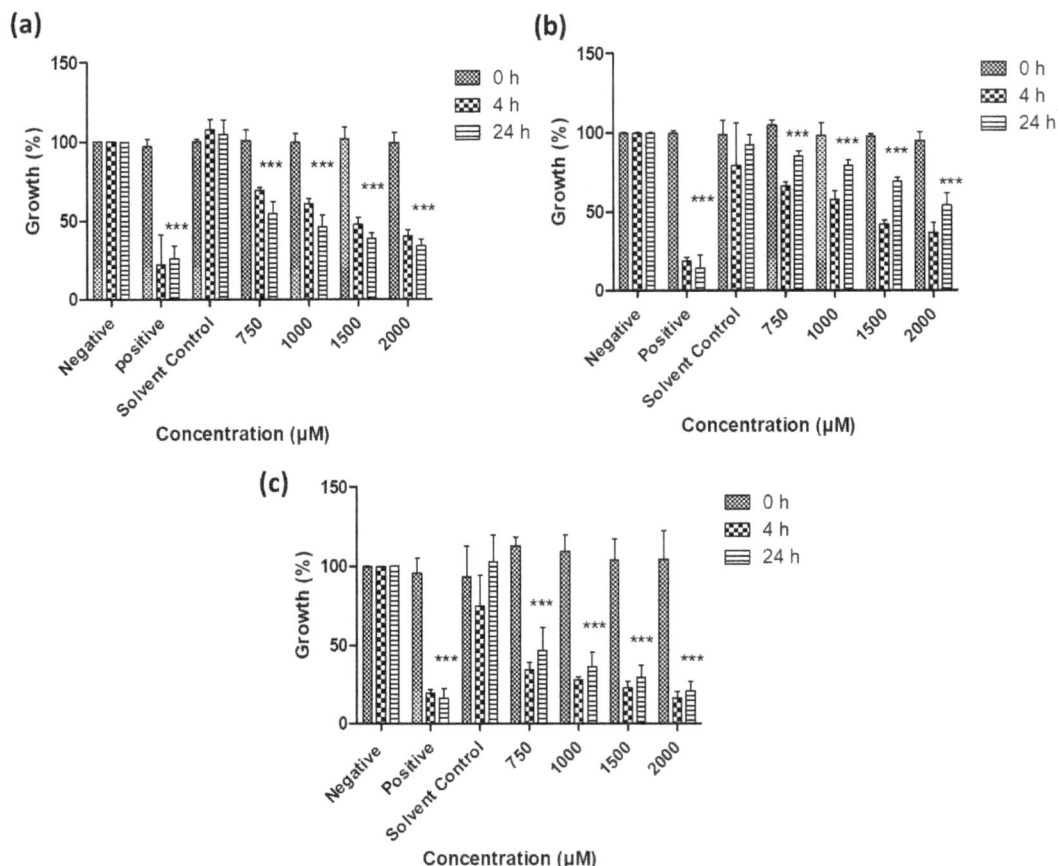

Figure 9. Impact of lyophilized nanosized particles of (**a**) sulfur, (**b**) selenium and (**c**) tellurium on the growth of *S. carnosus*. Values represent mean ± S.D. *** $p < 0.001$. See text for further details.

3.3. Activity against S. Feltiae

So far, the investigation has focused on the activity of the nanosuspensions against single cell organisms. In this, case, uptake, transport, metabolism and excretion differ considerably from multicellular organisms, which on the one side may be more protected against such particles yet, at the same time, may also become impaired by the particular particulate nature of such insoluble objects. The agricultural nematode *S. feltiae* has therefore been employed since it represents a readily available, easy to use, robust and fairly reliable model system to study toxicity against a small, yet multicellular organism [27–29]. The results for the different chalcogen particles are shown in Figure 10. In essence, they agree rather well with the previous findings in *C. albicans* and bacteria. It appears that the tellurium and selenium particles at concentrations from 25 µM upwards are more active when compared to the sulfur ones. After 4 h and at a concentration of 25 µM, a reduction in viability by 21%, 44% and 35% is observed for the sulfur, selenium and tellurium particles, respectively, which at 50 µM increases slightly to 28%, 46% and 37%, respectively. This toxicity, studied at lower concentrations due to a particular sensitivity of the nematodes against the chalcogens when compared to yeasts and bacteria, is indeed more pronounced as in the case of these microorganisms. Regardless of the chalcogen investigated, there seems to be some overall toxicity against the nematodes, which obviously needs to be investigated further and in considerably more detail, also with a sight on the impact of the stabilizers Plantacare® and mannitol which have been employed throughout as additional solvent controls.

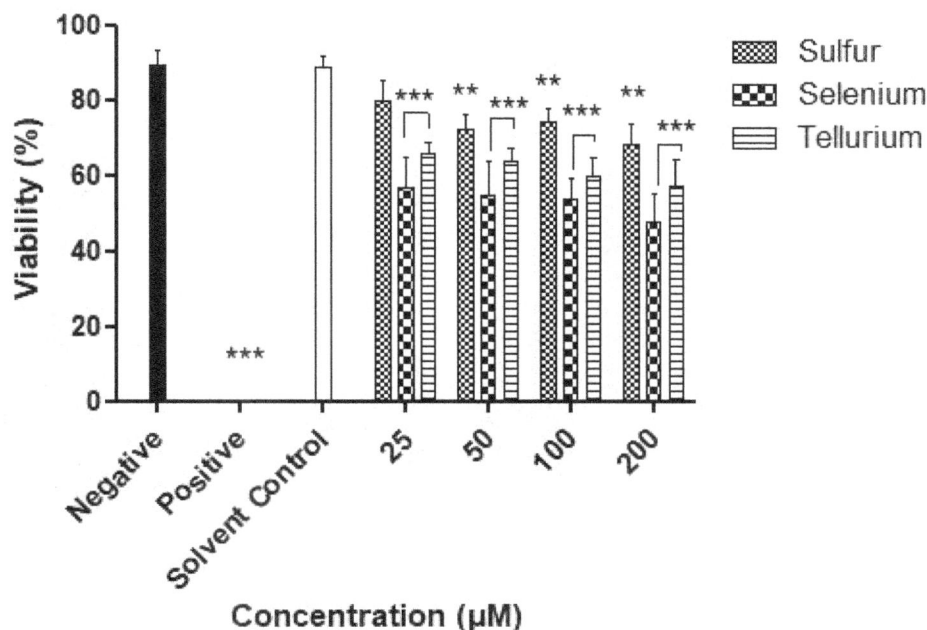

Figure 10. Impact of resuspended nanosized particles of sulfur, selenium and tellurium against *S. feltiae*. Values represent mean ± S.D. ** $p < 0.01$ and *** $p < 0.001$. See text for further details.

4. Discussion

Overall, the results obtained as part of this feasibility study demonstrate that a sequence of nanosizing and lyophilization leads to ready-to-use materials which can be resuspended easily by short manual shaking to nanosuspensions with improved bioavailability. In this study, such a NaLyRe sequence results in nanosuspensions of sulfur, selenium and tellurium, which are generally of a good physical quality and show impressive activity against a range of microorganisms, notably *C. albicans*, *E. coli* and *S. carnosus*. The results obtained along this NaLyRe avenue and their implications will now be discussed in more detail.

From the perspective of sample preparation and quality, formation of the various chalcogen nanosuspensions through mechanical techniques such as HPH was generally straightforward. Still there were also some notable differences (Figure 1). Sulfur was the least amenable of the three elements, its tendency to form cake-like materials and to sediment could be decreased by nanosizing, yet the average size of the sulfur particles could not be reduced much below 760 nm. Moving down the Periodic Table, the ability to nanosize seems to improve while applying the same experimental parameters. Under these conditions, selenium could be sized to an average particle diameter of 210 nm, while tellurium particles showed an average diameter of 170 nm. Similarly, the ability to lyophilize and to resuspend was most pronounced for the selenium and tellurium particles, while the resuspensions of the sulfur particles were stable, yet also rather "milky" (Figure 3).

From a more practical and applied perspective, these findings are rather intriguing as they represent a strategy to convert solid elemental sulfur, selenium and tellurium into powders of a similar elemental composition, yet with good suspension properties and hence applicability and activity in biological systems. Once lyophilized, the chalcogen nanoparticles form easy-to-handle fluffy cakes (Figure 3a) which require short manual resuspension times and maintain the size characteristics of the origin suspensions (Figures 3 and 4). Indeed, it appears that most particles retain their initial size and shape during the lyophilization/resuspension process, and that aggregation is not an encumbering issue. The respective ZPs, employed here as indicators of the stability of colloidal dispersions, also remain mostly unaffected by the lyophilization and resuspension procedure, and may even increase slightly. Unlike earlier liquid preparations, these lyophilized powders are considerably lighter, easier to store and to transport and do not need to be used up swiftly as they are dry and there is no danger of fouling. There is also no issue with leaks or spills which are common when handling liquid samples. Eventually, it is now feasible to prepare and store larger quantities of chalcogen nanoparticles of good quality and to resuspended them if, when and where desired for a range of possible applications, for instance in the fields of Medicine, Agriculture, Cosmetics and conceivably even in Nutrition, as may be applicable for selenium. Figure 11 provides a brief schematic illustration of the NaLyRe sequence and the potential medium-term applications associated with it.

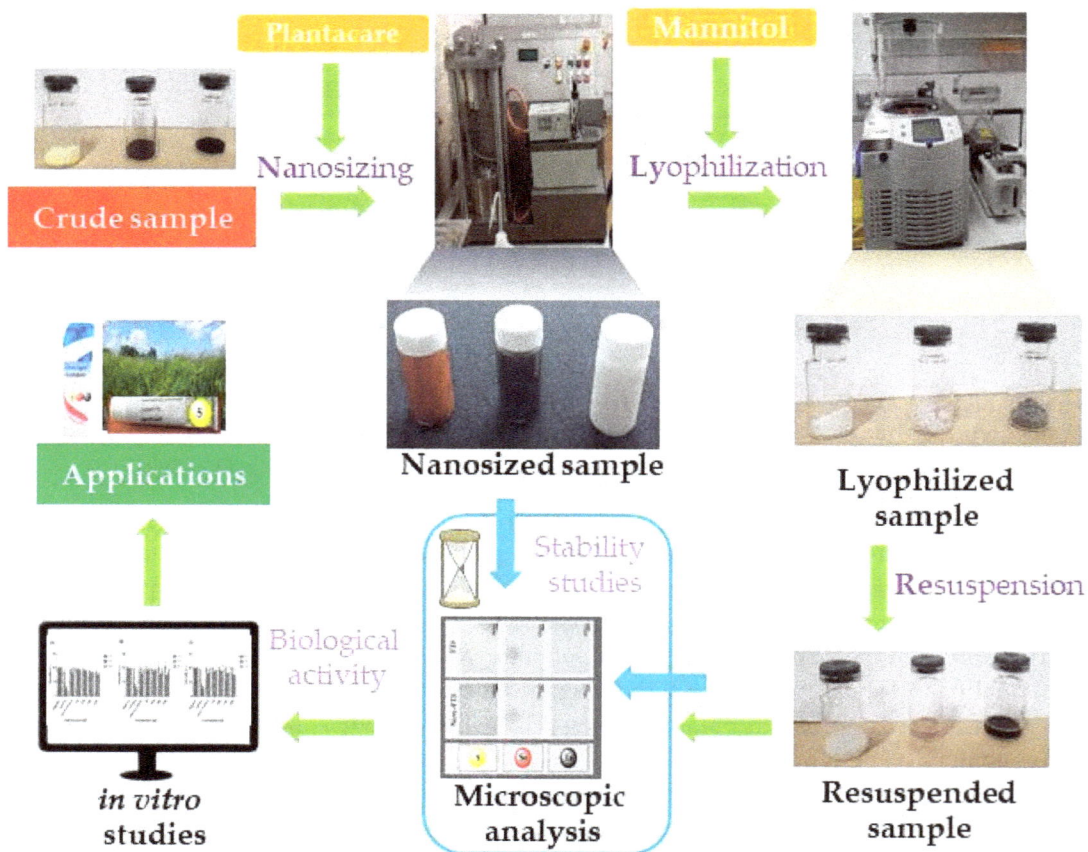

Figure 11. Schematic overview of the NaLyResequence to nanosize chalcogens and similar insoluble materials to nanosuspensions, to lyophilize these suspensions and store the resulting powders for possible practical applications. The biological activity associated with the resuspended samples promises possible applications in various areas, from Medicine to Agriculture.

Still, there are some issues which need to be addressed as part of subsequent studies. One of them is the use of stabilizers such as Plantacare® to prevent aggregation in solution and mannitol as "cryoprotectant". These components of the formulation are critical in providing protection against the stresses involved during the freeze-drying process. Indeed, without such stabilizers the formulation may be damaged in two ways. Firstly, particles at higher concentrations tend to agglomerate and to fuse. Secondly, the formation of ice crystals exerts mechanical stresses which destabilize the system [30]. These effects in the absence of protective materials were, in fact, observed in this study as illustrated in Figure 2. Here, the choice and concentration of protectant, as well as the size of particles affected are of importance. At concentrations of mannitol ranging from 1% to 5%, LD measurements show little impact of this apparent "cryoprotectant" on the agglomeration of larger particles. At higher concentrations of mannitol (e.g., at 20%), the integrity of the smaller size particles is maintained, and the agglomerations are also reduced. This can be explained by the properties of mannitol and similar cryoprotectants, which are able to form a protective matrix around the nanoparticles, isolating them as an unfrozen segment which in turn prevents the particles from agglomeration [31,32].

Eventually, the stabilizers employed in this study are well established in the literature along with other sugars [20]. Hence future studies may investigate the use of such agents in more detail and also consider alternatives. Trehalose, for instance, could possibly decrease the amount of cyroprotectant used, yet trehalose may complicate the composition and activity of the samples and is more expensive than common sugars, an economic aspect which may need to be considered as part of any practical application [20]. Notably, certain sugars may also serve as nutrients, and this may be counterproductive in the context of antimicrobial activity. It is, therefore, worthwhile to investigate alternative stabilizers which may be either more effective, less problematic and perhaps also more readily available. It may even be possible to identify "two-in-one" agents able to substitute simultaneously for both stabilizers, Plantacare® and mannitol, or to venture into agents which are "waste" or themselves biologically active for the additional "kick" [33]. In any case, the NaLyRe sequence represents a major improvement in the production and handling of otherwise insoluble or sparingly soluble materials and, indeed, one may now consider possible medical and agricultural applications in earnest.

From a biological perspective, the initial attempts with mannitol have already enabled lyophilization and resuspension with considerable biological activities observed for the resuspended samples against the microbes tested. Among the chalcogens, tellurium appears to be most toxic overall. It was least effective against *S. cerevisiae*, reducing the growth by just 20% at a formal concentration of 2000 μM (Figure 6). For *C. albicans* this activity was somewhat higher, with significant reductions already at a formal concentration of 1000 μM (Figure 7). The chalcogens were particularly effective against the two bacteria investigated, especially for Gram-positive *S. carnosus* where the growth was reduced by 50% in the presence of 2000 μM for selenium (Figures 8 and 9). In the case of the multicellular nematodes, tellurium was also active and, at a concentration of 200 μM, reduced growth to 60%. While the activity of selenium is often comparable to the one of tellurium, selenium was more active against the nematodes with a reduction of viability to below 50% of the control, while sulfur achieved a reduction to 70% (Figure 10).

In Medicine, such resuspended particles therefore may be employed against topical infections, for instance in the case of skin, mucous, nails and the gastrointestinal tract. Here, the activity of the more active tellurium particles is of special interest. Many organotellurium compounds, as well as simple tellurium salts, often show considerable activity against pathogenic organisms, in some instances even re-sensitizing drug resistant strains against common antibiotics [34]. Yet tellurium is also a fairly toxic element per se, and any application, even a topical one, clearly requires further investigations to exclude any unwanted side effects [35,36]. The particular particulate structure may actually be a benefit rather than drawback in this context, as it almost rules out the kind of systemic uptake and distribution characteristic of soluble, toxic organotellurium compounds and, at the same time, may provide a slowly releasing system for certain reactive tellurium species (RTeS).

General toxicity is less of an issue with the trace element selenium. While the selenium nanoparticles may be oxidized or reduced as well to release diverse reactive selenium species (RSeS), selenides (H_2Se), selenite (SeO_3^{2-}) and selenate (SeO_4^{2-}) are readily detoxified and even utilized by the human body. The activity of the selenium-based nanosuspensions is therefore rather stimulating, especially in the context of *C. albicans*, as yeasts are commonly known to be rather sensitive against this chalcogen and its diverse compounds. Here, the resuspended selenium particles, at a concentration of 2000 μM, reduce growth by 40%. Indeed, certain anti-dandruff shampoos contain selenium, and chemically speaking, the rather unusual mixed sulfur-selenium ring structures at the centre of such activity are not that different from the Se_8 rings found in the selenium nanoparticles [37–39]. Similarly, the resuspended selenium particles were also active against both strains of bacteria, at a formal concentration of 2000 μM reducing growth of *S. carnosus* to 55%.

In any case, the precise mode(s) of action of these particles, against microbes and also in more complex organisms—from *S. feltiae* to humans—needs to be studied in considerable detail as part of future investigations and also to rule out any undesired or detrimental side effects of this material. Based on the literature available to date and on previous studies, it is feasible that such chalcogen particles act via a combination of mechanisms, which may involve more general physical interactions of the particles with cells and organelles, rather specific surface interactions—such as binding of and to proteins and enzymes, a specific surface chemistry of the chalcogens as well as a slow release of chalcogen-based molecules, such as the kind of inorganic polysulfides ($S_x{}^{2-}$) mentioned in the Introduction.

From a wider perspective, and besides possible applications as antimicrobials in Medicine, resuspendable powders of selenium and sulfur may also be of interest in the field of Agriculture. As mentioned briefly in the Introduction, colloidal sulfur has a long tradition in the treatment of grapevines and a similar, perhaps more effective treatment could be envisaged for the nanosuspensions [13,14]. Similarly, selenium may also be applied, obviously under considerably more controlled conditions and in considerably lower amounts. Here, sulfur, as well as selenium, may not only protect the plant from (microbial, nematode) predators, these particles may also enrich the soil, and, by slowly degrading, may serve as a reservoir of an inorganic fertilizer and eventually, in the case of selenium, even as trace element enrichment which may be beneficial along the nutritional chain.

In the medium term, the choice of particles and stabilizers will depend on the specific applications under consideration, and native suspensions—which initially are also sterile due to the manufacturing process—as well as resuspended lyophilized preparations seem to be quite stable and may be considered.

5. Conclusions

In summary, and without much suspense, we have been able to demonstrate that resuspension of ready-to-use lyophilized powders of sulfur, selenium and tellurium nanosuspensions on demand results in biologically active suspensions, albeit not solutions. The focus of this investigation has been on the proof-of-principle, and to evaluate the general feasibility of the underlying NaLyRe sequence.

Subsequent studies obviously need to investigate the various aspects of production, stability and wider applications of this approach and its products in considerably more detail. The choice of stabilizers and "cryo-protectants" such as Plantacare® and mannitol, in particular, needs to be considered from the perspective of large-scale production, activity, side-effects, economy and environmental impact. Alternatives, for instance derived from agricultural waste or with specific, desirable biological activities may be of particular interest here [33]. The mode(s) of action also need to be considered in considerably more detail, since these materials may impact on living organisms in various, physical, chemical, biochemical and physiological aspects. Such interactions, or nanotoxicity itself, may result in possible limitations due to adverse side effects. Nonetheless, as the examples of certain anti-dandruff formulations and colloidal sulfur illustrate, there is considerable potential stowed away in the elemental forms of these chalcogens, and unlocking this potential may be possible using nanotechnology.

Admittedly, these elemental forms may appear as rather "primitive" in a more biological context, especially when considering the numerous biologically active sulfur, selenium and tellurium compounds already known. Still, elemental forms have the major advantage that they do not carry the ballast of organic groups which may become modified, released or otherwise problematic. Indeed, the considerable recent interest in biologically active polysulfides, such as the tetrasulfide ($S_4{}^{2-}$), demonstrates that "chalcogen only" substances can play a significant role in biological systems [12,40]. One may therefore speculate that S_8 or Se_8 rings exposed on the surface of a mighty, at the same time slowly moving and degrading and chalcogen-releasing particle might exhibit considerable activity. Eventually, and with the NaLyRe sequence now available, other materials, such as sparingly or insoluble natural materials or products, parts of plants and even waste, may be processed in the same manner, therefore widening the scope of this approach and providing access to an even wider field of materials and applications [33,41].

Acknowledgments: The authors would like to acknowledge the financial support of their respective Universities, namely The University of Saarland and the University of Marburg, the ZIM Project: TOPAS (Grant No. KZ16KN046424), the "Landesforschungsförderungsprogramm" of the State of Saarland (Grant No. WT/2–LFFP 16/01) and the INTERREG VA GR program (BIOVAL), Grant No. 4-09-21). The authors acknowledge the support of Rama Alhasan and express special thanks to Ken Rory, Ashfiq Al-Fakhim, Rosa Ponte, Vulgar Prol, Trafique Basel and many other colleagues of the "Academiacs International" network for helpful discussions and inspiration.

Author Contributions: Sharoon Griffin, Muhammad Sarfraz and Steffen F. Hartmann performed the experiments; Shashank Reddy Pinnapireddy performed scanning electron microscopy; Cornelia M. Keck, and Claus Jacob conceived and designed the experiments; Sharoon Griffin, Muhammad Sarfraz, Steffen F. Hartmann, Muhammad Jawad Nasim, Udo Bakowsky, Cornelia M. Keck and Claus Jacob analyzed and wrote the paper.

Conflicts of Interest: The authors declare no conflict of interest.

References

1. Jacob, C. A scent of therapy: Pharmacological implications of natural products containing redox-active sulfur atoms. *Nat. Prod. Rep.* **2006**, *23*, 851–863. [CrossRef] [PubMed]

2. Azad, G.K.; Tomar, R.S. Ebselen, a promising antioxidant drug: Mechanisms of action and targets of biological pathways. *Mol. Biol. Rep.* **2014**, *41*, 4865–4879. [CrossRef] [PubMed]

3. Jawad Nasim, M.; Ali, W.; Dominguez-Alvarez, E.; da Silva Junior, E.N.; Saleem, R.S.Z.; Jacob, C. Chapter 10 reactive selenium species: Redox modulation, antioxidant, antimicrobial and anticancer activities. In *Organoselenium Compounds in Biology and Medicine: Synthesis, Biological and Therapeutic Treatments*; The Royal Society of Chemistry: London, UK, 2018; pp. 277–302.

4. Pacula, A.J.; Kaczor, K.B.; Antosiewicz, J.; Janecka, A.; Dlugosz, A.; Janecki, T.; Wojtczak, A.; Scianowski, J. New chiral ebselen analogues with antioxidant and cytotoxic potential. *Molecules* **2017**, *22*, 492. [CrossRef] [PubMed]

5. Lima, C.B.C.; Arrais-Silva, W.W.; Cunha, R.L.O.R.; Giorgio, S. A novel organotellurium compound (RT-01) as a new antileishmanial agent. *Korean J. Parasitol.* **2009**, *47*, 213–218. [CrossRef] [PubMed]

6. Hachmo, Y.; Kalechman, Y.; Skornick, I.; Gafter, U.; Caspi, R.R.; Sredni, B. The small tellurium compound as101 ameliorates rat crescentic glomerulonephritis: Association with inhibition of macrophage caspase-1 activity via very late antigen-4 inactivation. *Front. Immunol.* **2017**, *8*, 240. [CrossRef] [PubMed]

7. Agata, J.P.; Francesca, M.; Luca, S.; Eder, J.L.; Jacek, Ś.; Claudio, S. An update on "selenium containing compounds from poison to drug candidates: A review on the GPx-like activity". *Curr. Chem. Biol.* **2015**, *9*, 97–112.

8. Mugesh, G.; du Mont, W.W.; Sies, H. Chemistry of biologically important synthetic organoselenium compounds. *Chem. Rev.* **2001**, *101*, 2125–2179. [CrossRef] [PubMed]

9. Mauro, J.C.; Loucks, R.J.; Balakrishnan, J.; Varshneya, A.K. Potential energy landscapes of elemental and heterogeneous chalcogen clusters. *Phys. Rev. A* **2006**, *73*. [CrossRef]

10. Moustafa, A.; Habara, Y. Cross talk between polysulfide and nitric oxide in rat peritoneal mast cells. *Am. J. Physiol. Cell Physiol.* **2016**, *310*, C894–C902. [CrossRef] [PubMed]

11. Kimura, H. Signaling molecules: Hydrogen sulfide and polysulfide. *Antioxid. Redox Signal.* **2015**, *22*, 362–376. [CrossRef] [PubMed]

12. Estevam, E.C.; Faulstich, L.; Griffin, S.; Burkholz, T.; Jacob, C. Polysulfides in biology: From intricate chemistry to an astonishing yet hidden biological activity. *Curr. Org. Chem.* **2016**, *20*, 211–217. [CrossRef]

13. Young, H.C. Colloidal sulphur as a spray material. *Ann. Mo. Bot. Gard.* **1925**, *12*, 133–143. [CrossRef]

14. Kwasniewski, M.T.; Sacks, G.L.; Wilcox, W.F. Persistence of elemental sulfur spray residue on grapes during ripening and vinification. *Am. J. Enol. Vitic.* **2014**, *65*, 453–462. [CrossRef]

15. Estevam, E.C.; Griffin, S.; Nasim, M.J.; Denezhkin, P.; Schneider, R.; Lilischkis, R.; Dominguez-Alvarez, E.; Witek, K.; Latacz, G.; Keck, C.; et al. Natural selenium particles from staphylococcus carnosus: Hazards or particles with particular promise? *J. Hazard Mater.* **2017**, *324*, 22–30. [CrossRef] [PubMed]

16. Schneider, T.; Baldauf, A.; Ba, L.A.; Jamier, V.; Khairan, K.; Sarakbi, M.B.; Reum, N.; Schneider, M.; Roseler, A.; Becker, K.; et al. Selective antimicrobial activity associated with sulfur nanoparticles. *J. Biomed. Nanotechnol.* **2011**, *7*, 395–405. [CrossRef] [PubMed]

17. Chacon, M.; Molpeceres, J.; Berges, L.; Guzman, M.; Aberturas, M.R. Stability and freeze-drying of cyclosporine loaded poly(D,L lactide-glycolide) carriers. *Eur. J. Pharm. Sci.* **1999**, *8*, 99–107. [CrossRef]

18. Sameti, M.; Bohr, G.; Ravi Kumar, M.N.; Kneuer, C.; Bakowsky, U.; Nacken, M.; Schmidt, H.; Lehr, C.M. Stabilisation by freeze-drying of cationically modified silica nanoparticles for gene delivery. *Int. J. Pharm.* **2003**, *266*, 51–60. [CrossRef]

19. Konan, Y.N.; Gurny, R.; Allemann, E. Preparation and characterization of sterile and freeze-dried sub-200 nm nanoparticles. *Int. J. Pharm.* **2002**, *233*, 239–252. [CrossRef]

20. Abdelwahed, W.; Degobert, G.; Stainmesse, S.; Fessi, H. Freeze-drying of nanoparticles: Formulation, process and storage considerations. *Adv. Drug Deliv. Rev.* **2006**, *58*, 1688–1713. [CrossRef] [PubMed]

21. Sis, H.; Birinci, M. Effect of nonionic and ionic surfactants on zeta potential and dispersion properties of carbon black powders. *Colloid Surf. A* **2009**, *341*, 60–67. [CrossRef]

22. Pyo, S.; Meinke, M.; Keck, C.; Müller, R. Rutin—Increased antioxidant activity and skin penetration by nanocrystal technology (smartcrystals). *Cosmetics* **2016**, *3*, 9. [CrossRef]

23. Mishra, P.R.; Al Shaal, L.; Muller, R.H.; Keck, C.M. Production and characterization of hesperetin nanosuspensions for dermal delivery. *Int. J. Pharm.* **2009**, *371*, 182–189. [CrossRef] [PubMed]

24. Pinnapireddy, S.R.; Duse, L.; Strehlow, B.; Schafer, J.; Bakowsky, U. Composite liposome-pei/nucleic acid lipopolyplexes for safe and efficient gene delivery and gene knockdown. *Colloid Surf. B* **2017**, *158*, 93–101. [CrossRef] [PubMed]

25. Faulstich, L.; Griffin, S.; Nasim, M.J.; Masood, M.I.; Ali, W.; Alhamound, S.; Omran, Y.; Kim, H.; Kharma, A.; Schafer, K.H.; et al. Nature's hat-trick: Can we use sulfur springs as ecological source for materials with agricultural and medical applications? *Int. Biodeterior. Biodegrad.* **2017**, *119*, 678–686. [CrossRef]

26. Kuhn, A.V.; Neubert, R.H.H. Characterization of mixtures of alkyl polyglycosides (plantacare) by liquid chromatography-electrospray ionization quadrupole time-of-flight mass spectrometry. *Pharm. Res.* **2004**, *21*, 2347–2353. [CrossRef] [PubMed]

27. Czepukojc, B.; Viswanathan, U.M.; Raza, A.; Ali, S.; Burkholz, T.; Jacob, C. Tetrasulfanes as selective modulators of the cellular thiolstat. *Phosphorus Sulfur* **2013**, *188*, 446–453. [CrossRef]

28. Griffin, S.; Tittikpina, N.K.; Al-Marby, A.; Alkhayer, R.; Denezhkin, P.; Witek, K.; Gbogbo, K.A.; Batawila, K.; Duval, R.E.; Nasim, M.J.; et al. Turning waste into value: Nanosized natural plant materials of *Solanum incanum* L. and pterocarpus erinaceus poir with promising antimicrobial activities. *Pharmaceutics* **2016**, *8*, 11. [CrossRef] [PubMed]

29. Al-Marby, A.; Ejike, C.E.C.C.; Nasim, M.J.; Awadh-Ali, N.A.; Al-Badani, R.A.; Alghamdi, G.M.A.; Jacob, C. Nematicidal and antimicrobial activities of methanol extracts of 17 plants, of importance in ethnopharmacology, obtained from the arabian peninsula. *J. Intercult. Ethnopharmacol.* **2016**, *5*, 114–121. [CrossRef] [PubMed]

30. De Jaeghere, F.; Allemann, E.; Feijen, J.; Kissel, T.; Doelker, E.; Gurny, R. Freeze-drying and lyopreservation of diblock and triblock poly(lactic acid)-poly(ethylene oxide) (PLA-PEO) copolymer nanoparticles. *Pharm. Dev. Technol.* **2000**, *5*, 473–483. [CrossRef] [PubMed]

31. Tang, X.; Pikal, M.J. Design of freeze-drying processes for pharmaceuticals: Practical advice. *Pharm. Res.* **2004**, *21*, 191–200. [CrossRef] [PubMed]

32. Allison, S.D.; Molina, M.C.; Anchordoquy, T.J. Stabilization of lipid/DNA complexes during the freezing step of the lyophilization process: The particle isolation hypothesis. *Biochim. Biophys. Acta* **2000**, *1468*, 127–138. [CrossRef]

33. Griffin, S.; Sarfraz, M.; Farida, V.; Nasim, M.J.; Ebokaiwe, A.P.; Keck, C.M.; Jacob, C. No time to waste organic waste: Nanosizing converts remains of food processing into refined materials. *J. Environ. Manag.* **2018**, *210*, 114–121. [CrossRef] [PubMed]

34. Castellucci Estevam, E.; Witek, K.; Faulstich, L.; Nasim, M.J.; Latacz, G.; Dominguez-Alvarez, E.; Kiec-Kononowicz, K.; Demasi, M.; Handzlik, J.; Jacob, C. Aspects of a distinct cytotoxicity of selenium salts and organic selenides in living cells with possible implications for drug design. *Molecules* **2015**, *20*, 13894–13912. [CrossRef] [PubMed]

35. Pessoa-Pureur, R.; Heimfarth, L.; Rocha, J.B. Signaling mechanisms and disrupted cytoskeleton in the diphenyl ditelluride neurotoxicity. *Oxid. Med. Cell. Longev.* **2014**, *2014*, 458601. [CrossRef] [PubMed]

36. Heimfarth, L.; Loureiro, S.O.; Reis, K.P.; de Lima, B.O.; Zamboni, F.; Gandolfi, T.; Narvaes, R.; da Rocha, J.B.T.; Pessoa-Pureur, R. Cross-talk among intracellular signaling pathways mediates the diphenyl ditelluride actions on the hippocampal cytoskeleton of young rats. *Chem. Res. Toxicol.* **2011**, *24*, 1754–1764. [CrossRef] [PubMed]

37. Cummins, L.M.; Kimura, E.T. Safety evaluation of selenium sulfide antidandruff shampoos. *Toxicol. Appl. Pharm.* **1971**, *20*, 89–96. [CrossRef]

38. Lin, Z.; Wang, Z.; Chen, W.; Lir, L.; Li, G.; Liu, Z.; Han, H.; Wang, Z. Absorption and Raman spectra of Se8-ring clusters in zeolite 5A. *Solid State Commun.* **1996**, *100*, 841–843. [CrossRef]

39. Steudel, R.; Laitinen, R. Cyclic selenium sulfides. *Top. Curr. Chem.* **1982**, *102*, 177–197. [PubMed]

40. Kimura, H. Hydrogen sulfide and polysulfides as signaling molecules. *Nitric Oxide Biol. Chem.* **2015**, *47*, S6. [CrossRef]

41. Griffin, S.; Masood, M.I.; Nasim, M.J.; Sarfraz, M.; Ebokaiwe, A.P.; Schafer, K.H.; Keck, C.M.; Jacob, C. Natural nanoparticles: A particular matter inspired by nature. *Antioxidants* **2017**, *7*, 3. [CrossRef] [PubMed]

7

Modulation of the Oxidative Stress and Lipid Peroxidation by Endocannabinoids and their Lipid Analogues

Cristina Anna Gallelli [1,†] (iD), Silvio Calcagnini [1,†] (iD), Adele Romano [1],
Justyna Barbara Koczwara [1] (iD), Marialuisa de Ceglia [1] (iD), Donatella Dante [1], Rosanna Villani [2],
Anna Maria Giudetti [3] (iD), Tommaso Cassano [4,*] (iD) and Silvana Gaetani [1] (iD)

[1] Department of Physiology and Pharmacology "V. Erspamer", Sapienza University of Rome,
Piazzale Aldo Moro 5, 00185 Rome, Italy; cristinaanna.gallelli@uniroma1.it (C.A.G);
silvio.calcagnini@uniroma1.it (S.C.); adele.romano@uniroma1.it (A.R.);
justynabarbara.koczwara@uniroma1.it (J.B.K); marialuisa.deceglia@uniroma1.it (M.d.C.);
donatella.dante@uniroma1.it (D.D.); silvana.gaetani@uniroma1.it (S.G.)

[2] C.U.R.E. University Centre for Liver Disease Research and Treatment, Department of Medical and Surgical
Sciences, Institute of Internal Medicine, University of Foggia, 71122 Foggia, Italy; rosanna.villani@unifg.it

[3] Department of Biological and Environmental Sciences and Technologies, University of Salento,
Via Monteroni, 73100 Lecce, Italy; anna.giudetti@unisalento.it

[4] Department of Clinical and Experimental Medicine, University of Foggia, Via Luigi Pinto,
c/o Ospedali Riuniti, 71122 Foggia, Italy

* Correspondence: tommaso.cassano@unifg.it

† These authors contributed equally to this study.

Abstract: Growing evidence supports the pivotal role played by oxidative stress in tissue injury development, thus resulting in several pathologies including cardiovascular, renal, neuropsychiatric, and neurodegenerative disorders, all characterized by an altered oxidative status. Reactive oxygen and nitrogen species and lipid peroxidation-derived reactive aldehydes including acrolein, malondialdehyde, and 4-hydroxy-2-nonenal, among others, are the main responsible for cellular and tissue damages occurring in redox-dependent processes. In this scenario, a link between the endocannabinoid system (ECS) and redox homeostasis impairment appears to be crucial. Anandamide and 2-arachidonoylglycerol, the best characterized endocannabinoids, are able to modulate the activity of several antioxidant enzymes through targeting the cannabinoid receptors type 1 and 2 as well as additional receptors such as the transient receptor potential vanilloid 1, the peroxisome proliferator-activated receptor alpha, and the orphan G protein-coupled receptors 18 and 55. Moreover, the endocannabinoids lipid analogues N-acylethanolamines showed to protect cell damage and death from reactive aldehydes-induced oxidative stress by restoring the intracellular oxidants-antioxidants balance. In this review, we will provide a better understanding of the main mechanisms triggered by the cross-talk between the oxidative stress and the ECS, focusing also on the enzymatic and non-enzymatic antioxidants as scavengers of reactive aldehydes and their toxic bioactive adducts.

Keywords: oxidative stress; lipid peroxidation; reactive aldehydes; reactive oxygen and nitrogen species; free radicals; endocannabinoids; cannabinoid receptors; peroxisome proliferator-activated receptors; transient receptor potential vanilloid; G protein-coupled receptors

1. Introduction

Oxidative stress and lipid peroxidation are the consequences of a deregulated redox homeostasis that results in the accumulation of highly reactive molecules and cellular injury, especially in those tissues with a high oxygen consumption, such as heart, kidney, and brain, thus leading to cardiovascular [1,2], renal [3], and neurodegenerative diseases [4–6], just to mention a few. Examples of the possible repercussions of free radical damage are provided in this review with special emphasis on lipid peroxidation-derived reactive aldehydes including acrolein (ACR), malondialdehyde (MDA), and 4-hydroxy-2-nonenal (4-HNE), among others [7].

To get a deeper insight into the cellular pathways that regulate reactive oxygen and nitrogen species (ROS/RNS) as well as reactive aldehydes formation, there is a growing interest in identifying free radical scavenging molecules that can prevent cell death following oxidative stress-induced damage of cellular membranes. In this perspective, over the last few years, the endocannabinoid system (ECS) has attracted significant attention because of the existing cross-talk between endocannabinoids (ECs) as well as their lipid analogues and various redox-dependent processes. Therefore, the pathways by which the ECs and their lipid-related mediators contribute to the modulation of oxidative stress and lipid peroxidation represent a significant research area that will yield novel pharmaceutical strategies for the treatment of diseases characterized by a redox imbalance.

The cannabinoid receptors type 1 (CB1) and 2 (CB2), together with additional ECs receptor targets, take part in the complex ECS and, because of their wide distribution, they may play a role in mediating the antioxidant properties of ECs [8–10]. However, the great diversity of results in this field discloses the requirement of a better understanding on the pathways by which these receptors are involved in regulating oxidative stress and lipid peroxidation processes.

In this review, we will provide an overview of the role of the ECS in pathological conditions related to a redox status imbalance, leading to a better comprehension of the intricate routes that are associated to the antioxidant properties exerted by the ECs, thus enhancing the research in finding a therapeutic benefit for cannabinoid-based drugs in various redox-dependent disorders.

2. Oxidative Stress and Lipid Peroxidation

Oxidative stress can be described as an imbalance between the production of oxidant species and the antioxidant defenses, which may affect cellular redox homeostasis leading to molecular alterations and thus resulting in cell and tissue damage [11]. The term "oxidants" is a general term used to identify several groups of reactive molecules among which ROS and RNS are considered the most interesting from a biological point of view. ROS/RNS are natural byproducts of aerobic metabolism and are produced by all living multicellular organisms. ROS include free oxygen radicals and non-radical molecules, such as superoxide anion ($O_2\bullet^-$), hydroxyl ($\bullet OH$), peroxyl, alkyl, and alkoxyl radicals, as well as singlet oxygen ($^1O_2$), hydrogen peroxide (H_2O_2), ozone (O_3), and hypochlorous acid (HClO), while RNS include nitrogen compounds such as nitric oxide ($\bullet NO$), nitrogen dioxide ($NO_2\bullet$), nitrate (NO_3^-), nitrite (NO_2^-), and peroxynitrite ($ONOO^-$) [12,13].

In mammals, the main cellular sources of ROS/RNS are the mitochondrial and microsomal electron transport chains [14], the NADPH oxidase enzymes (NOXs), which consist of seven isoforms with various tissue distributions and mechanisms of activation [15,16], the flavoenzyme endoplasmic reticulum oxireductin 1 [17], nitric oxide synthase (NOS) [18], cytochrome P450 enzymes [19], cyclooxygenases (COXs), lipoxygenases (LOXs) [20], xanthine oxidase [21], diamine oxidase [22], and prostaglandin synthase [23]. In addition to these endogenous sources, the ionizing radiation, ultraviolet rays, pathogens, xenobiotics (e.g., drugs, herbicides, fungicides, trace metals, etc.), and environmental pollutants (e.g., smog, cigarette smoke, smoke from wood combustion, etc.) are identified as exogenous sources of ROS/RNS [24], which may seriously alter the fundamental oxidants-antioxidants balance.

To date, growing evidence confirms that ROS/RNS are produced by healthy cells in a highly regulated fashion in order to maintain the intracellular redox homeostasis. Moreover, ROS/RNS regulate several cellular functions ranging from immune defense to gene expression regulation, thus acting as reactive molecules secreted against circulating pathogens [25] or as second messengers of specific signaling pathways [26]. The crucial role played by ROS/RNS in immune defense was demonstrated by the discovery of the chronic granulomatous disorder (CGD), a hereditary disease characterized by NOX type 2 (NOX2)-defective phagocytes [27] which are unable to produce ROS/RNS. This genetic defect leads CGD patients in developing a primary immunodeficiency due to the inability of host innate defense to kill and digest ingested pathogens such as bacterial and fungal cells [28–31]. Moreover, ROS/RNS play also an important role in the cardiovascular system because of their ability to regulate blood pressure. In particular, the endothelial NOX2 isoform regulates the release of $\bullet$NO, the endothelium-derived relaxing factor, which modulates the caliber of blood vessels, through the production of $O_2\bullet^-$. In hypertension and other vascular pathologies, NOX2 seems to be up-regulated leading to a reduced $\bullet$NO bioavailability and to the consequent oxidants-antioxidants imbalance in the endothelium, further worsening the oxidative state [32–34]. Moreover, in vivo studies of single nephron function and in vitro studies performed on perfused juxtaglomerular apparatus preparation demonstrated that also the normal renal functions are modulated by ROS/RNS. In particular, $O_2\bullet^-$ and $\bullet$NO, which are generated by NOX type 3 (NOX3) and NOS type 1 (NOS1) enzymes, respectively, modulate afferent arteriolar tone and control Na^+ reabsorption and renal oxygenation by regulating the tubuloglomerular feedback response [35–37]. Furthermore, in the loop of Henle, ROS/RNS increase the absorption of NaCl by modulating the activity of the Na^+/H^+ exchanger [38,39]. In airway and pulmonary artery smooth muscle cells of the lung, NOX2-generated ROS/RNS act as signaling intermediates, which regulate the proliferation and differentiation by the activation of the nuclear factor-κB (NF-κB) and NOS2, and they further show an important role in O_2 sensing [39–41].

Moreover, ROS/RNS formation by mucosal cells of the colon seems to modulate the serotonin production by enterochromaffin cells through a NOXs-dependent system, thus contributing to the regulation of serotonin secretion as well as intestinal motility [42]. ROS/RNS have also a fundamental role in the central nervous system (CNS), in particular in central autonomic neurons. To this regard, ROS/RNS produced by NOX2 in the nucleus of the solitary tract, in the hypothalamic paraventricular nucleus, and in the subfornical organ modulate angiotensin II signaling, thus contributing to the regulation of cardiovascular homeostasis [43,44]. Moreover, in microglia but not in astrocytes, H_2O_2 formation by NOX2 enzyme is involved in the regulation of cell proliferation [45].

Beyond the role as signaling molecules, it has been shown that the aberrant ROS/RNS formation is the leading cause of cell and tissue oxidative stress-induced damage. Indeed, it is well known that excessive levels of ROS/RNS may directly damage lipids containing carbon-carbon double bounds such as cholesterol, glycolipids, phospholipids, and polyunsatured fatty acids (PUFAs), which are abundant within cellular membranes. To this regard, free radical–mediated lipid peroxidation of PUFAs is one of the main mechanisms by which ROS/RNS induce the generation of reactive aldehydes [46]. Due to their abundance of reactive hydrogens, PUFAs are more oxidation-prone lipids compared to monounsatured fatty acids. PUFAs include the ω-3 (e.g., linolenic acid, eicosapentaenoic acid and docosahexaenoic acid) and ω-6 (e.g., linoleic acid and arachidonic acids) fatty acids.

Lipid peroxidation is a chain reaction, which, once started, proceeds through three main steps referred to initiation, propagation and termination [47]. Moreover, lipid peroxidation may occur by several mechanisms: (1) free radical-mediated oxidation [47], (2) enzymatic oxidation, and (3) spontaneous oxidation [48]. In this review, we will focus mainly on the free radical–mediated mechanisms that lead to the formation of reactive aldehydes from PUFAs. In particular, the free radical-mediated oxidation of PUFAs occurs through the following reactions: (1) During the initiation phase, ROS/RNS free radicals attack PUFAs ripping off one hydrogen atom, leading to lipid radicals formation. (2) During the propagation phase, lipid radicals react with oxygen molecules, thus producing peroxyl radicals, which, in turn, react with nearby lipids resulting in the formation of new lipid radicals and lipid hydroperoxides. Due to their high instability, lipid hydroperoxides are further degraded into reactive secondary products, such as ACR, MDA, 4-HNE and other reactive aldehydes [7]. (3) During the termination phase, peroxyl radicals may react with other radicals thus generating less reactive compounds, which block the propagation phase (Figure 1) [49].

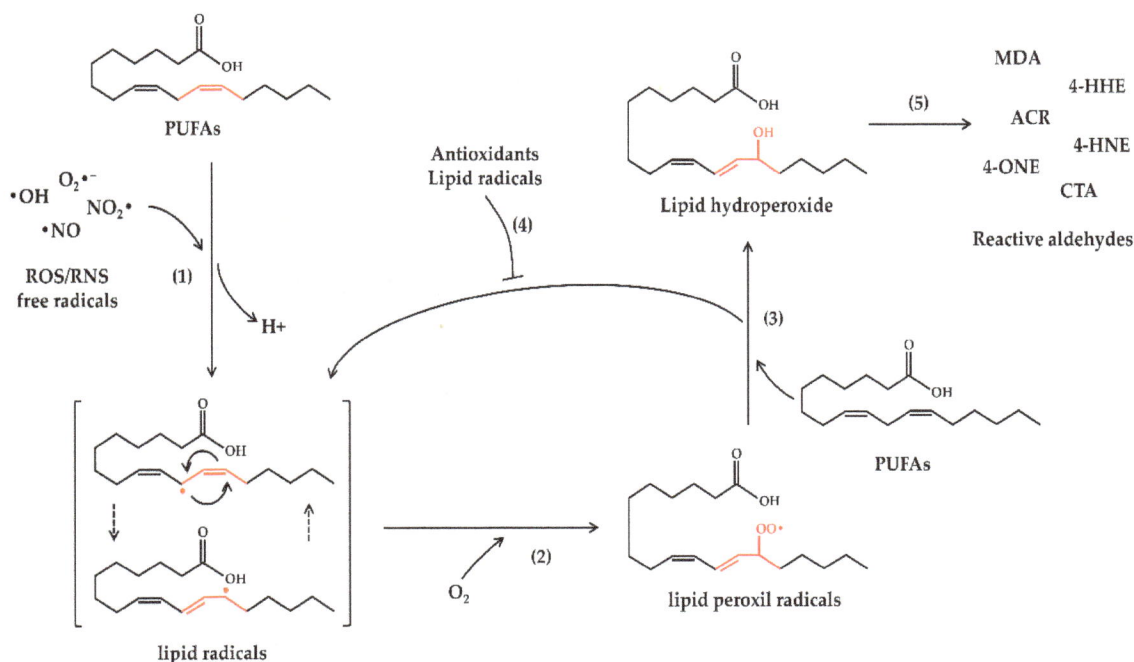

Figure 1. Schematic diagram of the free radicals-mediated peroxidation of polyunsatured fatty acids (PUFAs). ROS/RNS: reactive oxygen and nitrogen species; ACR: acrolein; MDA: malondialdehyde; CTA: crotonaldehyde; 4-HNE: 4-hydroxy-2-nonenal; 4-HHE: 4-hydroxy-hexanal; 4-ONE: 4-oxo-nonenal. During the initiation phase (1), ROS/RNS free radicals react with PUFAs and rip off an allylic hydrogen thus forming lipid radicals. Generally, lipid radicals tend to be stabilized by a molecular rearrangement. (2) In the propagation phase, lipid radicals react with oxygen to form lipid peroxyl radicals, which in turn react with PUFAs or other nearby lipids resulting in the formation of new lipid radicals and lipid hydroperoxides (3). During the termination phase (4), antioxidants or lipid radicals block the propagation phase by donating a hydrogen atom to lipid peroxyl radicals resulting in the formation of non-radical products. Nevertheless, lipid hydroperoxides are highly unstable therefore they are further degraded into reactive secondary products such as ACR, MDA, 4-HNE, and other reactive aldehydes (5).

Today, it is well accepted that oxidative stress and lipid peroxidation are key features in the pathogenesis of several disorders. Indeed, it has been reported that lipid peroxidation products may interfere in vivo with several biological processes, such as substrate-receptor interaction, signal transduction, gene expression, and homeostatic responses to intracellular and environmental stimuli [50–53]. Currently, the main objective of research focused on oxidative stress, lipid peroxidation, and reactive aldehydes is the characterization of the pathogenic mechanisms in several disorders as well as the identification of specific biomarkers for diseases.

Among the reactive aldehydes, the most frequently studied are ACR, MDA, 4-HNE, 4-hydroxy-hexanal (4-HHE), 4-oxo-nonenal (4-ONE), and crotonaldehyde (CTA) (Figure 2).

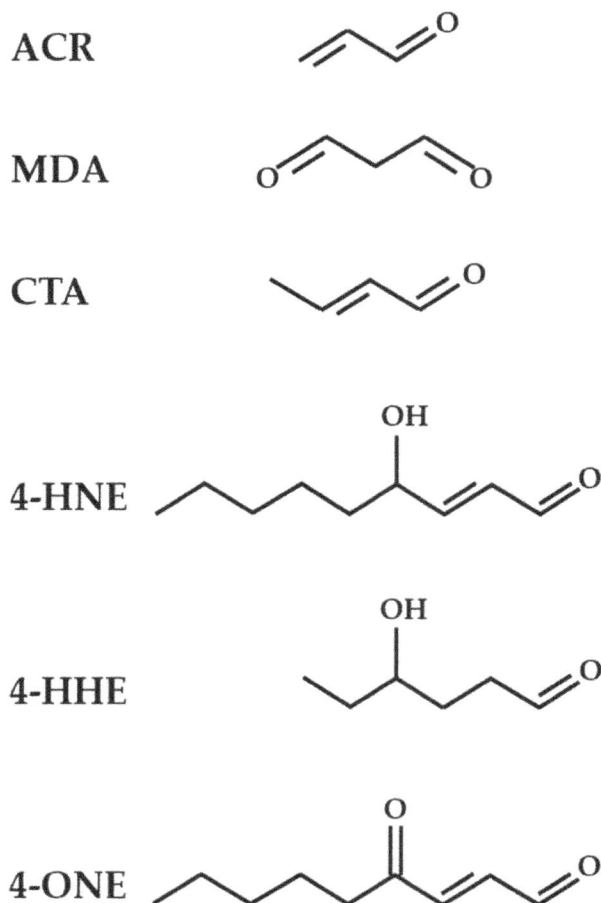

Figure 2. Chemical structures of the main reactive aldehydes produced by lipid peroxidation. ACR: acrolein; MDA: malondialdehyde; CTA: crotonaldehyde; 4-HNE: 4-hydroxy-2-nonenal; 4-HHE: 4-hydroxy-hexanal; 4-ONE: 4-oxo-nonenal.

Some of these compounds are known to contribute to the pathogenesis of several diseases, such as atherosclerosis, rheumatoid arthritis, neuropsychiatric disorders, heart disease, cellular reperfusion injury, cancer, and metabolic disorders such as diabetes and hepatic diseases [4,5,7,12,54]. Reactive aldehydes are a group of electrophilic molecules with different features: some of them are very unstable, characterized by a short half-life, while others are long-lived and highly reactive. In the past years, the endogenous formation of reactive aldehydes has drawn great interest. The ability of aldehydes to easily diffuse across biological membranes [55], and to form adducts with macromolecules such as phospholipids, nucleic acids and proteins [7,46,56–58], is of particular concern. Adducts consist of covalent modifications, which involve the formation of Schiff bases or Michael addition reactions. To this regard, the reactive aldehydes toxicity against peptides and proteins is due to their ability to alter their structure and/or function through the formation of cross-links between different amino acid chains, thus potentially leading to the production of aberrant protein aggregates (Figure 3) [59]. Concerning the toxicity of reactive aldehydes against DNA, it has been shown that these compounds may react against nucleobases, among which the most affected is guanine, due to its chemical structure prone to oxidative modifications. The most studied DNA modifications caused by reactive aldehydes are the exocyclic adducts (Figure 4) [57,58,60].

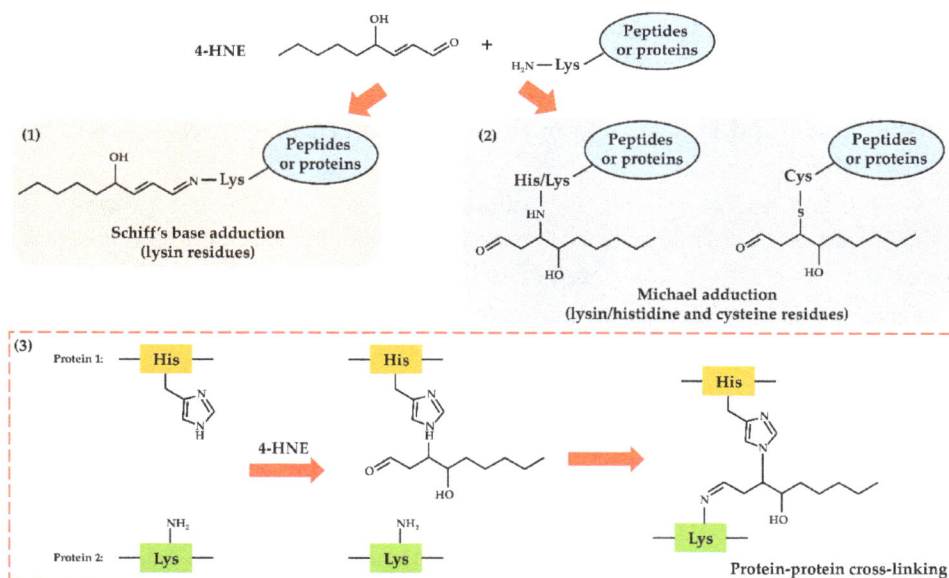

Figure 3. Schematic representation of protein adducts formation and protein-protein cross-linking by 4-HNE. Reactive aldehydes are able to modify peptides/proteins by the formation of toxic adducts which may alter the structure and/or the function of targeted peptides/proteins. These adducts consist of covalent modifications which occur through the formation of Schiff bases or through Michael addition reactions: (1) Schiff base formation on primary amine (lysine residue) through the reaction between peptides/proteins and 4-HNE, (2) Michael addition of 4-HNE on amino groups (lysine/histidine residues) or thiols (cysteine residue) through the reaction between peptides/proteins and 4-HNE, and (3) Protein-protein cross-linking through the reaction between 4-HNE with histidine and lysine residues from different peptides/proteins.

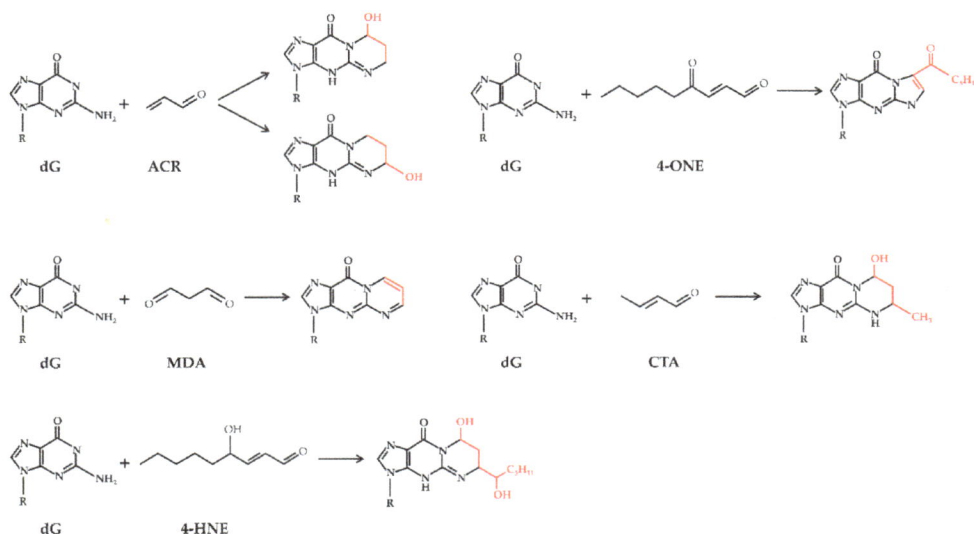

Figure 4. Hypothetical DNA adducts produced by reactive aldehydes. By reacting with DNA, in particular with the deoxyguanosine nucleobases, several reactive aldehydes such as ACR, MDA, 4-HNE, 4-ONE and CTA produce DNA modifications named exocyclic adducts that alter the DNA structure and, if not correctly repaired, may produce carcinogenic effects.

4-HNE and 4-ONE are generated from lipid peroxidation of ω-6 PUFAs (e.g., arachidonic acid and linoleic acid) [61]. Among reactive aldehydes, 4-HNE is the most studied, and its toxic effects can be explained by its ability to form protein adducts by reacting with thiols and amino groups of cysteine, histidine, and lysine amino acid residues [62]. For a detailed explanation of the main 4-HNE-modified proteins, see the following publication [63]. 4-ONE is an electrophilic compound that reacts both in vitro and in vivo with nucleobases, in particular with 2'-deoxyadenosine and 2'-deoxycytidine [64–67].

Unlike 4-HNE and 4-ONE, 4-HHE is generated from ω-3 PUFAs (e.g., docoshexaenoic acid, eicosapentaenoic acid and linolenic acid) and, because of its chemical structure, it is considered a soft electrophil with a lower reactivity compared to 4-HNE [7].

MDA, which is widely used as a marker of lipid peroxidation [68], contains at least two unsaturations [7] and is generally produced by PUFAs. Regarding its toxicity, MDA modifies target proteins through the formation of Schiff base complexes, which occur on the amino groups of lysine, histidine, arginine, glutamine, and asparagine amino acid residues as well as on the N-terminal of peptide chains [69]. For a detailed explanation of the main MDA-modified proteins, see the following publication [63]. Moreover, in vitro mutagenicity of MDA has been observed by several authors using the Salmonella tiphimurium assay [70–72]. Several studies showed the presence of both MDA and MDA-protein adducts in rheumatoid arthritis patients compared to healthy controls [73–76]. Moreover, high levels of circulating autoantibodies against MDA-modified epitopes have been detected in serum or plasma of patients affected by rheumatoid arthritis [77–79]. CTA or 2-butenal is a carcinogenic aldehyde formed by lipid peroxidation, which is also commonly found in air pollution, in cigarette smoke and in other combustion processes. CTA is able to form adducts with DNA [80–83] and proteins. In accordance with in vitro mutagenesis assay with Salmonella typhimorium, CTA is a mutagenic compound [84] able to induce hepatocellular carcinoma in rats [85]. About protein modifications, CTA reacts preferentially with lysine and histidine amino acid residues, thus forming β-substituted butanal adducts [86].

ACR or propenal is a metabolite of PUFAs lipid peroxidation, but it is also a ubiquitous environmental pollutant by-product derived by incomplete combustion of organic matter and plastic, cigarette smoke, overheated cooking oils, as well as by anticancer treatment with cyclophosphamide [87,88]. Among reactive aldehydes, ACR is the strongest electrophile, which shows a high reactivity with cysteine, histidine, and lysine amino acid residues. Moreover, ACR forms cyclic adducts with nucleosides in vitro, and is recognized as a potent mutagen [89].

Despite their harmful properties, growing evidence has also demonstrated the hormetic effects of reactive aldehydes [51,63,90–93]. The term "hormesis" refers to a highly conserved and dose-dependent response of biological systems in which low doses of noxious stimuli activate an adaptive response that increases the functionality and/or resistance of the systems to more severe stress. Conversely, high doses of noxious stimuli cause inhibition or detrimental effects [94]. To this regard, low levels of reactive aldehydes may modulate cell signaling, cellular proliferation and many other processes [7,61,89,95]. A typical example is represented by 4-HNE, which may also act as a signaling molecule by modulating the activity of different stress-related transcription factors, such as nuclear factor-erythroid 2-related factor 2 (Nrf2), activating protein-1, NF-κB, and peroxisome proliferator-activated receptors (PPARs) [96–100]. Moreover, low levels of 4-HNE may stimulate the activity of protein kinase C (PKC), may increase cell proliferation, and the expression of cyclooxygenase type 2 (COX-2) and prostaglandin E2 (PGE2) [51].

3. The Endocannabinoid System: Endocannabinoids, Their Lipid Analogues, and the Receptors

Over the last years, the ECS has attracted considerable attention as a signaling system because of its emerging regulatory functions in health and disease.

Several components jointly make up the ECS, and they specifically consist of (1) the ECs, endogenous bioactive lipid mediators generated in the brain and in several peripheral tissues; (2) two membrane G-protein-coupled receptors (GPCRs) referred to as CB1 and CB2, and others, not yet identified, receptors; and (3) several proteins implicated in the biosynthesis, release, transport, and degradation of these lipid mediators [101].

N-arachidonoyl-ethanolamine or anandamide (AEA) and 2-arachidonoyl-glycerol (2-AG), both derived from the arachidonic acid, are the best characterized members of the main families of ECs (N-acylethanolamines (NAEs) and monoacylglycerols (MAG), respectively) and exert their biological effects by interacting with CB1 and/or CB2 receptors [102]. AEA, an endogenous eicosanoid derivative isolated from pig brain in 1992, was the first EC to be identified [103], and it is well known to modulate several physiological functions being present in the autonomic and in the CNS as well as in the gastrointestinal tract and in the cardiovascular, immune and reproductive systems [104,105].

The second EC ligand to be discovered was 2-AG [106], which has been identified in brain and reproductive tissues in higher concentrations compared to AEA [107–109]. Moreover, 2-AG has also been found in the heart, endothelial cells and circulating cells such as macrophages and platelets [104].

Even though AEA and 2-AG interact with both CB1 and CB2 [110], they show different affinity and efficacy. In particular, depending of on the specific tissue, AEA can be either a partial or a full agonist of CB1, whereas it shows a low overall efficacy for CB2, for which it is a relatively weak ligand [111]. On the contrary, 2-AG appears to be a full agonist of both receptors [112] showing higher CB1 and CB2 efficacy than AEA.

Unlike what has been thought for many years, CB1 expression is not restricted to the brain, where it represents the most abundant of all GPCRs [113,114], but it has been also identified, albeit at much lower concentrations, in various peripheral tissues and cell types including adipose tissue, liver, skeletal muscle, kidney, bone, pancreas, myocardium, human coronary artery endothelial and smooth muscle cells and inflammatory cells (macrophages, lymphocytes) [104,115,116].

In the brain, CB1 is widely present in cerebral cortex, hippocampus, caudate-putamen, substantia nigra pars reticulata, globus pallidus, entopeduncular nucleus, and cerebellum [117]. Interestingly, accumulating evidence supports a new mechanism of action of CB1 signalling in the brain, since it has been found in mitochondria, where it probably modulates neuronal energy homeostasis [118]. On the other hand, the CB2, also known as the "immune cannabinoid receptor", is primarily expressed in immune and hematopoietic cells. However, its presence has also been established at lower, although functionally relevant, levels in the brain, liver, gut, exocrine and endocrine pancreas, reproductive cells, bone, myocardium, human coronary endothelial and smooth muscle cells, and inflammatory cells (e.g., lymphocytes, macrophages, neutrophils) [104,115,119].

CB1 and CB2 are seven-transmembrane-domain proteins both coupled with $G_{\alpha i/o}$ proteins, which inhibit adenylyl cyclase (AC) leading to a reduced protein kinase A (PKA) and PKC activity and to the consequent inhibition of voltage-gated Ca^{2+} channels and activation of inwardly rectifying K^+ currents [120]. Furthermore, through a common pathway mediated by $G_{\alpha o}$ proteins, CB1 and CB2 are also able to modulate Ras-related protein (Rap) (a member of the Ras small G protein family) and, in particular, it has been postulated that the activation of $G_{\alpha o}$ would release Rap1 guanosine triphosphatase (GTPase) activating protein (Rap1 GAP), which then would be free to inhibit the activity of Rap [121]. Moreover, several observations demonstrated that, depending on the CB1 agonist, this receptor could also interact with $G_{\alpha s}$ proteins [122,123].

On the basis of the cell type, the signaling of CB1 and CB2 may also involve G protein independent mechanisms, leading to the activation of mitogen-activated protein kinases (MAPKs) including p38- and p44/42-MAPKs, c-Jun N-terminal kinase (JNK), PKA and PKC, COX-2, and ceramide signaling [124–126].

However, beyond binding the CB1 and CB2 there is increasing pharmacological evidence for additional receptor targets for ECs [127], such as the transient receptor potential vanilloid 1 (TRPV1) [127–129], the PPARs family [130,131] and the orphan G protein-coupled receptors 119 (GPR119), 55 (GPR55) and 18 (GPR18) [132]. TRPV1 is a member of the vanilloid transient receptor potential cation channel subfamily, abundantly expressed in the cardiovascular system, peripheral nervous system, CNS and in epithelial cells of the bladder and the gastrointestinal tract. It is known to act by activating PKA and the endothelial nitric oxide synthase (eNOS), thus stimulating the production of •NO and the release of calcitonin gene-related peptide and substance P [133,134], which, in turn, lead to the altered ion permeability [135].

The finding that some pharmacological actions of AEA can be mediated by the activation of TRPV1 suggests the capability of this endogenous lipid compound to act as an "endovanilloid" [136,137], although AEA induces typical TRPV1-mediated effects with a lower affinity compared to CB1 [127].

PPARs are a family of transcription factors constituted by three different isoforms (α, β/δ, and γ), widely expressed in tissues with a higher oxidative capacity such as the cardiovascular system and, in particular, cardiomyocytes, endothelial cells, and vascular smooth muscle cells [104], but also in several brain areas and in peripheral tissues such as kidney and liver [138].

After being activated by a ligand, PPARs stimulate gene expression by creating heterodimers with the retinoid X receptor (RXR), thereby binding to specific peroxisome proliferator response elements (PPREs) in the promotor region of target genes [139]. They are involved in different biological processes, such as energy homeostasis, lipid and lipoprotein metabolism, cell proliferation and inflammation, blood pressure control and hypertensive-related complications, such as stroke and renal damage [140,141]. Furthermore, among the different members of the PPARs family, PPAR-α is recently attracting great attention for its anti-oxidative properties [142].

Moreover, AEA has been shown to exert anti-inflammatory and analgesic actions, and to control feeding behavior by activating the isoform α and γ of PPARs receptors [130,143,144]. Unlike AEA, 2-AG has no affinity for TRPV1 and is only able to activate PPARs [144,145].

As above mentioned, additional GPCRs were suggested to participate in non-CB1/CB2-mediated actions of ECs including the GPR18, GPR119 and GPR55 [146].

The GPR18, widely expressed in the cardiovascular system, CNS, spleen, and testis, is coupled with $G_{\alpha i/o}$ proteins whose activation results in the AC inhibition and in the modulation of the PI3K/Akt and extracellular signal-related kinases (ERK 1/2) pathways [104]. The $G_{\alpha s}$ coupled-GPR119, primarily expressed in human and rodent pancreas, foetal liver, gastrointestinal tract and in rodent brain, stimulates AC leading to increased intracellular adenosine 3',5'-cyclic monophosphate (cAMP) levels, thus regulating incretin and insulin hormone secretion [147].

Finally, the GPR55, which is expressed in human brain and liver, but also in rat spleen, vasculature, intestine, foetal tissues, decidua, and placenta, is coupled with $G_{\alpha 12/13}$ proteins and increases intracellular Ca^{2+} via the activation of RhoGTPase nucleotide exchange factors (RhoGEFs) [148].

Different from the classical neurotransmitters, the ECs are not stored in intracellular vesicles but are synthesized "on demand" from membrane phospholipid precursors in response to stimuli that trigger an increase in intracellular Ca^{2+} levels [131], and then released from postsynaptic neurons to act on presynaptic CB1/CB2 through a retrograde mechanism [149,150]. However, recent findings suggested that AEA could be stored inside the cell into adiposomes, which are thought to connect plasma membrane to internal organelles along the metabolic route of this EC [151].

Although 2-AG and AEA are both derived from arachidonic acid, they do not share the same anabolic and catabolic enzymes [126]. Depending on the available precursors and the distinct physiological or pathological conditions [131], AEA can be synthesized by multiple routes. The main pathway for AEA biosynthesis consists of the enzymatic cleavage of the precursor N-acyl-phosphatidylethanolamine (NAPE), which is mediated by the NAPE-phospholipase D (NAPE-PLD) [152], whereas the biosynthesis of 2-AG begins with the hydrolysis of 2-arachidonoyl-phosphatidylinositol that occurs through the activity of diacylglycerol lipase (DAGL) and phospholipase Cβ [153].

ECs have a short duration of action, being rapidly metabolized by intracellular enzymes such as fatty acid amide hydrolase (FAAH), the main enzyme responsible for AEA degradation [154–156], and monoacylglycerol lipase (MAGL), which favors 2-AG catabolism [157].

Additional oxidative enzymes, including COX-2, LOXs and cytochrome P450 may also play a role in the metabolism of both AEA and 2-AG by transforming them in bioactive eicosanoids [158,159], which may activate cannabinoid receptor-independent mechanisms [160].

Beyond the ECs, several other endogenous mediators have attracted considerable attention, despite some of them showed poor affinity for CB1 and CB2 [126]. Among them, palmitoylethanolamide (PEA), stearoylethanolamide (SEA), and oleoylethanolamide (OEA), belonging to the family of NAEs, are the best characterized. However, other lipid analogues have recently been discovered and include N-arachidonoyldopamine (NADA), Cis-9,10-octadecanoamide (oleamide or ODA), and N-arachidonoylglycine (NAGly) [161], commonly referred to as endovanilloids because of their ability to activate TRPV1. Additionally, 2-arachidonoylglyceryl ether (noladin ether, 2-AGE), O-rachidonoylethanolamine (virodhamine), and arachidonoyl-L-serine (ARA-S) have also been identified [105].

Although still debated, NAEs are generally thought to be cannabinoid-receptor inactive, and they appeared to be responsible for enhancing AEA activity through the so-called "entourage effect", which consists in the inhibition of FAAH leading to an increase of AEA tissue levels [162].

PEA and OEA, shorter and fully saturated analogues of AEA, are well-documented high affinity PPAR-α and TRPV1 endogenous ligands and have been shown to exert roles in many physiological and pathological conditions such as satiety, inflammation, pain and memory consolidation [163–168]. Furthermore, due to their high expression in the CNS, growing evidence established their protective effects in neurodegenerative and neuropsychiatric disorders [169–172]. Moreover, PEA is also an endogenous agonist of GPR55, while OEA can bind GPR119.

As already mentioned, NADA belongs to the endovanilloid class of ECs and is an endogenous ligand of CB1, TRPV1 and PPAR-γ [105]. Since this compound is widely distributed in the brain, particularly in the striatum, hippocampus, cerebellum, and dorsal root ganglia, it has been shown to exert a role in neuronal pain and inflammation [105]. Interestingly, NADA also showed antioxidative and anti-inflammatory effects on glial cells [105].

2-AGE is an endogenous analogue of 2-AG, able to bind to CB1, PPAR-α and very weakly to CB2 [143,173]. Moreover, thanks to its chemical structure, 2-AGE is more stable compared to AEA and 2-AG, which are rapidly hydrolysed in vivo [102].

Virodhamine is the ester of arachidonic acid and ethanolamine and is more expressed in the periphery compared to the brain, where it is rapidly converted to AEA, due to its chemical instability. Virodhamine has been shown to act as a full agonist of CB2 and a partial agonist of CB1, whereas at higher concentrations it can be also a CB1 antagonist [174]. Furthermore, it appeared to activate also PPAR-α [143] and GPR55 [175].

NAGly is an efficacious ligand of the orphan GPR18, with no CB1, CB2, or TRPV1 activity, and shows analgesic, anti-inflammatory, and vasorelaxant properties [176].

AraS is another ECs-like compound structurally similar to AEA, which was demonstrated to produce endothelium-dependent arterial vasodilatation and to activate p44/42 MAPKs in cultured endothelial cells, effects also observed after ECs treatment [105]. To date, AraS has been shown to be a low efficacy agonist to GPR18 without binding CB1/CB2 or additional ECs receptors [105].

Lastly, ODA is a full agonist of cannabinoid receptors with selectivity for the CB1, whose activation is the primary responsible for ODA effects [105].

As suggested by the wide range and distribution of the cannabinoid receptors and by the several compounds that take part in the ECS, the latter is now considered as a complex signaling system that may play a key role in physiological and pathological conditions. Thus, targeting these intricate pathways can represent a challenge in finding a therapeutic benefit for cannabinoid-based drugs in various disorders.

4. Modulation of Oxidative Stress and Lipid Peroxidation through Cannabinoid Receptors by Endocannabinoids and Their Lipid Analogues

It is well documented that there is an important cross-talk between the ECS and various redox-dependent processes. Indeed, the ECS has been reported as a novel therapeutic target against free radical-induced lipid peroxidation. In fact, it has been shown that ECS is implicated in the development of a growing number of diseases linked with redox homeostasis deregulation, including those associated with metabolic disorders, such as type 2 diabetes and obesity, cardiovascular diseases, as well as various neuropsychiatric and neurodegenerative disorders, ischemia/reperfusion (I/R) injury, and renal diseases [2,4,5,54,177].

In the past decade, various and complex pathways have been studied to clarify the role of ECs in the modulation of redox imbalance, whose knowledge is the specific aim of this review.

There is accumulating evidence that shows the ability of ECs to alter the expression and/or the activity of enzymes implicated in the generation of these reactive small molecules (such as NOX2 and NOX4), and to modulate the production of cellular ROS/RNS by controlling mitochondrial-derived ROS/RNS generation [177].

Alternatively, ECs and their lipid analogues may modulate oxidative stress and lipid peroxidation either by conveying beneficial free radical scavenging effects or through targeting CB1 and CB2 [8–10]. Furthermore, CB1 and CB2 are differentially involved in oxidative stress modulation. In fact, several studies highlight that the activation of CB1 results in a redox imbalance enhancement, whereas CB2 stimulation is responsible for lowering ROS/RNS formation [9]. The beneficial or detrimental effects of ECs may be cell- and injury-type-specific and may depend on the stage of the disease progression as well [8].

This aspect was further investigated by Han and colleagues, who demonstrated a different role of CB1 and CB2 in regulating macrophage activity, and, in particular, the former appeared to be directly involved in the induction of intracellular ROS/RNS formation with consequent pro-inflammatory macrophage response, while the latter, after being activated by AEA, was able to negatively regulate CB1-stimulated ROS/RNS generation, through a pathway involving the small G protein, Rap1 [9]. The authors further showed that blocking CB1 while selectively activating CB2 might suppress pro-inflammatory responses of macrophages.

These data are consistent with other studies using cisplatin-induced renal dysfunction [178–181], in which it was observed that blocking the CB1 [179], or activating the CB2 [180,181], led to the attenuation of the cisplatin-induced increase of renal 4-HNE and ROS/RNS-generating enzymes (NOX2 and NOX4) expression, thus protecting against tubular damage.

Other examples of the opposite effects of CB1 and CB2 come from studies conducted in animal models of obesity and type 1 and 2 diabetes mellitus, where an increase of oxidative stress is observed [182–184]. In fact, in these models, increased levels of ECs in various renal cells contribute to the development of oxidative stress, as a result of renal CB1 activation, whereas inhibition of CB1 or activation of CB2 are able to ameliorate such effects (Figure 5) [185].

Overall, the over activation of the ECS that occurs in many type of tissue injury may induce oxidative stress, inflammatory cell infiltration, and the consequent cell death through CB1 activation [8,179], while it may also serve as an endogenous compensatory mechanism to limit early inflammatory response and interrelated oxidative stress-cell death through the activation of CB2 [186].

Interestingly, a cross-talk between redox homeostasis and ECS is particularly involved in the regulation of the cardiovascular system and metabolic tissues (i.e., liver, skeletal muscle and adipose tissue) [187,188], where CB1 and CB2 are widely distributed. Furthermore, previous studies have suggested increased ECs levels in many cardiovascular disorders, such as cardiomyopathies, atherosclerosis, and hypertension [189].

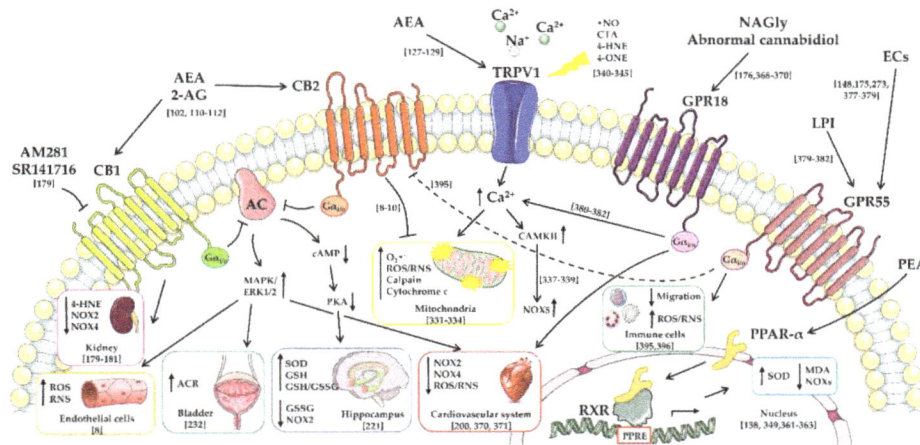

Figure 5. Role of endocannabinoids (ECs) and their lipid analogues in modulating reactive oxygen and nitrogen species (ROS/RNS) and reactive aldehydes formation. AM281: 1-(2,4-dichlorophenyl)-5-(4-iodophenyl)-4-methyl-N-4-morpholinyl-1H-pyrazole-3-carboxamide; SR141716: rimonabant; CB: can nabinoid receptors; AEA: anandamide; 2-AG: 2-arachidonoyl-glycerol; TRPV: transient receptor potential vanilloid; CTA: crotonaldehyde; NAGly: N-arachidonoylglycine; GPR18: G protein-coupled receptor 18; GPR55: G protein-coupled receptor 55; LPI: L-α-lysophosphatidylinositol; ECs: endocannabinoids; PEA: palmitoylethanolamide; PPARs: peroxisome proliferator-activated receptors; SOD: Cu^{2+}/Zn^{2+}-superoxide dismutase; MDA: malondialdehyde; PPRE: peroxisome proliferator response element; RXR: retinoid X receptor; NOX: NADPH oxidase enzyme; GSH: glutathione; GSSG: oxidized glutathione; ACR: acrolein; MAPK/ERK1/2: mitogen-activated protein kinases/extracellular signal-regulated kinases; PKA: protein kinase A; cAMP: adenosine 3′,5′-cyclic monophosphate; CAMKII: Ca^{2+}/calmodulin-dependent protein kinase; AC: adenylyl cyclase.

It is well known that cardiovascular diseases are associated with oxidative stress, which leads to the accumulation of lipid peroxidation-derived reactive aldehydes and may consequently cause an increase in the formation of ROS/RNS and/or a decrease in the antioxidant defense [2].

In this regard, it has been demonstrated that, after being activated by AEA, CB1 expressed in endothelial cells [190] and in cardiomyocytes in a murine model of doxorubicin-induced cardiomyopathy [8], induce the activation of the p38-JNK-MAPK pathway and increase the generation of ROS/RNS. These effects lead to cell death and resulted to be partially attenuated by the pharmacological inhibition of CB1 [9].

In contrast to CB1, the activation of CB2 appeared to exert cardioprotective effects by reducing $O_2\bullet^-$ production and decreasing endothelial cell activation. These findings are in agreement with recent studies showing that CB2 activation, by ECs and their analogue lipid mediators, protects against oxidative stress-induced tissue damage in experimental models of I/R injury [191–195], cardiovascular inflammation, and/or atherosclerosis [191,196,197].

Among the cardiovascular diseases, atherosclerosis is due to altered homeostatic redox processes with progressive ROS/RNS over production, which leads to the generation and deposition of toxic oxidized low-density lipoproteins (oxLDL) in the vessel wall. It has been clearly demonstrated that OxLDL promote the activation of NOXs and the synthesis of $O_2\bullet^-$ by a cluster of differentiation 36 (CD36) scavenger receptor-mediated method, effects that can be counteracted by several compensatory mechanisms including the involvement of the ECS [198].

Support for this comes from the observation that increased production of $O_2\bullet^-$ and enhanced NOXs activation in atherosclerosis correlated with increased rates of 2-AG biosynthesis in the vessel wall, which may be a compensatory response to oxidative stress via CB2 signaling [199].

In agreement with these results, it has been observed that the genetic disruption of CB2 in Apolipoprotein E-deficient mice (ApoE$^{-/-}$), a murine model of atherosclerosis, is the cause of boosted $O_2\bullet^-$ generation, whereas its stimulation reduced vascular $O_2\bullet^-$ release, resulting in the suppression of ROS/RNS generation and a subsequent reduction in the size of atherosclerotic lesions (Figure 5) [200].

Further evidence of the protective effects of ECs in atherosclerosis comes from the demonstration that CB1 inhibition in ApoE$^{-/-}$ mice is able to promote the down-regulation of vascular angiotensin II type 1 receptor (AT1), which is responsible for NOXs activation when stimulated by angiotensin II [201]. Consequently, the decreased expression of AT1, mediated by CB1 inhibition, leads to the reduction of NOXs activity and oxidative stress, thereby improving endothelial function and exerting beneficial direct vascular effects [201].

Since the discovery that the levels of NAEs are higher in several pathological conditions linked with redox homeostasis impairment, these compounds are attracting great attention as a survival response toward oxidative damage [202].

Indeed, it has been clearly shown that NAEs, particularly 16:0 and 18:0, exert protective effects in many diseases by the inhibition of free radical-induced lipid peroxidation [203], which is considered one of the main causes of cell damage and death [204].

In particular, previous findings discovered an involvement of two long-chain NAEs, PEA and SEA, in the inhibition of lipid peroxidation in liver mitochondria membranes of acute hypoxic hypoxia animal model [203], a pathological condition associated with an increase in partially reduced oxygen products, which represent the main cause of lipid oxidation-induced formation of reactive aldehydes [205]. The authors suggested that the inhibitory effect of NAEs on lipid peroxidation depends on the length of acyl chain and is related to their ability to protect membranes [206].

These results are in good agreement with other data showing that OEA treatment of rat heart mitochondria is able to reduce the production of MDA, which is one of the end products of lipid peroxidation in cell membrane [203].

Among NAEs, OEA, PEA, and AEA appeared to inhibit Cu^{2+}-induced in vitro lipid peroxidation in plasma lipoproteins [202] and cardiac mitochondria [207], consequently showing antioxidant properties in the pathogenesis of atherosclerosis. Moreover, Zolese and collaborators demonstrated that, depending on its concentration of incubation, PEA exerts both anti-oxidative and pro-oxidative effects on radical-induced oxidation of plasma LDL [208]. The authors showed that higher PEA concentrations could be responsible for its pro-oxidant effect, whereas PEA at lower levels is able to suppress reactive aldehydes, generated by lipid peroxidation, and to decrease the consumption rate of LDL endogenous anti-oxidants, thereby showing anti-oxidant properties [208].

In the context of cardiovascular diseases is also interesting to mention hypertension, which is characterized by (1) deregulation of ECS with increased activity of FAAH and MAGL, (2) increased levels of AEA, 2-AG, and NADA, and (3) increased expression of CB1 [209], effects that are accompanied by an imbalance of redox homeostasis (decreased activities of glutathione peroxidase (GPx), glutathione reductase (GR) and the antioxidant enzymes Cu^{2+}/Zn^{2+}-superoxide dismutase (SOD) and catalase (CAT)).

It has been demonstrated that increased levels of AEA, following chronic administration of the FAAH inhibitor URB597 in a rat model of hypertension [210], significantly enhanced the expression of the CB1, thus preventing the hypertension-induced decrease of SOD, glutathione (GSH) and glutathione transferase (GT) activities and consequently lowering ROS generation and inducing hypotension. However, it has been postulated that the enhanced AEA levels are responsible for the perturbation of membrane phospholipid metabolism resulting in PUFAs chain cyclization or fragmentation. This causes an increase in the formation of α,β-unsaturated reactive aldehydes such as 4-HNE, MDA, and 4-ONE in the liver of hypertensive rats [209].

It is well documented that ECS and oxidative stress may also play a role in the pathophysiology of liver diseases [188,211]. For instance, DeLeve and collaborators [212] reported that CB1 activation is responsible for liver inflammation and, therefore, induces non-alcoholic liver disease, whereas the CB2 stimulation appeared to have protective effects in liver damage through reducing liver oxidative stress [213].

Accumulating evidence supports the involvement of ECS as a therapeutic potential in many neurodegenerative pathologies such as Alzheimer's and Parkinson's diseases, in which oxidative stress has been recognized as one of the hallmarks of the pathology [4,171,172,214–217].

Indeed, the brain is a tissue with a high oxygen consumption whose cell membranes are particularly rich in PUFA side-chains and, therefore, highly sensitive to lipid peroxidation and oxidative damage [54,183,218].

NOXs enzymes have been shown to be significant sources of ROS/RNS during tissue injury and, in particular, it has been observed that the activation of NOX2 contributes to oxidative imbalance–induced CNS damage [219], while its inhibition is able to ameliorate cerebral oxidative stress injury [220].

A recent study conducted by Jia and collaborators defined AEA as a promising candidate for the treatment of oxidative stress–related neurological disorders [221]. In particular, AEA has been found to protect a mouse hippocampal neuron cell line from H_2O_2-induced redox imbalance by increasing SOD and GSH intracellular levels, reducing oxidized glutathione (GSSG), increasing the GSH/GSSG ratio, and lowering NOX2 expression. All of these effects were completely abolished by both CB1 antagonist administration and CB1-siRNA, suggesting that the ability of AEA to ameliorate oxidative stress in hippocampal neurons may be mediated by CB1 activation (Figure 5) [221].

Similarly, it has been also reported that the stimulation of CB1 is able to reduce intracellular ROS/RNS generation and NOX2 expression thus enhancing nigrostriatal dopaminergic neurons survival in a mouse model of Parkinson's disease [222].

These findings supporting the beneficial effects of CB1 activation against ROS/RNS formation in the brain seem to be controversial in comparison to what above mentioned for the cardiovascular and renal tissues. An explanation for this argument comes from growing evidence suggesting that the pathways underlying the interplay between cannabinoid receptors and oxidative stress modulation may be cell type–specific [177].

Notably, as well as responses mediated by CB1, further data showed that the modulation of CB2 signaling, either by using specific CB2 agonists [223–225] or by inhibiting 2-AG degrading enzyme MAGL [226], can ameliorate the morphological changes induced by oxidative stress and attenuate cerebral β-amyloid plaque accumulation in a mouse model of Alzheimer's disease carrying mutated human APPswe and PS1dE9 genes [227,228].

Interestingly, in vitro studies revealed that a selective CB1 agonist, arachidonyl-2-chloroethylamide, decreased the Fe^{2+}-induced lipid peroxidation in the brain, through a metal-chelating mechanism, as well as the •OH radicals generated by the Fenton system [229].

Moreover, the activation of the recently discovered mitochondrial CB1 by arachidonyl-2-chloroethylamide has been demonstrated to reduce oxidative stress, thereby exerting neuroprotective effects in I/R injury [227]. To this regard, CB2 activation also appeared to have a role in attenuating I/R damage through lowering ROS/RNS production and lipid peroxidation [227].

The involvement of CB2 in I/R injury has also been investigated in a context of propofol cardioprotection in an in vivo model of myocardial I/R injury, in which it has been observed that CB2 inactivation reverses propofol cardioprotective and anti-oxidative effects [230]. These findings imply that the enhancement of ECs release and the subsequent activation of CB2 signaling are responsible for the reduced oxidative stress mediated by propofol cardioprotection in myocardial I/R injury [230].

Furthermore, CB2 are expressed in the bladder [231] and are involved in the treatment of hemorrhagic cystitis, a common side effect of Cyclophosphamide, an antineoplastic alkylating agent usually metabolized by the liver to ACR, which is accumulated in urine and therefore is considered to be the main responsible for Cyclophosphamide-induced cystitis [232]. The findings of this study revealed that, following stimulation, CB2 attenuated ACR-induced cystitis through modulating ERK1/2 MAPK pathways (Figure 5) [232].

AEA and 2-AG are also involved in the progression of cancer, where they were shown to exert protective effects against increased ROS/RNS production–induced tumor [233], leading to apoptosis in normal and cancer cells by modulating ERK and ROS/RNS pathways [234].

5. Modulation of Oxidative Stress and Lipid Peroxidation through the Transient Receptor Potential Vanilloid Channels by Endocannabinoids and Their Lipid Analogues

The transient receptor potential (TRP) channels superfamily is a wide group of tetrameric channels formed by six transmembrane domains and a cation-selective pore. On the basis of its amino acid sequence homology, TRP superfamily, in mammals, is organized into six subfamilies, which include TRP canonical, TRP melastatin, TRP ankyrin, TRP mucolipin, TRP vanilloid, and TRP polycistin channels. TRP channels are ubiquitously expressed in most mammalian cells [235,236] and they depolarize cells by altering membrane potential or intracellular Ca^{2+} concentration. With the exception of some TRP channels, most of them are non-selective and weakly voltage-sensitive [237]. TRP channels are fundamental players of sensory physiology as they respond to environmental stimuli such as taste, light, sound, smell, touch, temperature, and osmolarity [238]. Today, only a few endogenous ligands are known to activate TRP channels, and it is not yet clear how they are activated in vivo [237]. However, several experiments performed on knockout mice are revealing the complexity and the different functions of TRP channels [238–240].

In this review, we will focus mainly on the vanilloid TRP (TRPV) channels subfamily and how they respond to oxidative stress and lipid peroxidation-induced cell damage. Currently, six TRPV channels (TRPV1-6) have been identified and divided into two subgroups: TRPV1-4 and TRPV5-6, based on their amino acid sequence, functions, and cation selectivity. A detailed review on TRPV channels pharmacology has been provided by Vriens and colleagues [241]. Briefly, TRPV1 is expressed in primary sensory neurons, in few brain regions (hypothalamus, intrafascicular, supramammillary and rostral raphe nuclei, entorhinal cortex, hippocampus, and periaqueductal gray), as well as in smooth muscle cells of several thermoregulatory tissues (skin, dura, tongue, trachea, cremaster muscle, and ear) [242]. TRPV1 seem to be activated by heat above 43 °C, by low pH [243–245], by vanilloid compounds (e.g., capsaicin and capsinate) [243,246], by ethanol [247,248], as well as by several endogenous compounds such as AEA [127], OEA [249], NADA [250], N-oleoyldopamine (OLDA) [251], and arachidonic acid-derived metabolites released by LOXs [252]. Moreover, TRPV1 activity is modulated by various intracellular molecules and signals including calmodulin [253,254], ATP [255], phosphatidylinositol 4,5-bisphosphate (PIP2) and phosphatidylinositol 3,4,5-trisphosphate (PIP3) [256], PKC [257], PKA [258], as well as protein phosphatase calcineurin [259].

Among the main functions, in addition to acting as a thermoreceptor, TRPV1 regulates the normal functioning of urinary bladder [260], controls the gut afferent sensitivity to distension and acids [261] and it also allows the taste perception of sodium chloride [262]. From a physiopathological point of view, TRPV1 has a direct role in the behavioral response to ethanol [247,248,263], as well as in inflammatory airway diseases [264]. Moreover, TRPV1 is also involved in vascular dementia as well as in Huntington's disease, where its activation promotes neuroprotection, increase learning and memory, and reduce oxidative stress [265–267].

Differently, TRPV2 is a weakly Ca^{2+}-selective channel, which seems to be activated by thermal stimuli above 53 °C but not by low pH or vanilloid compounds [268]. TRPV2 is expressed in different tissues including brain, spinal cord, spleen, and intestine, as well as in vas deferens, bladder, heart, kidney [269], and immune cells such as monocytes and dendritic cells [270]. It is noteworthy that TRPV2 signaling plays an important role in the endosomal pathway, where TRPV2 modulates the fusion between endosomal membranes by releasing Ca^{2+} from early endosomes [271,272] as well as in phagocytosis [273,274].

TRPV3 is a non-selective cation channel activated by temperatures of 33–39 °C, which showed a marked sensitization following repeated heat stimuli [275,276]. Moreover, TRPV3 could be activated by several vegetable-derived molecules, such as eugenol, thymol, camphor and carvacrol [277,278]. Furthermore, other agents such as PIP2/PIP3, calmodulin, ATP, and inflammatory mediators like histamine, bradykinin, and PGE2 are able to sensitize TRPV3 function [278–281]. Moreover, it was hypothesized that, in rodent skin cells, heat-induced TRPV3 signaling could mediate an autonomous response to heat stimulation, thus acting as thermoreceptors in keratinocytes [275,282]. In support of this evidence, TRPV3 knock-out mice showed strong deficits in response to heat stimulation [277]. Likewise, TRPV4 is also activated by heat, in particular by temperatures of 27–34 °C, as well as by osmotic and mechanical stimuli [283,284]. Among putative endogenous ligands, it was observed that AEA, 2-AG, and arachidonic acid indirectly activate TRPV4 by epoxyeicosatrienoic acids released from cytochrome P450 epoxygenases [285,286]. As for TRPV1 and TRPV3, TRPV4 activity is modulated by PIP2/PIP3, calmodulin and ATP [287–289] and by several protein kinases, such as PKA, PKC, Src family kinases (SFKs), and serum glucocorticoid-induced protein kinase-1 (SGK1) [290–293]. TRPV4 channels are widely expressed in epithelial cells of the renal convoluted tubule, trachea, submucosal glands, as well as in neutrophils, in autonomic nerve fibers, in peripheral sensory ganglia, in hair cells of the inner ear, and brain structures such as vascular organ of the lamina terminalis and the hypothalamic median preoptic region [283,294,295]. Due to its widespread expression, TRPV4 is involved in several physiological functions. In particular, it mediates temperature sensation in skin keratinocytes, anterior hypothalamus, and sensory ganglia [275,283,284]. TRPV4 is also involved in mechanosensation [296] and contribute to the normal functioning of the urinary bladder [297,298] and pulmonary alveoli [299,300] and to the development of mechanical hyperalgesia in inflammatory states [301].

TRPV5 and TRPV6 share a high sequence homology (74% of identity) and form highly Ca^{2+}-selective channels, which are not activated by heat [302–304]. As for the other TRPV family members, the activity of TRPV5 and TRPV6 is modulated by a variety of second messengers, including Ca^{2+}, Mg^{2+}, ATP, PIP2, calmodulin, and PKC [302,303,305–313]. TRPV5 is expressed in several tissues but is mostly abundant in renal tubules, where it regulates transcellular transport and reabsorption of Ca^{2+} [314]. Furthermore, TRPV5 is also involved in bone remodeling [315,316]. TRPV6 is widely expressed [305,317,318] but is mostly distributed in the intestine, kidney, and placenta, where it respectively modulates the Ca^{2+} transcellular entry, reabsorption, and transfer to fetus [319–322].

Among endogenous ligands of TRPV, or endovanilloids, there are leukotriene B4 and 12-hydroperoxyeicosatetraenoic acid that belong to the eicosanoid family, produced by lipoxygenase-mediated oxidation of PUFAs (especially arachidonic acid), which are potent activators of TRPV1 [252,323]. Other lipid-derived mediators of TRPV are epoxyeicosatrienoic acids, such as 5',6'-epoxyeicosatrienoic acid, which are synthesized from arachidonic acid by cytochrome P450 epoxygenases and may activate TRPV1 and TRPV4 [286,324].

As AEA is structurally similar to arachidonic acid as well as to PUFAs, it can be metabolized by COX-2 and LOXs. In particular, COX-2 converts AEA into prostaglandin-ethanolamides, which are endoperoxide molecules also known as prostamides [325,326]. On the other hand, LOXs convert AEA into hydroperoxy fatty acids, such as 12- and 15-hydroperoxyeicosatetraenoylethanolamide, which are, respectively, synthesized by 12-LOX and 15-LOX [327,328]. In guinea-pig bronchi, these oxidized lipid mediators seem to act as TRPV1 agonists and are also responsible, at least partially, for the contractile action of AEA [329].

Growing evidence supports a key role for TRPV, especially TRPV1, in the modulation of oxidative stress and lipid peroxidation mediated by endocannabinoids, their lipid analogues, and other lipid-related mediators. As known, AEA is considered an endovanilloid because of its ability to activate TRPV1 [127,136,330]: several in vitro analyses performed on human and rat cell lines have shown that AEA induces apoptotic effects via a TRPV1-mediated mechanism, which induces and increase in intracellular Ca^{2+} levels, mitochondrial uncoupling, oxidative stress due to increased $O_2 \bullet^-$ formation, cytochrome c release as well as calpain and caspase-3 activation [331–333]. Similarly, another in vitro study performed on human bladder cancer T24 cells showed that TRPV1 activation by capsaicin was correlated in a dose-dependent manner with an increase of cytosolic Ca^{2+} levels, with mithocondrial membrane depolarization and a marked ROS/RNS generation, which reduced T24 cells viability (Figure 5) [334].

Other studies showed that AEA was able to increase ROS/RNS production by targeting TRPV1, [335,336], which lead to the activation of the Ca^{2+}/calmodulin-dependent protein kinase II (CAMKII), and to the upregulation of NOX5 [337–339].

Moreover, it was observed, in the human esophageal epithelial cell line Het1A, that acid- or capsaicine-induced activation of TRPV1 leads to an increased production of intracellular ROS/RNS levels as well as to increased ROS/RNS- or HNE-modified proteins. In the same study, immunoprecipitation analyses of 4-HNE-stimulated Het1A cells revealed, also, that TRPV1 was modified by 4-HNE [340]. In addition to 4-HNE, TRPV1 is directly activated by •NO, oxidants and other chemical agents through the modification of cysteine free sulfhydryl groups [341]. Moreover, functional assays with mutated TRPV showed that cysteine residues 553 and 558, between the fifth and sixth transmembrane domains, are essential for •NO-induced activation of TRPV1, TRPV3, and TRPV4 and thus are potential targets of nitrosylation [342]. In addition, TRPV1 nitrosylation by •NO increased the intracellular Ca^{2+} levels and thus enhanced the channel sensitivity to H^+ and heat. These sensitizing effects induced by nitrosylation of cysteine residues were further supported by the use of oxidizing agents such as diamide and chloramine-T [343]. Furthermore, several studies reported that TRPV1 is also responsive to other electrophilic compounds generated during oxidative stress. To this regard, in TRPV1 channel-expressing human embryonic kidney (HEK) cells, a modest TRPV1 activation was observed following 4-ONE treatment (100 µM) [344]. Another TRPV1 activator is CTA. In particular, an in vitro study performed on murine cardiomyocytes incubated with CTA showed an increase in TRPV1 and NOXs levels, in ROS/RNS formation, in apoptotic events, and a decrease in the activity of mithocondrial proteins such as aconytase, uncoupling protein 2, and peroxisome proliferator-activated receptor-gamma coactivator-1alpha [345].

6. Modulation of Oxidative Stress and Lipid Peroxidation through the Peroxisome Proliferator-Activated Receptors-Alpha by Endocannabinoids and Their Lipid Analogues

Because of the high expression of PPAR-α in kidney, liver, heart, and brain, it is well documented that the activation of these transcription factors exerts protective roles in cardiovascular as well as renal, hepatic, and neurodegenerative diseases [138,346–349].

There is rising acknowledgment that the beneficial effects of PPAR-α stimulation could be explained by its ability to dampen oxidative stress in several pathological conditions linked to the redox impairment. A number of reports point to the involvement of various mechanisms through which PPAR-α agonists can modulate antioxidants.

In particular, the identification of PPREs elements in promoter regions of CAT and SOD genes in rat [347] additionally supported the involvement of these nuclear receptors in lowering ROS/RNS formation and lipid peroxidation products.

Nevertheless, PPAR-α is not only involved in suppressing ROS/RNS generation, but it can also play a role in modulating enzymes involved in ROS/RNS synthesis and/or scavenging. Consistently, the decrease in striatal SOD expression, which resulted in the 6-hydroxydopamine (6-OHDA)-induced Parkinson disease mouse model, was completely counteracted by PPAR-α agonists confirming the ability of this nuclear receptor to regulate the transcription of antioxidant enzymes (Figure 5) [138,346,350].

For instance, Diep and colleagues reported that the PPAR-α -induced suppression of oxidative stress in cardiovascular diseases is mediated by the ability of PPAR-α activators to inhibit angiotensin II-induced activation of NOXs in the vascular wall [348] and to increase scavenging enzymes as well.

Among the PPAR-α ligands, ECs and their lipids analogues have been shown to play a prominent role in affecting redox homeostasis in several oxidative stress-related pathologies, through a PPAR-α dependent mechanism. Consistently, it has been shown that PPAR-α stimulation by PEA lowers blood pressure and prevents hypertension-induced renal damage in hypertensive rats by inhibiting the subunit p47phox of NOXs (a key regulatory subunit essential for NOXs functioning) [349], and by significantly reducing the hypertension-induced increased levels of MDA in urine and renal tissues (Figure 5) [348].

Moreover, through PPAR-α activation, PEA appeared to simultaneously enhance the antioxidant defense by increasing SOD expression in the kidney [348], thus protecting from renal damage. In agreement with these results, other studies further support the potential beneficial effects of PEA activated-PPAR-α on kidney diseases [351]. For instance, it has been demonstrated that PEA, by targeting PPAR-α, is able to prevent kidney damage induced by I/R injury through dampening the lipid peroxidation products in the kidney, thereby leading to a reduction of neutrophil recruitment [352].

Moreover, because of the high expression of PPAR-α and its endogenous lipid agonists in the CNS, it has been demonstrated that PPAR-α activation can exert neuroprotective properties in several neuropathological conditions, especially in neurodegenerative disorders [169], by modulating the redox balance that resulted altered in these situations.

Further support for this comes from the observation that the brain areas that display the highest PPAR-α expression exhibit an overlapping expression pattern with key enzymes involved in ROS/RNS synthesis and/or scavenging including CAT, SOD1 and acyl-CoA oxidase 1 (ACOX1) [353–355], whose genes are known to be under the control of PPAR-α [356,357].

Thanks to its anti-oxidative properties, PPAR-α protects against normal brain aging and regulates the onset and progression of neurodegenerative disorders [358,359]. Interestingly, evidence suggests that in conditions of neurodegeneration, oxidative stress itself is responsible for the induction of PPAR-α expression. As a matter of fact, in hippocampal CA1 pyramidal cells of a transgenic mouse model of Alzheimer's disease, an increase in the levels of PPAR-α simultaneously with the production of ACR and 8-hydroxy(de)oxyguanosine, which represent markers of oxidative imbalance, was observed [360]. Such increase in hippocampal PPAR-α expression could trigger the induction of its target genes encoding for peroxisomal membrane protein-70 (PMP70) and ACOX1, which are involved in fatty acyl-CoA transport across peroxisomal membranes and peroxisomal β-oxidation respectively, by evoking a compensatory response to Aβ-mediated mitochondrial insult that occurs in early stage of Alzheimer's disease [4–6,360].

In this context, PEA was demonstrated to protect neurons and glia from oxidative stress by reducing MDA formation, thereby restoring a proper cellular redox state, and this effect appeared to be PPAR-α-dependent [171,172,361,362]. It has also been established that PEA neuroprotective effects are mediated, at least in part, through the de novo synthesis of neurosteroids (particularly allopregnanolone), which is triggered by PPAR-α activation [362].

The abovementioned findings, coupled with a recent report demonstrating that PEA treatment (through binding PPAR-α) is able to induce SOD and dampen ROS/RNS-induced oxidative damage in 6-OHDA-induced mouse model of Parkinson disease, additionally suggest the neuroprotective scavenging effects of this lipid compound (Figure 5) [363]. Beyond the ECs, several other synthetic ligands of PPAR-α have been shown to exert antioxidative properties. For instance, Wy14643 through binding PPAR-α is able to protect rabbit hearts from I/R injury by increasing the expression of the oxidative stress-inducible isoform of heme oxygenase and to preserve hippocampal neurons from H_2O_2 challenge by modulating mitochondrial fusion and fission events [360].

Moreover, it should be noted that the production of PPAR-α endogenous ligands, PEA and OEA as the mostly characterized, could be differently affected by physiological and pathological oxidative stress-related conditions. For instance, the ROS/RNS metabolism imbalance, which is responsible for oxidative stress-induced brain aging and neurodegeneration, can quantitatively and qualitatively modify the production of PPAR-α agonists and thus differently modulate PPAR-α-mediated pathways in neuronal and astroglial cells [169].

Additionally, the interplay between PPAR-α and oxidative-stress-induced lipid peroxidation comes also from the observation that NOXs activated-4-HNE is able to act as an endogenous PPAR-α activator leading to the discovery of the so called "lipid peroxidation products–PPARs–NOXs axis" [364]. The regulation of this axis, which represents an alternative pathway mediating ROS/RNS production, could ensure additional strategies to counteract oxidative-stress-related disorders.

7. Modulation of Oxidative Stress and Lipid Peroxidation through Other Receptors by Endocannabinoids and Their Lipid Analogues

Recently, in addition to PPAR-α and TRPV1, the orphan receptors GPR18, GPR55 and GPR119 were assessed as novel cannabinoid-related receptors [365]. Structurally, GPRs are GPCRs and, among them, GPR18, GPR55 and GPR119 share a limited primary sequence homology with CB1 and CB2.

GPR18 was discovered for the first time in 1997 by Gantz and colleagues [366]. GPR18 is widely expressed in testis and spleen, and in lesser extent in several other tissues such as thymus, lymph nodes, peripheral blood leukocytes, small intestine, and appendix, thus suggesting a regulatory role for GPR18 in the immune system [366]. Moreover, GPR18 was also found in several brain regions such as hypothalamus, brainstem, cerebellum, and striatum as well as in lung, thyroid and ovary [367]. Several studies reported that NAGly is the endogenous ligand of GPR18 that induces an elevation of intracellular Ca^{2+} levels [176]. The same authors demonstrated also that GPR18 activation was pertussis toxin-sensitive, suggesting the involvement of a $G_{\alpha i/o}$ protein in this response [176]. Despite these first evidence, several authors reported variable responses of GPR18 following the administration of NAGly [368,369].

For the first time Penumarti and colleagues demonstrated that GPR18 is expressed in the rostral ventrolateral medulla of rats and exerts tonic restraining influence on blood pressure [370]. In particular, authors observed that the systemic administration of abnormal cannabidiol, a synthetic agonist of GPR18, induced a dose-dependent reduction of blood pressure and increased heart rate. In addition, GPR18 activation increased neuronal adiponectin and •NO, and finally reduced neuronal ROS/RNS levels. These findings suggested for the first time a sympathoinhibitory role of GPR18 (Figure 5) [370].

More recently, another study confirmed that chronic GPR18 activation with its agonist abnormal cannabidiol produced hypotension, suppressed the cardiac sympathetic dominance, and improved left ventricular function in conscious rats [371]. In the same study, ex vivo analysis of plasma, heart, and vascular tissues of treated rats revealed an increase in cardiac and plasmatic adiponectin levels, an increase in aortic eNOS expression, augmented levels of vascular and serum •NO, high levels of myocardial and plasmatic guanosine 3',5'-cyclic monophosphate (cGMP), an increase of myocardial Akt and ERK1/2 phosphorylation, and, more importantly, reduced myocardial ROS/RNS formation [371]. These results suggest a protective role of GPR18 in cardiovascular diseases, in particular highlights the possibility to consider GPR18 as a viable molecular target for developing new antihypertensive drugs which are able to improve also the cardiac function.

Human GPR55 receptor was identified for the first time in 1999, through in silico studies, and was subsequently cloned [372]. GPR55 receptor is widely expressed, and therefore its activity was correlated with multiple physiological processes. In particular, GPR55 is expressed in the frontal cortex, striatum, hippocampus, hypothalamus, cerebellum, and brainstem [372,373]. Moreover, GPR55 was also found in peripheral organs and cells such as dorsal root ganglion [148], spleen, adrenal glands, jejunum, ileum [373], pancreas [374], bones [375] and microglia [376]. The GPR55 pharmacology and its downstream signaling are not yet certain. Nevertheless, some authors reported that ECs such as AEA, 2-AG, and virodhamine can activate both etherologous and native GPR55-expressing cells [148,273,377], while other groups reported that ECs are weak ligands [378,379], may act as partial agonists [175], or are not able to activate GPR55 receptors [380,381]. Another open debate regards the ability of PEA to activate [373] or not the GPR55 receptors [148,382]. Despite the controversial results about the ability of ECs to activate GPR55, it is well accepted that the endogenous lipid L-α-lysophosphatidylinositol (LPI) and its analogue 2-arachidonoyl-sn-glycero-3-phosphoinositol are endogenous ligand of GPR55 [379–382]. However, it is necessary to specify that LPI is not selective only for GPR55 [383]. Moreover, GPR55 may also heterodimerize with other receptors, such as CB2 [384], thus further confounding the results obtained so far.

About the mechanisms of downstream signaling, GPR55 activation was associated with an increase of intracellular Ca^{2+} levels, with the activation of RhoA and ERK1/2 pathway, and with the activation of several transcription factors, such as the nuclear factor of activated T-cells and the cAMP response element binding protein (CREB) [380,382].

The human orphan receptor GPR119 was identified for the first time in 2003 by sequence alignment tools analysis [385]. GPR119 is expressed mainly in pancreas and gut, in particular in β-cells and pancreatic polypeptide-producing PP cells, where its activity modulates the glucose-dependent insulin secretion [386,387], as well as in enteroendocrine L-cells, where it regulates the secretion of glucagon-like peptide 1 [388,389]. GPR119 is also expressed in liver [390] and skeletal muscle [Cornall et al., 2013]. In normal-weight and healthy patients it was observed that gut GPR119 expression rapidly increased following acute fat exposure [391], thus suggesting a potential involvement of GPR119 in type 2 dyabetes, metabolic disorder, and obesity.

The main endogenous ligands of GPR119 are, in order of potency, OLDA, OEA, PEA, and AEA [392,393]. Other endogenous GPR119 agonists are 2-oleoylglycerol [394] and oleoyl-lysophosphatidylcholine [386]. Clearly, also in this case, further studies are required to better characterize the pharmacological profile of GPR119.

Increasing evidence suggests that ECs may regulate ROS/RNS levels and thus reactive aldehydes formation by targeting GPR55. In this regard, Balenga and colleagues showed that GPR55 activity modulates RhoA-dependent neutrophil migration, and it may prevent oxidative damage [395]. In particular, this study, performed on neutrophils, demonstrated that 2-AG-induced ROS/RNS production, which was mediated by a CB2-dependent mechanism, appeared to be significantly decreased following the co-treatment with the GPR55 agonist LPI [395]. This negative interaction between GPR55 and CB2 was observed during neutrophil respiratory burst. Therefore, after an initial synergism in inducing chemotaxis, GPR55 and CB2 disengaged and, by a functional repression, GPR55 decreased CB2-induced oxidative damage by blocking CB2 downstream signaling [395]. Conversely, a recent study performed on human natural killer cells and monocytes unveiled a proinflammatory role of GPR55 activation (Figure 5) [396], which could be potentially correlated with an increase of ROS/RNS production and thus with oxidative stress.

8. The Role of Antioxidant System as Scavenger of ROS/RNS and Reactive Aldehydes

The "endogenous antioxidant system" relies on several enzymes, peptides, cofactors, and other molecules that are essential for the maintenance of a physiological redox homeostasis. Overall, endogenous antioxidants may be divided into two main groups, formed by enzymatic and non-enzymatic antioxidants [6,397]. The enzymatic group include CAT [398], SOD [399,400], GPx, GR, GT [401], thioredoxin (Trx) and thioredoxin reductase (TrxR) [402] while the non-enzymatic group include several antioxidant molecules such as GSH, GSSG, [403], vitamin A (retinol) [404], vitamin C (L-ascorbic acid) [405], vitamin E (tocopherols) [406], coenzyme Q10 (CoQ10) [407], carotenoids [408], flavonoids, polyphenols [409–411], minerals such as Se^{2+} [412], Cu^{2+}, and Zn^{2+} [413], as well as metabolites such as uric acid, bilirubin [414] and melatonin [415], which also possess antioxidant properties.

Briefly, CATs are Cu^{2+}/Zn^{2+}-dependent enzymes present in peroxisomes that catalyze the conversion of H_2O_2 in water and oxygen [398]. Among SOD enzymes, cytolosic SOD are Cu^{2+}/Zn^{2+}-dependent enzymes, while mitochondrial SODs are Mn^{2+}-dependent enzymes that metabolize $O_2\bullet^-$ into H_2O_2 and oxygen. Therefore, SOD represents the first line of defense against reactive aldehydes formation [400]. GPx, GR and GT are Se^{2+}-dependent enzymes that, together with GSH and GSSG, constitute the glutathione system, which contributes to eliminate H_2O_2 and other reactive molecules [403]. Similarly, Trx, TrxR, and NADPH constitute the thioredoxin system, which is critical for redox regulation of protein function and signaling via thiol redox control [402].

Vitamin A is produced in the liver, derives from β-carotene and acts as a lipid peroxidation blocker by preventing the chaining process in the propagation phase [404]. Similarly, also vitamin E acts as a lipid peroxidation blocker by donating a hydrogen atom to peroxyl radicals, thus forming tocopheroxyl radicals which are unable to continue the propagation phase of lipid peroxidation [416]. Vitamin C is effective in scavenging several ROS/RNS as well as in the detoxification of peroxyl and hydroxyl radicals [405]. CoQ10 is involved in the neutralization of the damages induced by peroxyl radicals and also in the regeneration of vitamin E [407]. Uric acid is known to prevent protein nitrosylation, as well as lipid and protein peroxidation, and therefore it is considered as a protectant agent of the CNS [417]. Melatonin is a natural scavenger derived from tryptophan, which is involved in the neutralization of several ROS/RNS and thus reduces the generation of reactive aldehydes [415]. Finally, flavonoids and polyphenols are ubiquitous plant-derived molecules, which act as chelators and scavengers of ROS/RNS as well as of hydroxyl and peroxyl radicals [418,419].

9. Conclusions

Oxidative stress represents an underlying disturbance that is involved in many pathophysiological conditions. Increasing evidence suggests that tissues with a high oxygen consumption, such as brain and heart among others, are particularly sensitive to lipid peroxidation products and free radical accumulation, which are responsible for oxidative stress–induced damages with consequent cell death [2,4–6,218].

Thus, acting on the cellular processes that suppress the generation of these reactive small molecules or altering the expression and/or activity of enzymes involved in their formation may be crucial for the treatment of a growing number of diseases linked with redox homeostasis deregulation.

In this scenario, there is rising acknowledgment about a cross-talk between the ECS and various redox-dependent processes. Indeed, it has been observed that the redox impairment induces the enhancement of AEA and 2-AG levels, as a consequence of phospholipid hydrolysis [420,421], and the upregulation of CB1 and CB2 expression [422,423], as well as the downregulation of FAAH [422].

A large number of reports point to the involvement of ECs and their lipid analogues in regulating ROS/RNS and reactive aldehydes generation through targeting CB1 and CB2 [8–10] and thereby exerting protective effects in cardiovascular as well as renal, hepatic, neuropsychiatric, and neurodegenerative diseases.

Moreover, it has been observed that, depending on the type of cell and/or injury, cannabinoid receptors show opposite effects in oxidative stress modulation, since CB1 activation results in a redox imbalance enhancement, while CB2 stimulation is responsible for lowering oxidative stress [9,223] and may convey beneficial free radical scavenging effects.

Overall, the mechanisms by which CB2 receptors, following ECs-mediated activation, are involved in the reduction of oxidative injury seem to be primarily mediated by the reduction of NOX2 and NOX4, and the simultaneous induction of the antioxidant defense through the increase of the SOD scavenging enzymes [180,181].

Emerging evidence indicates that the neuroprotective, cardioprotective and renoprotective effects of ECs and NAEs are additionally mediated by CB1/CB2-independent mechanisms and involve the contribution of alternative intracellular targets such as PPAR-α, TRPV1, GPR55, and GPR18 [169,348,349,370,371,395].

In particular, an interplay between PPAR-α and oxidative stress has been suggested from the observation that an imbalance in the redox state may modulate several signaling pathways, including PPAR-α signaling, via transcriptional regulation and post-translational modification.

Among the PPAR-α ligands, PEA appeared to exert beneficial effects by simultaneously enhancing the antioxidant defense through the increase of SOD expression and inhibiting NOXs activity with a consequent reduction of the lipid peroxidation products such as MDA [138].

Although the huge amount of knowledge has been gained about the effects of the ECs on oxidative stress and lipid peroxidation in several pathological conditions, many ECS compounds fail during clinical trials due to inefficacy or unforeseeable safety concerns. For the treatment of the cardiovascular diseases, for instance, no cannabinoid-based drugs have been approved so far, except for those acting as PPARs agonists [348]. Among the limitations that play a role in restricting the translation of ECs studies into clinical trials, the different animal paradigms as well as the route of administration used (central vs peripheral) and the differences between species seem to be primarily involved.

Moreover, most of the studies have focused on the role of CB1, CB2, TRPV1, PPARs and less is known about other candidates such as GPR18, GPR55 and GPR119.

Despite promising goals have been achieved over the last years on ECS research, there is an urgent necessity to expand the knowledge on the ECs complex signalling in order to better identify an explanation of the serious side-effects observed in clinical studies. Lessons from clinical experience should encourage the scientific community to better clarify how to modulate the ECS thus leading to major breakthroughs in the treatment of many diseases.

Overall, the findings discussed in this review may further elucidate the complex interaction existing between ECS, oxidative stress, and lipid peroxidation, resulting in a better understanding of the multiple beneficial effects of this signaling system in several pathological conditions related to a redox status impairment.

Author Contributions: The project idea was developed by S.G., T.C. and A.M.G.; C.A.G., S.C., T.C., and A.R. wrote the first draft of the manuscript. C.A.G, S.C., A.R., J.B.K., M.d.C., T.C., S.G., D.D., R.V., and A.M.G. conducted the literature review and revised the manuscript. S.C., C.A.G., and D.D. created the figures.

Funding: This project was supported by the Italian Ministry for Education, University and Research (PRIN20153NBRS3_003 to S.G.).

Conflicts of Interest: The authors declare no conflict of interest.

Abbreviations

•NO = nitric oxide; •OH = hydroxyl radical; $^1O_2$ = oxygen singlet; 2-AG = 2-arachidonoyl-glycerol; 2-AGE = 2-arachidonoylglyceryl ether or noladin ether; 4-HHE = 4-hydroxy-hexanal; 4-HNE = 4-hydroxy-2-nonenal; 4-ONE = 4-oxo-nonenal; 6-OHDA = 6-hydroxydopamine; AC = adenylyl cyclase; ACOX1 = acyl-CoA oxidase 1; ACR = acrolein; AEA = N-arachidonoyl-ethanolamine or anandamide; ApoE$^{-/-}$ = Apolipoprotein E-deficient mice; ARA-S = arachidonoyl-L-serine; AT1 = angiotensin II type 1 receptor; CAMKII = Ca^{2+}/calmodulin-dependent protein kinase II; cAMP = adenosine 3′,5′-cyclic monophosphate; CAT = catalase; CB1 = cannabinoid receptor type 1; CB2 = cannabinoid receptor type 2; CD36 = cluster of differentiation 36; CGD = chronic granulomatous disorder; cGMP = guanosine 3′,5′-cyclic monophosphate; CNS = central nervous system; CoQ10 = coenzyme Q10; COX-2 = cyclooxygenase type 2; COXs = cyclooxygenases; CREB = cAMP response element binding protein; CTA = crotonaldehyde; DAGL = diacylglycerol lipase; dG = deoxyguanosine; ECS = endocannabinoid system; ECs = endocannabinoids; eNOS = endothelial nitric oxide synthase; ERK1/2 = extracellular signal-related kinases; FAAH = fatty acid amide hydrolase; GPCRs = G-protein-coupled receptors; GPR18 = G protein-coupled receptor 18; GPR55 = G protein-coupled receptor 55; GPR119 = G protein-coupled receptor 119; GPx = glutathione peroxidase; GR = glutathione reductase; GSH = glutathione; GSSG = oxidized glutathione; GT = glutathione transferase; GTPase = guanosine triphosphatase; H_2O_2 = hydrogen peroxide; HClO = hypochlorous acid; HEK = human embryonic kidney; I/R = ischemia/reperfusion; JNK = c-Jun N-terminal kinase; LOXs = lipooxygenases; LPI = L-α-lysophosphatidylinositol; MAG = monoacylglycerols; MAGL = monoacylglycerol lipase; MAPKs = mitogen-activated protein kinases; MAPK/ERK1/2 = mitogen-activated protein kinases/extracellular signal-regulated kinases; MDA = malondialdehyde; NADA = N-arachidonoyldopamine; NAEs = N-acylethanolamines; NAGLy = N-arachidonoylglycine; NAPE = N-acyl-phosphatidylethanolamine; NAPE-PLD = NAPE-phospholipase D; NF-κB = nuclear factor-κB; NO_2 = nitric dioxide; NO_2^- = nitrite; NO_3^- = nitrate; NOS = nitric oxide synthase; NOS1 = NOS type 1; NOX2 = NOX type 2; NOX3 = NOX type 3; NOXs = NADPH oxidase enzymes; Nrf2 = nuclear factor-erythroid 2-related factor 2; O_2•$^-$ = superoxide anion; O_3 = ozone; ODA = Cis-9,10-octadecanoamide or oleamide; OEA = oleoylethanolamide; OLDA = N-oleoyldopamine; ONOO$^-$ = peroxynitrite; oxLDL = oxidized low-density lipoproteins; PEA = palmitoylethanolamide; PGE2 = prostaglandin E2; PIP2 = phosphatidylinositol 4,5-bisphosphate; PIP3 = phosphatidylinositol 3,4,5-trisphosphate; PKA = protein kinase A; PKC = protein kinase C; PMP70 = peroxisomal membrane protein-70; PPARs = peroxisome proliferator-activated receptors; PPRES = peroxisome proliferator response elements; PUFAs = polyunsatured fatty acids; Rap = Ras-related protein; Rap1GAP = Rap1 GTPase activating protein; RhoGEFs = RhoGTPase nucleotide exchange factors; ROS/RNS = reactive oxygen and nitrogen species; RXR = retinoid X receptor; SEA = stearoylethanolamide; SFKs = Src family kinases; SGK1 = serum glucocorticoid-induced protein kinase-1; SOD = superoxide dismutase; TRP = transient receptor potential; TRPV = transient receptor potential vanilloid; TRPV1 = transient receptor potential vanilloid 1; Trx = thioredoxin; TrxR = thioredoxin reductase.

References

1. Pomara, C.; Cassano, T.; D'Errico, S.; Bello, S.; Romano, A.D.; Riezzo, I.; Serviddio, G. Data available on the extent of cocaine use and dependence: Biochemistry, pharmacologic effects and global burden of disease of cocaine abusers. *Curr. Med. Chem.* **2012**, *19*, 5647–5657. [CrossRef] [PubMed]

2. Matthews, A.T.; Ross, M.K. Oxyradical Stress, Endocannabinoids, and Atherosclerosis. *Toxics* **2015**, *3*, 481–498. [CrossRef] [PubMed]

3. Sureshbabu, A.; Ryter, S.W.; Choi, M.E. Oxidative stress and autophagy: Crucial modulators of kidney injury. *Redox Biol.* **2015**, *4*, 208–214. [CrossRef] [PubMed]

4. Cassano, T.; Serviddio, G.; Gaetani, S.; Romano, A.; Dipasquale, P.; Cianci, S.; Bellanti, F.; Laconca, L.; Romano, A.D.; Padalino, I.; et al. Glutamatergic alterations and mitochondrial impairment in a murine model of Alzheimer disease. *Neurobiol. Aging* **2012**, *33*, 1121-e1. [CrossRef] [PubMed]

5. Cassano, T.; Pace, L.; Bedse, G.; Lavecchia, A.M.; De Marco, F.; Gaetani, S.; Serviddio, G. Glutamate and Mitochondria: Two Prominent Players in the Oxidative Stress-Induced Neurodegeneration. *Curr. Alzheimer Res.* **2016**, *13*, 185–197. [CrossRef] [PubMed]

6. Serviddio, G.; Romano, A.D.; Cassano, T.; Bellanti, F.; Altomare, E.; Vendemiale, G. Principles and therapeutic relevance for targeting mitochondria in aging and neurodegenerative diseases. *Curr. Pharm. Des.* **2011**, *17*, 2036–2055. [CrossRef] [PubMed]

7. Guéraud, F.; Atalay, M.; Bresgen, N.; Cipak, A.; Eckl, P.M.; Huc, L.; Jouanin, I.; Siems, W.; Uchida, K. Chemistry and biochemistry of lipid peroxidation products. *Free Radic. Res.* **2010**, *44*, 1098–1124. [CrossRef] [PubMed]

8. Mukhopadhyay, P.; Rajesh, M.; Bátkai, S.; Patel, V.; Kashiwaya, Y.; Liaudet, L.; Evgenov, O.V.; Mackie, K.; Haskó, G.; Pacher, P. CB1 cannabinoid receptors promote oxidative stress and cell death in murine models of doxorubicin-induced cardiomyopathy and in human cardiomyocytes. *Cardiovasc. Res.* **2010**, *85*, 773–784. [CrossRef] [PubMed]

9. Han, K.H.; Lim, S.; Ryu, J.; Lee, C.W.; Kim, Y.; Kang, J.H.; Kang, S.S.; Ahn, Y.K.; Park, C.S.; Kim, J.J. CB1 and CB2 cannabinoid receptors differentially regulate the production of reactive oxygen species by macrophages. *Cardiovasc. Res.* **2009**, *84*, 378–386. [CrossRef] [PubMed]

10. Hao, X.; Chen, J.; Luo, Z.; He, H.; Yu, H.; Ma, L.; Ma, S.; Zhu, T.; Liu, D.; Zhu, Z. TRPV1 activation prevents high-salt diet-induced nocturnal hypertension in mice. *Pflügers Arch. Eur. J. Physiol.* **2011**, *461*, 345–353. [CrossRef] [PubMed]

11. Sies, H. Oxidative stress: A concept in redox biology and medicine. *Redox Biol.* **2015**, *4*, 180–183. [CrossRef] [PubMed]

12. Di Meo, S.; Reed, T.T.; Venditti, P.; Victor, V.M. Role of ROS and RNS Sources in Physiological and Pathological Conditions. *Oxid. Med. Cell. Longev.* **2016**, *2016*, 1245049. [CrossRef] [PubMed]

13. Weidinger, A.; Kozlov, A.V. Biological Activities of Reactive Oxygen and Nitrogen Species: Oxidative Stress versus Signal Transduction. *Biomolecules* **2015**, *5*, 472–484. [CrossRef] [PubMed]

14. Liu, Y.; Fiskum, G.; Schubert, D. Generation of reactive oxygen species by the mitochondrial electron transport chain. *J. Neurochem.* **2002**, *80*, 780–787. [CrossRef] [PubMed]

15. Aguirre, J.; Lambeth, J.D. Nox enzymes from fungus to fly to fish and what they tell us about Nox function in mammals. *Free Radic. Biol. Med.* **2010**, *49*, 1342–1353. [CrossRef] [PubMed]

16. Panday, A.; Sahoo, M.K.; Osorio, D.; Batra, S. NADPH oxidases: An overview from structure to innate immunity-associated pathologies. *Cell. Mol. Immunol.* **2015**, *12*, 5–23. [CrossRef] [PubMed]

17. Sevier, C.S.; Kaiser, C.A. Ero1 and redox homeostasis in the endoplasmic reticulum. *Biochim. Biophys. Acta* **2008**, *1783*, 549–556. [CrossRef] [PubMed]

18. Wang, W.; Wang, S.; Yan, L.; Madara, P.; Del Pilar Cintron, A.; Wesley, R.A.; Danner, R.L. Superoxide production and reactive oxygen species signaling by endothelial nitric-oxide synthase. *J. Biol. Chem.* **2000**, *275*, 16899–16903. [CrossRef] [PubMed]

19. Hrycay, E.G.; Bandiera, S.M. Involvement of Cytochrome P450 in Reactive Oxygen Species Formation and Cancer. *Adv. Pharmacol.* **2015**, *74*, 35–84. [CrossRef] [PubMed]

20. Nathan, C.; Cunningham-Bussel, A. Beyond oxidative stress: An immunologist's guide to reactive oxygen species. *Nat. Rev. Immunol.* **2013**, *13*, 349–361. [CrossRef] [PubMed]

21. Vergeade, A.; Mulder, P.; Vendeville, C.; Ventura-Clapier, R.; Thuillez, C.; Monteil, C. Xanthine oxidase contributes to mitochondrial ROS generation in an experimental model of cocaine-induced diastolic dysfunction. *J. Cardiovasc. Pharmacol.* **2012**, *60*, 538–543. [CrossRef] [PubMed]

22. McGrath, A.P.; Hilmer, K.M.; Collyer, C.A.; Shepard, E.M.; Elmore, B.O.; Brown, D.E.; Dooley, D.M.; Guss, J.M. Structure and inhibition of human diamine oxidase. *Biochemistry* **2009**, *48*, 9810–9822. [CrossRef] [PubMed]

23. Marnett, L.J. Prostaglandin synthase-mediated metabolism of carcinogens and a potential role for peroxyl radicals as reactive intermediates. *Environ. Health Perspect.* **1990**, *88*, 5–12. [CrossRef] [PubMed]

24. Schröder, P.; Krutmann, J. Environmental Oxidative Stress—Environmental Sources of ROS. In *Reactions, Processes*; Grune, T., Ed.; Springer: Berlin/Heidelberg, Germany, 2005; Volume 2, ISBN 3540235876.

25. Dupré-Crochet, S.; Erard, M.; Nüße, O. ROS production in phagocytes: Why, when, and where? *J. Leukoc. Biol.* **2013**, *94*, 657–670. [CrossRef] [PubMed]

26. Görlach, A.; Bertram, K.; Hudecova, S.; Krizanova, O. Calcium and ROS: A mutual interplay. *Redox Biol.* **2015**, *6*, 260–271. [CrossRef] [PubMed]

27. Winkelstein, J.A.; Marino, M.C.; Johnston, R.B., Jr.; Boyle, J.; Curnutte, J.; Gallin, J.I.; Malech, H.L.; Holland, S.M.; Ochs, H.; Quie, P.; et al. Chronic granulomatous disease. Report on a national registry of 368 patients. *Medicine* **2000**, *79*, 155–169. [CrossRef]

28. Quie, P.G.; White, J.G.; Holmes, B.; Good, R.A. In vitro bactericidal capacity of human polymorphonuclear leukocytes: Diminished activity in chronic granulomatous disease of childhood. *J. Clin. Investig.* **1967**, *46*, 668–679. [CrossRef] [PubMed]

29. Holmes, B.; Quie, P.G.; Windhorst, D.B.; Good, R.A. Fatal granulomatous disease of childhood. An inborn abnormality of phagocytic function. *Lancet* **1966**, *1*, 1225–1228. [CrossRef]

30. Bylund, J.; Goldblatt, D.; Speert, D.P. Chronic granulomatous disease: From genetic defect to clinical presentation. *Adv. Exp. Med. Biol.* **2005**, *568*, 67–87. [CrossRef] [PubMed]

31. Quinn, M.T.; Ammons, M.C.; Deleo, F.R. The expanding role of NADPH oxidases in health and disease: No longer just agents of death and destruction. *Clin. Sci.* **2006**, *111*, 1–20. [CrossRef] [PubMed]

32. Cifuentes, M.E.; Pagano, P.J. Targeting reactive oxygen species in hypertension. *Curr. Opin. Nephrol. Hypertens.* **2006**, *15*, 179–186. [CrossRef] [PubMed]

33. Moncada, S.; Higgs, E.A. The discovery of nitric oxide and its role in vascular biology. *Br. J. Pharmacol.* **2006**, *147* (Suppl. 1), S193–S201. [CrossRef] [PubMed]

34. Drummond, G.R.; Sobey, C.G. Endothelial NADPH oxidases: Which NOX to target in vascular disease? *Trends Endocrinol. Metab.* **2014**, *25*, 452–463. [CrossRef] [PubMed]

35. Wilcox, C.S. Redox regulation of the afferent arteriole and tubuloglomerular feedback. *Acta Physiol. Scand.* **2003**, *179*, 217–223. [CrossRef] [PubMed]

36. Wilcox, C.S. Oxidative stress and nitric oxide deficiency in the kidney: A critical link to hypertension? *Am. J. Physiol. Regul. Integr. Comp. Physiol.* **2005**, *289*, R913–R935. [CrossRef] [PubMed]

37. Zou, A.P.; Cowley, A.W., Jr. Reactive oxygen species and molecular regulation of renal oxygenation. *Acta Physiol. Scand.* **2003**, *179*, 233–241. [CrossRef] [PubMed]

38. Juncos, R.; Hong, N.J.; Garvin, J.L. Differential effects of superoxide on luminal and basolateral Na^+/H^+ exchange in the thick ascending limb. *Am. J. Physiol. Regul. Integr. Comp. Physiol.* **2006**, *290*, R79–R83. [CrossRef] [PubMed]

39. Hoidal, J.R.; Brar, S.S.; Sturrock, A.B.; Sanders, K.A.; Dinger, B.; Fidone, S.; Kennedy, T.P. The role of endogenous NADPH oxidases in airway and pulmonary vascular smooth muscle function. *Antioxid. Redox Signal.* **2003**, *5*, 751–758. [CrossRef] [PubMed]

40. Brar, S.S.; Kennedy, T.P.; Sturrock, A.B.; Hueckstedt, T.P.; Quinn, M.T.; Murphy, T.M.; Chitano, P.; Hoidal, J.R. NADPH oxidase promotes NF-kappaB activation and proliferation in human airway smooth muscle. *Am. J. Physiol. Lung Cell. Mol. Physiol.* **2002**, *282*, L782L795. [CrossRef] [PubMed]

41. Piao, Y.J.; Seo, Y.H.; Hong, F.; Kim, J.H.; Kim, Y.J.; Kang, M.H.; Kim, B.S.; Jo, S.A.; Jo, I.; Jue, D.M.; et al. Nox 2 stimulates muscle differentiation via NF-kappaB/iNOS pathway. *Free Radic. Biol. Med.* **2005**, *38*, 989–1001. [CrossRef] [PubMed]

42. Kojim, S.; Ikeda, M.; Shibukawa, A.; Kamikawa, Y. Modification of 5-hydroxytryptophan-evoked 5-hydroxytryptamine formation of guinea pig colonic mucosa by reactive oxygen species. *Jpn. J. Pharmacol.* **2002**, *88*, 114–118. [CrossRef] [PubMed]

43. Wang, G.; Anrather, J.; Huang, J.; Speth, R.C.; Pickel, V.M.; Iadecola, C. NADPH oxidase contributes to angiotensin II signaling in the nucleus tractus solitarius. *J. Neurosci.* **2004**, *24*, 5516–5524. [CrossRef] [PubMed]

44. Erdös, B.; Broxson, C.S.; King, M.A.; Scarpace, P.J.; Tümer, N. Acute pressor effect of central angiotensin II is mediated by NAD(P)H-oxidase-dependent production of superoxide in the hypothalamic cardiovascular regulatory nuclei. *J. Hypertens.* **2006**, *24*, 109–116. [CrossRef] [PubMed]

45. Mander, P.K.; Jekabsone, A.; Brown, G.C. Microglia proliferation is regulated by hydrogen peroxide from NADPH oxidase. *J. Immunol.* **2006**, *176*, 1046–1052. [CrossRef] [PubMed]

46. Fritz, K.S.; Petersen, D.R. An overview of the chemistry and biology of reactive aldehydes. *Free Radic. Biol. Med.* **2013**, *59*, 85–91. [CrossRef] [PubMed]

47. Yin, H.; Xu, L.; Porter, N.A. Free radical lipid peroxidation: Mechanisms and analysis. *Chem. Rev.* **2011**, *111*, 5944–5972. [CrossRef] [PubMed]

48. Niki, E.; Yoshida, Y.; Saito, Y.; Noguchi, N. Lipid peroxidation: Mechanisms, inhibition, and biological effects. *Biochem. Biophys. Res. Commun.* **2005**, *338*, 668–676. [CrossRef] [PubMed]

49. Porter, N.A.; Caldwell, S.E.; Mills, K.A. Mechanisms of free radical oxidation of unsaturated lipids. *Lipids* **1995**, *30*, 277–290. [CrossRef] [PubMed]

50. Forman, H.J.; Fukuto, J.M.; Miller, T.; Zhang, H.; Rinna, A.; Levy, S. The chemistry of cell signaling by reactive oxygen and nitrogen species and 4-hydroxynonenal. *Arch. Biochem. Biophys.* **2008**, *477*, 183–195. [CrossRef] [PubMed]

51. Poli, G.; Schaur, R.J.; Siems, W.G.; Leonarduzzi, G. 4-hydroxynonenal: A membrane lipid oxidation product of medicinal interest. *Med. Res. Rev.* **2008**, *28*, 569–631. [CrossRef] [PubMed]

52. Noguchi, N. Role of oxidative stress in adaptive responses in special reference to atherogenesis. *J. Clin. Biochem. Nutr.* **2008**, *43*, 131–138. [CrossRef] [PubMed]

53. Zmijewski, J.W.; Landar, A.; Watanabe, N.; Dickinson, D.A.; Noguchi, N.; Darley-Usmar, V.M. Cell signalling by oxidized lipids and the role of reactive oxygen species in the endothelium. *Biochem. Soc. Trans.* **2005**, *33*, 1385–1389. [CrossRef] [PubMed]

54. Romano, A.; Serviddio, G.; Calcagnini, S.; Villani, R.; Giudetti, A.M.; Cassano, T.; Gaetani, S. Linking lipid peroxidation and neuropsychiatric disorders: Focus on 4-hydroxy-2-nonenal. *Free Radic. Biol. Med.* **2017**, *111*, 281–293. [CrossRef] [PubMed]

55. Negre-Salvayre, A.; Coatrieux, C.; Ingueneau, C.; Salvayre, R. Advanced lipid peroxidation end products in oxidative damage to proteins. Potential role in diseases and therapeutic prospects for the inhibitors. *Br. J. Pharmacol.* **2008**, *153*, 6–20. [CrossRef] [PubMed]

56. Winczura, A.; Zdżalik, D.; Tudek, B. Damage of DNA and proteins by major lipid peroxidation products in genome stability. *Free Radic. Res.* **2012**, *46*, 442–459. [CrossRef] [PubMed]

57. Winter, C.K.; Segall, H.J.; Haddon, W.F. Formation of cyclic adducts of deoxyguanosine with the aldehydes trans-4-hydroxy-2-hexenal and trans-4-hydroxy-2-nonenal in vitro. *Cancer Res.* **1986**, *46*, 5682–5686. [PubMed]

58. Chung, F.L.; Young, R.; Hecht, S.S. Formation of cyclic $1,N^2$-propanodeoxyguanosine adducts in DNA upon reaction with acrolein or crotonaldehyde. *Cancer Res.* **1984**, *44*, 990–995. [PubMed]

59. Cohn, J.A.; Tsai, L.; Friguet, B.; Szweda, L.I. Chemical characterization of a protein-4-hydroxy-2-nonenal cross-link: Immunochemical detection in mitochondria exposed to oxidative stress. *Arch. Biochem. Biophys.* **1996**, *328*, 158–164. [CrossRef] [PubMed]

60. Seto, H.; Okuda, T.; Takesue, T.; Ikemura, T. Reaction of malonaldehyde with nucleic acid. I. Formation of fluorescent pyrimido[1,2-a]purin-10-one nucleosides. *Bull. Chem. Soc. Jpn.* **1983**, *56*, 1799–1802. [CrossRef]

61. Esterbauer, H. Cytotoxicity and genotoxicity of lipid-oxidation products. *Am. J. Clin. Nutr.* **1993**, *57*, 779S–785S. [CrossRef] [PubMed]

62. Schaur, R.J. Basic aspects of the biochemical reactivity of 4-hydroxynonenal. *Mol. Asp. Med.* **2003**, *24*, 149–159. [CrossRef]

63. Zarkovic, N.; Cipak, A.; Jaganjac, M.; Borovic, S.; Zarkovic, K. Pathophysiological relevance of aldehydic protein modifications. *J. Proteom.* **2013**, *92*, 239–247. [CrossRef] [PubMed]

64. Rindgen, D.; Nakajima, M.; Wehrli, S.; Xu, K.; Blair, I.A. Covalent modifications to 2'-deoxyguanosine by 4-oxo-2-nonenal, a novel product of lipid peroxidation. *Chem. Res. Toxicol.* **1999**, *12*, 1195–1204. [CrossRef] [PubMed]

65. Lee, S.H.; Rindgen, D.; Bible, R.H., Jr.; Hajdu, E.; Blair, I.A. Characterization of 2'-deoxyadenosine adducts derived from 4-oxo-2-nonenal, a novel product of lipid peroxidation. *Chem. Res. Toxicol.* **2000**, *13*, 565–574. [CrossRef] [PubMed]

66. Pollack, M.; Oe, T.; Lee, S.H.; Silva Elipe, M.V.; Arison, B.H.; Blair, I.A. Characterization of 2'-deoxycytidine adducts derived from 4-oxo-2-nonenal, a novel lipid peroxidation product. *Chem. Res. Toxicol.* **2003**, *16*, 893–900. [CrossRef] [PubMed]

67. Williams, M.V.; Lee, S.H.; Pollack, M.; Blair, I.A. Endogenous lipid hydroperoxide-mediated DNA-adduct formation in min mice. *J. Biol. Chem.* **2006**, *281*, 10127–10133. [CrossRef] [PubMed]

68. Del Rio, D.; Stewart, A.J.; Pellegrini, N. A review of recent studies on malondialdehyde as toxic molecule and biological marker of oxidative stress. *Nutr. Metab. Cardiovasc. Dis.* **2005**, *15*, 316–328. [CrossRef] [PubMed]

69. Zhao, J.; Chen, J.; Zhu, H.; Xiong, Y.L. Mass spectrometric evidence of malonaldehyde and 4-hydroxynonenal adductions to radical-scavenging soy peptides. *J. Agric. Food Chem.* **2012**, *60*, 9727–9736. [CrossRef] [PubMed]

70. Mukai, F.H.; Goldstein, B.D. Mutagenicity of malonaldehyde, a decomposition product of peroxidized polyunsaturated fatty acids. *Science* **1976**, *191*, 868–869. [CrossRef] [PubMed]

71. Basu, A.K.; Marnett, L.J. Unequivocal demonstration that malondialdehyde is a mutagen. *Carcinogenesis* **1983**, *4*, 331–333. [CrossRef] [PubMed]

72. Marnett, L.J.; Hurd, H.K.; Hollstein, M.C.; Levin, D.E.; Esterbauer, H.; Ames, B.N. Naturally occurring carbonyl compounds are mutagens in Salmonella tester strain TA104. *Mutat. Res.* **1985**, *148*, 25–34. [CrossRef]

73. Vasanthi, P.; Nalini, G.; Rajasekhar, G. Status of oxidative stress in rheumatoid arthritis. *Int. J. Rheum. Dis.* **2009**, *12*, 29–33. [CrossRef] [PubMed]

74. Mishra, R.; Singh, A.; Chandra, V.; Negi, M.P.; Tripathy, B.C.; Prakash, J.; Gupta, V. A comparative analysis of serological parameters and oxidative stress in osteoarthritis and rheumatoid arthritis. *Rheumatol. Int.* **2012**, *32*, 2377–2382. [CrossRef] [PubMed]

75. Mateen, S.; Moin, S.; Khan, A.Q.; Zafar, A.; Fatima, N. Increased Reactive Oxygen Species Formation and Oxidative Stress in Rheumatoid Arthritis. *PLoS ONE* **2016**, *11*, e0152925. [CrossRef] [PubMed]

76. Shah, D.; Wanchu, A.; Bhatnagar, A. Interaction between oxidative stress and chemokines: Possible pathogenic role in systemic lupus erythematosus and rheumatoid arthritis. *Immunobiology* **2011**, *216*, 1010–1017. [CrossRef] [PubMed]

77. Liao, C.C.; Chang, Y.S.; Cheng, C.W.; Chi, W.M.; Tsai, K.L.; Chen, W.J.; Kung, T.S.; Tai, C.C.; Lin, Y.F.; Lin, H.T.; et al. Isotypes of autoantibodies against differentially expressed novel malondialdehyde-modified peptide adducts in serum of Taiwanese women with rheumatoid arthritis. *J. Proteom.* **2018**, *170*, 141–150. [CrossRef] [PubMed]

78. Cvetkovic, J.T.; Wållberg-Jonsson, S.; Ahmed, E.; Rantapää-Dahlqvist, S.; Lefvert, A.K. Increased levels of autoantibodies against copper-oxidized low density lipoprotein, malondialdehyde-modified low density lipoprotein and cardiolipin in patients with rheumatoid arthritis. *Rheumatology* **2002**, *41*, 988–995. [CrossRef] [PubMed]

79. Wållberg-Jonsson, S.; Cvetkovic, J.T.; Sundqvist, K.G.; Lefvert, A.K.; Rantapää-Dahlqvist, S. Activation of the immune system and inflammatory activity in relation to markers of atherothrombotic disease and atherosclerosis in rheumatoid arthritis. *J. Rheumatol.* **2002**, *29*, 875–882. [PubMed]

80. Chung, F.L.; Chen, H.J.; Nath, R.G. Lipid peroxidation as a potential endogenous source for the formation of exocyclic DNA adducts. *Carcinogenesis* **1996**, *17*, 2105–2111. [CrossRef] [PubMed]

81. Chung, F.L.; Nath, R.G.; Nagao, M.; Nishikawa, A.; Zhou, G.D.; Randerath, K. Endogenous formation and significance of $1,N^2$-propanodeoxyguanosine adducts. *Mutat. Res.* **1999**, *424*, 71–81. [CrossRef]

82. Wang, M.Y.; Chung, F.L.; Hecht, S.S. Identification of crotonaldehyde as a hepatic microsomal metabolite formed by alpha-hydroxylation of the carcinogen *N*-nitrosopyrrolidine. *Chem. Res. Toxicol.* **1988**, *1*, 28–31. [CrossRef] [PubMed]

83. Wang, M.; McIntee, E.J.; Cheng, G.; Shi, Y.; Villalta, P.W.; Hecht, S.S. Identification of paraldol-deoxyguanosine adducts in DNA reacted with crotonaldehyde. *Chem. Res. Toxicol.* **2000**, *13*, 1065–1074. [CrossRef] [PubMed]

84. International Agency for Research on Cancer. IARC Monographs on the Evaluation of Carcinogenic Risks to Humans. In *Dry Cleaning, Some Chlorinated Solvents and Other Industrial Chemicals*; International Agency for Research on Cancer: Lyon, France, 1995; Volume 63, pp. 373–391.

85. Chung, F.L.; Tanaka, T.; Hecht, S.S. Induction of liver tumors in F344 rats by crotonaldehyde. *Cancer Res.* **1986**, *46*, 1285–1289. [PubMed]

86. Ichihashi, K.; Osawa, T.; Toyokuni, S.; Uchida, K. Endogenous formation of protein adducts with carcinogenic aldehydes: Implications for oxidative stress. *J. Biol. Chem.* **2001**, *276*, 23903–23913. [CrossRef] [PubMed]

87. Furuhata, A.; Nakamura, M.; Osawa, T.; Uchida, K. Thiolation of protein-bound carcinogenic aldehyde. An electrophilic acrolein-lysine adduct that covalently binds to thiols. *J. Biol. Chem.* **2002**, *277*, 27919–27926. [CrossRef] [PubMed]

88. Uchida, K.; Kanematsu, M.; Morimitsu, Y.; Osawa, T.; Noguchi, N.; Niki, E. Acrolein is a product of lipid peroxidation reaction. Formation of free acrolein and its conjugate with lysine residues in oxidized low density lipoproteins. *J. Biol. Chem.* **1998**, *273*, 16058–16066. [CrossRef] [PubMed]

89. Esterbauer, H.; Schaur, R.J.; Zollner, H. Chemistry and biochemistry of 4-hydroxynonenal, malonaldehyde and related aldehydes. *Free Radic. Biol. Med.* **1991**, *11*, 81–128. [CrossRef]

90. Cohen, G.; Riahi, Y.; Sunda, V.; Deplano, S.; Chatgilialoglu, C.; Ferreri, C.; Kaiser, N.; Sasson, S. Signaling properties of 4-hydroxyalkenals formed by lipid peroxidation in diabetes. *Free Radic. Biol. Med.* **2013**, *65*, 978–987. [CrossRef] [PubMed]

91. Higdon, A.; Diers, A.R.; Oh, J.Y.; Landar, A.; Darley-Usmar, V.M. Cell signalling by reactive lipid species: New concepts and molecular mechanisms. *Biochem. J.* **2012**, *442*, 453–464. [CrossRef] [PubMed]

92. Riahi, Y.; Cohen, G.; Shamni, O.; Sasson, S. Signaling and cytotoxic functions of 4-hydroxyalkenals. *Am. J. Physiol. Endocrinol. Metab.* **2010**, *299*, E879–E886. [CrossRef] [PubMed]

93. Schaur, R.J.; Siems, W.; Bresgen, N.; Eckl, P.M. 4-Hydroxy-nonenal-A Bioactive Lipid Peroxidation Product. *Biomolecules* **2015**, *5*, 2247–2337. [CrossRef] [PubMed]

94. Calabrese, E.J.; Bachmann, K.A.; Bailer, A.J.; Bolger, P.M.; Borak, J.; Cai, L.; Cedergreen, N.; Cherian, M.G.; Chiueh, C.C.; Clarkson, T.W.; et al. Biological stress response terminology: Integrating the concepts of adaptive response and preconditioning stress within a hormetic dose-response framework. *Toxicol. Appl. Pharmacol.* **2007**, *222*, 122–128. [CrossRef] [PubMed]

95. Pizzimenti, S.; Barrera, G.; Dianzani, M.U.; Brüsselbach, S. Inhibition of D1, D2, and A-cyclin expression in HL-60 cells by the lipid peroxydation product 4-hydroxynonenal. *Free Radic. Biol. Med.* **1999**, *26*, 1578–1586. [CrossRef]

96. Huang, Y.; Li, W.; Kong, A.N. Anti-oxidative stress regulator NF-E2-related factor 2 mediates the adaptive induction of antioxidant and detoxifying enzymes by lipid peroxidation metabolite 4-hydroxynonenal. *Cell Biosci.* **2012**, *2*, 40. [CrossRef] [PubMed]

97. Zhang, Y.; Sano, M.; Shinmura, K.; Tamaki, K.; Katsumata, Y.; Matsuhashi, T.; Morizane, S.; Ito, H.; Hishiki, T.; Endo, J.; et al. 4-hydroxy-2-nonenal protects against cardiac ischemia-reperfusion injury via the Nrf2-dependent pathway. *J. Mol. Cell. Cardiol.* **2010**, *49*, 576–586. [CrossRef] [PubMed]

98. Siow, R.C.; Ishii, T.; Mann, G.E. Modulation of antioxidant gene expression by 4-hydroxynonenal: Atheroprotective role of the Nrf2/ARE transcription pathway. *Redox Rep.* **2007**, *12*, 11–15. [CrossRef] [PubMed]

99. Tanito, M.; Agbaga, M.P.; Anderson, R.E. Upregulation of thioredoxin system via Nrf2-antioxidant responsive element pathway in adaptive-retinal neuroprotection in vivo and in vitro. *Free Radic. Biol. Med.* **2007**, *42*, 1838–1850. [CrossRef] [PubMed]

100. Ishii, T.; Itoh, K.; Ruiz, E.; Leake, D.S.; Unoki, H.; Yamamoto, M.; Mann, G.E. Role of Nrf2 in the regulation of CD36 and stress protein expression in murine macrophages: Activation by oxidatively modified LDL and 4-hydroxynonenal. *Circ. Res.* **2004**, *94*, 609–616. [CrossRef] [PubMed]

101. De Petrocellis, L.; Cascio, M.G.; Di Marzo, V. The endocannabinoid system: A general view and latest additions. *Br. J. Pharmacol.* **2004**, *141*, 765–774. [CrossRef] [PubMed]

102. Mechoulam, R.; Fride, E.; Di Marzo, V. Endocannabinoids. *Eur. J. Pharmacol.* **1998**, *359*, 1–18. [CrossRef]

103. Devane, W.A.; Hanus, L.; Breuer, A.; Pertwee, R.G.; Stevenson, L.A.; Griffin, G.; Gibson, D.; Mandelbaum, A.; Etinger, A.; Mechoulam, R. Isolation and structure of a brain constituent that binds to the cannabinoid receptor. *Science* **1992**, *258*, 1946–1949. [CrossRef] [PubMed]

104. Sierra, S.; Luquin, N.; Navarro-Otano, J. The endocannabinoid system in cardiovascular function: Novel insights and clinical implications. *Clin. Auton Res.* **2018**, *28*, 35–52. [CrossRef] [PubMed]

105. Fonseca, B.M.; Costa, M.A.; Almada, M.; Correia-da-Silva, G.; Teixeira, N.A. Endogenous cannabinoids revisited: A biochemistry perspective. *Prostaglandins Other Lipid Mediat.* **2013**, *102–103*, 13–30. [CrossRef] [PubMed]

106. Sugiura, T.; Kondo, S.; Sukagawa, A.; Nakane, S.; Shinoda, A.; Itoh, K.; Yamashita, A.; Waku, K. 2-Arachidonoylglycerol: A possible endogenous cannabinoid receptor ligand in brain. *Biochem. Biophys. Res. Commun.* **1995**, *215*, 89–97. [CrossRef] [PubMed]

107. Stella, N.; Schweitzer, P.; Piomelli, D. A second endogenous cannabinoid that modulates long-term potentiation. *Nature* **1997**, *388*, 773–778. [CrossRef] [PubMed]

108. Fonseca, B.M.; Correia-da-Silva, G.; Taylor, A.H.; Lam, P.M.; Marczylo, T.H.; Bell, S.C.; Konje, J.C.; Teixeira, N.A. The endocannabinoid 2-arachidonoylglycerol (2-AG) and metabolizing enzymes during rat fetoplacental development: A role in uterine remodelling. *Int. J. Biochem. Cell Biol.* **2010**, *42*, 1884–1892. [CrossRef] [PubMed]

109. Fonseca, B.M.; Correia-da-Silva, G.; Taylor, A.H.; Lam, P.M.; Marczylo, T.H.; Konje, J.C.; Bell, S.C.; Teixeira, N.A. *N*-acylethanolamine levels and expression of their metabolizing enzymes during pregnancy. *Endocrinology* **2010**, *151*, 3965–3974. [CrossRef] [PubMed]

110. Di Marzo, V. The endocannabinoid system: Its general strategy of action, tools for its pharmacological manipulation and potential therapeutic exploitation. *Pharmacol. Res.* **2009**, *60*, 77–84. [CrossRef] [PubMed]

111. Gonsiorek, W.; Lunn, C.; Fan, X.; Narula, S.; Lundell, D.; Hipkin, R.W. Endocannabinoid 2-arachidonyl glycerol is a full agonist through human type 2 cannabinoid receptor: Antagonism by anandamide. *Mol. Pharmacol.* **2000**, *57*, 1045–1050. [PubMed]

112. Pertwee, R.G. The pharmacology of cannabinoid receptors and their ligands: An overview. *Int. J. Obes.* **2006**, *30* (Suppl. 1), S13–S18. [CrossRef] [PubMed]

113. Matsuda, L.A.; Lolait, S.J.; Brownstein, M.J.; Young, A.C.; Bonner, T.I. Structure of a cannabinoid receptor and functional expression of the cloned cDNA. *Nature* **1990**, *346*, 561–564. [CrossRef] [PubMed]

114. Freund, T.F.; Katona, I.; Piomelli, D. Role of endogenous cannabinoids in synaptic signaling. *Physiol. Rev.* **2003**, *83*, 1017–1066. [CrossRef] [PubMed]

115. Pacher, P.; Steffens, S. The emerging role of the endocannabinoid system in cardiovascular disease. *Semin. Immunopathol.* **2009**, *31*, 63–77. [CrossRef] [PubMed]

116. Tam, J.; Hinden, L.; Drori, A.; Udi, S.; Azar, S.; Baraghithy, S. The therapeutic potential of targeting the peripheral endocannabinoid/CB$_1$ receptor system. *Eur. J. Intern. Med.* **2018**, *49*, 23–29. [CrossRef] [PubMed]

117. Hu, S.S.; Mackie, K. Distribution of the Endocannabinoid System in the Central Nervous System. *Handb. Exp. Pharmacol.* **2015**, *231*, 59–93. [CrossRef] [PubMed]

118. Bénard, G.; Massa, F.; Puente, N.; Lourenço, J.; Bellocchio, L.; Soria-Gómez, E.; Matias, I.; Delamarre, A.; Metna-Laurent, M.; Cannich, A.; et al. Mitochondrial CB$_1$ receptors regulate neuronal energy metabolism. *Nat. Neurosci.* **2012**, *15*, 558–564. [CrossRef] [PubMed]

119. Pacher, P.; Kunos, G. Modulating the endocannabinoid system in human health and disease—Successes and failures. *FEBS J.* **2013**, *280*, 1918–1943. [CrossRef] [PubMed]

120. Pertwee, R.G. Cannabinoid receptor ligands: Clinical and neuropharmacological considerations, relevant to future drug discovery and development. *Expert Opin. Investig. Drugs* **2000**, *9*, 1553–1571. [CrossRef] [PubMed]

121. Jordan, J.D.; Carey, K.D.; Stork, P.J.; Iyengar, R. Modulation of rap activity by direct interaction of Galpha(o) with Rap1 GTPase-activating protein. *J. Biol. Chem.* **1999**, *274*, 21507–21510. [CrossRef] [PubMed]

122. Glass, M.; Felder, C.C. Concurrent stimulation of cannabinoid CB1 and dopamine D2 receptors augments cAMP accumulation in striatal neurons: Evidence for a G$_s$ linkage to the CB1 receptor. *J. Neurosci.* **1997**, *17*, 5327–5333. [CrossRef] [PubMed]

123. Maneuf, Y.P.; Brotchie, J.M. Paradoxical action of the cannabinoid WIN 55, 212–212 in stimulated and basal cyclic AMP accumulation in rat globus pallidus slices. *Br. J. Pharmacol.* **1997**, *120*, 1397–1398. [CrossRef] [PubMed]

124. Howlett, A.C. Cannabinoid receptor signaling. *Handb. Exp. Pharmacol.* **2005**, *168*, 53–79. [CrossRef]

125. Turu, G.; Hunyady, L. Signal transduction of the CB1 cannabinoid receptor. *J. Mol. Endocrinol.* **2010**, *44*, 75–85. [CrossRef] [PubMed]

126. Pacher, P.; Batkai, S.; Kunos, G. The endocannabinoid system as an emerging target of pharmacotherapy. *Pharmacol. Rev.* **2006**, *58*, 389–462. [CrossRef] [PubMed]

127. Zygmunt, P.M.; Petersson, J.; Andersson, D.A.; Chuang, H.; Sørgård, M.; Di Marzo, V.; Julius, D.; Högestätt, E.D. Vanilloid receptors on sensory nerves mediate the vasodilator action of anandamide. *Nature* **1999**, *400*, 452–457. [CrossRef] [PubMed]

128. Starowicz, K.; Nigam, S.; Di Marzo, V. Biochemistry and pharmacology of endovanilloids. *Pharmacol. Ther.* **2007**, *114*, 13–33. [CrossRef] [PubMed]

129. Di Marzo, V.; De Petrocellis, L. Endocannabinoids as regulators of transient receptor potential (TRP) channels: A further opportunity to develop new endocannabinoid-based therapeutic drugs. *Curr. Med. Chem.* **2010**, *17*, 1430–1449. [CrossRef] [PubMed]

130. O'Sullivan, S.E. Cannabinoids go nuclear: Evidence for activation of peroxisome proliferator-activated receptors. *Br. J. Pharmacol.* **2007**, *152*, 576–582. [CrossRef] [PubMed]

131. Lu, H.C.; Mackie, K. An introduction to the endogenous cannabinoid system. *Biol. Psychiatry* **2016**, *79*, 516–525. [CrossRef] [PubMed]

132. Haugh, O.; Penman, J.; Irving, A.J.; Campbell, V.A. The emerging role of the cannabinoid receptor family in peripheral and neuro-immune interactions. *Curr. Drug Targets* **2016**, *17*, 1834–1840. [CrossRef] [PubMed]

133. Yang, D.; Luo, Z.; Ma, S.; Wong, W.T.; Ma, L.; Zhong, J.; He, H.; Zhao, Z.; Cao, T.; Yan, Z.; et al. Activation of TRPV1 by dietary capsaicin improves endothelium-dependent vasorelaxation and prevents hypertension. *Cell Metab.* **2010**, *12*, 130–141. [CrossRef] [PubMed]

134. Poblete, I.M.; Orliac, M.L.; Briones, R.; Adler-Graschinsky, E.; Huidobro-Toro, J.P. Anandamide elicits an acute release of nitric oxide through endothelial TRPV1 receptor activation in the rat arterial mesenteric bed. *J. Physiol.* **2005**, *568*, 539–551. [CrossRef] [PubMed]

135. Randhawa, P.K.; Jaggi, A.S. TRPV1 channels in cardiovascular system: A double edged sword? *Int. J. Cardiol.* **2017**, *228*, 103–113. [CrossRef] [PubMed]

136. Di Marzo, V.; Bisogno, T.; De Petrocellis, L. Anandamide: Some like it hot. *Trends Pharmacol. Sci.* **2001**, *22*, 346–349. [CrossRef]

137. Starowicz, K.; Makuch, W.; Osikowicz, M.; Piscitelli, F.; Petrosino, S.; Di Marzo, V.; Przewlocka, B. Spinal anandamide produces analgesia in neuropathic rats: Possible CB_1- and TRPV1-mediated mechanisms. *Neuropharmacology* **2012**, *62*, 1746–1755. [CrossRef] [PubMed]

138. Mattace Raso, G.; Simeoli, R.; Russo, R.; Santoro, A.; Pirozzi, C.; d'Emmanuele di Villa Bianca, R.; Mitidieri, E.; Paciello, O.; Pagano, T.B.; Orefice, N.S.; et al. *N*-Palmitoylethanolamide protects the kidney from hypertensive injury in spontaneously hypertensive rats via inhibition of oxidative stress. *Pharmacol. Res.* **2013**, *76*, 67–76. [CrossRef] [PubMed]

139. Zoete, V.; Grosdidier, A.; Michielin, O. Peroxisome proliferator-activated receptor structures: Ligand specificity, molecular switch and interactions with regulators. *Biochim. Biophys. Acta* **2007**, *1771*, 915–925. [CrossRef] [PubMed]

140. Shin, S.J.; Lim, J.H.; Chung, S.; Youn, D.Y.; Chung, H.W.; Kim, H.W.; Lee, J.-H.; Chang, Y.S.; Park, C.W.; et al. Peroxisome proliferator-activated receptor-alpha activator fenofibrate prevents high-fat diet-induced renal lipotoxicity in spontaneously hypertensive rats. *Hypertens. Res.* **2009**, *32*, 835–845. [CrossRef] [PubMed]

141. Gelosa, P.; Banfi, C.; Gianella, A.; Brioschi, M.; Pignieri, A.; Nobili, E.; Castiglioni, L.; Cimino, M.; Tremoli, E.; Sironi, L. Peroxisome proliferator-activated receptor α agonism prevents renal damage and the oxidative stress and inflammatory processes affecting the brains of stroke-prone rats. *J. Pharmacol. Exp. Ther.* **2010**, *335*, 324–331. [CrossRef] [PubMed]

142. Rosenson, R.S.; Wolff, D.A.; Huskin, A.L.; Helenowski, I.B.; Rademaker, A.W. Fenofibrate therapy ameliorates fasting and postprandial lipoproteinemia, oxidative stress, and the inflammatory response in subjects with hypertriglyceridemia and the metabolic syndrome. *Diabetes Care* **2007**, *30*, 1945–1951. [CrossRef] [PubMed]

143. Sun, Y.; Alexander, S.P.H.; Kendall, D.A.; Bennett, A.J. Cannabinoids and PPARalpha signalling. *Biochem. Soc. Trans.* **2006**, *34*, 1095–1097. [CrossRef] [PubMed]

144. Bouaboula, M.; Hilairet, S.; Marchand, J.; Fajas, L.; Le Fur, G.; Casellas, P. Anandamide induced PPARgamma transcriptional activation and 3T3-L1 preadipocyte differentiation. *Eur. J. Pharmacol.* **2005**, *517*, 174–181. [CrossRef] [PubMed]

145. Du, H.; Chen, X.; Zhang, J.; Chen, C. Inhibition of COX-2 expression by endocannabinoid 2-arachidonoylglycerol is mediated via PPAR-γ. *Br. J. Pharmacol.* **2011**, *163*, 1533–1549. [CrossRef] [PubMed]

146. Baker, D.; Pryce, G.; Davies, W.L.; Hiley, C.R. In silico patent searching reveals a new cannabinoid receptor. *Trends Pharmacol. Sci.* **2006**, *27*, 1–4. [CrossRef] [PubMed]

147. Shah, U.; Kowalski, T.J. GPR119 agonists for the potential treatment of type 2 diabetes and related metabolic disorders. *Vitam. Horm.* **2010**, *84*, 415–448. [CrossRef] [PubMed]

148. Lauckner, J.E.; Jensen, J.B.; Chen, H.Y.; Lu, H.C.; Hille, B.; Mackie, K. GPR55 is a cannabinoid receptor that increases intracellular calcium and inhibits M current. *Proc. Natl. Acad. Sci. USA* **2008**, *105*, 2699–2704. [CrossRef] [PubMed]

149. Ohno-Shosaku, T.; Maejima, T.; Kano, M. Endogenous cannabinoids mediate retrograde signals from depolarized postsynaptic neurons to presynaptic terminals. *Neuron* **2001**, *29*, 729–738. [CrossRef]

150. Hashimotodani, Y.; Ohno-Shosaku, T.; Kano, M. Endocannabinoids and synaptic function in the CNS. *Neuroscientist* **2007**, *13*, 127–137. [CrossRef] [PubMed]

151. Oddi, S.; Fezza, F.; Pasquariello, N.; De Simone, C.; Rapino, C.; Dainese, E.; Finazzi-Agrò, A.; Maccarrone, M. Evidence for the intracellular accumulation of anandamide in adiposomes. *Cell. Mol. Life Sci.* **2008**, *65*, 840–850. [CrossRef] [PubMed]

152. Di Marzo, V.; Fontana, A.; Cadas, H.; Schinelli, S.; Cimino, G.; Schwartz, J.C.; Piomelli, D. Formation and inactivation of endogenous cannabinoid anandamide in central neurons. *Nature* **1994**, *372*, 686–691. [CrossRef] [PubMed]

153. Wang, J.; Ueda, N. Biology of endocannabinoid synthesis system. *Prostaglandins Other Lipid Mediat.* **2009**, *89*, 112–119. [CrossRef] [PubMed]

154. Cravatt, B.F.; Giang, D.K.; Mayfield, S.P.; Boger, D.L.; Lerner, R.A.; Gilula, N.B. Molecular characterization of an enzyme that degrades neuromodulatory fatty-acid amides. *Nature* **1996**, *384*, 83–87. [CrossRef] [PubMed]

155. Seillier, A.; Advani, T.; Cassano, T.; Hensler, J.G.; Giuffrida, A. Inhibition of fatty-acid amide hydrolase and CB1 receptor antagonism differentially affect behavioural responses in normal and PCP-treated rats. *Int. J. Neuropsychopharmacol.* **2010**, *13*, 373–386. [CrossRef] [PubMed]

156. Bedse, G.; Colangeli, R.; Lavecchia, A.M.; Romano, A.; Altieri, F.; Cifani, C.; Cassano, T.; Gaetani, S. Role of the basolateral amygdala in mediating the effects of the fatty acid amide hydrolase inhibitor URB597 on HPA axis response to stress. *Eur. Neuropsychopharmacol.* **2014**, *24*, 1511–1523. [CrossRef] [PubMed]

157. Di Marzo, V. Targeting the endocannabinoid system: To enhance or reduce? *Nat. Rev. Drug Discov.* **2008**, *7*, 438–455. [CrossRef] [PubMed]

158. Ueda, N.; Tsuboi, K.; Uyama, T. *N*-acylethanolamine metabolism with special reference to *N*-acylethanolamine-hydrolyzing acid amidase (NAAA). *Prog. Lipid Res.* **2010**, *49*, 299–315. [CrossRef] [PubMed]

159. Ueda, N.; Tsuboi, K.; Uyama, T.; Ohnishi, T. Biosynthesis and degradation of the endocannabinoid 2-arachidonoylglycerol. *Biofactors* **2011**, *37*, 1–7. [CrossRef] [PubMed]

160. Rouzer, C.A.; Marnett, L.J. Endocannabinoid oxygenation by cyclooxygenases, lipoxygenases, andcytochromes P450: Cross-talk between the eicosanoid and endocannabinoid signaling pathways. *Chem. Rev.* **2011**, *111*, 5899–5921. [CrossRef] [PubMed]

161. Bradshaw, H.B.; Walker, J.M. The expanding field of cannabimimetic and related lipid mediators. *Br. J. Pharmacol.* **2009**, *144*, 459–465. [CrossRef] [PubMed]

162. Berdyshev, E.V.; Schmid, P.C.; Krebsbach, R.J.; Hillard, C.J.; Huang, C.; Chen, N.; Dong, Z.; Schmid, H.H. Cannabinoid-receptor-independent cell signalling by *N*-acylethanolamines. *Biochem. J.* **2001**, *360*, 67–75. [CrossRef] [PubMed]

163. Azari, E.K.; Ramachandran, D.; Weibel, S.; Arnold, M.; Romano, A.; Gaetani, S.; Langhans, W.; Mansouri, A. Vagal afferents are not necessary for the satiety effect of the gut lipid messenger oleoylethanolamide. *Am. J. Physiol. Regul. Integr. Comp. Physiol.* **2014**, *307*, R167–R178. [CrossRef] [PubMed]

164. Provensi, G.; Coccurello, R.; Umehara, H.; Munari, L.; Giacovazzo, G.; Galeotti, N.; Nosi, D.; Gaetani, S.; Romano, A.; Moles, A.; et al. Satiety factor oleoylethanolamide recruits the brain histaminergic system to inhibit food intake. *Proc. Natl. Acad. Sci. USA* **2014**, *111*, 11527–11532. [CrossRef] [PubMed]

165. Romano, A.; Cassano, T.; Tempesta, B.; Cianci, S.; Dipasquale, P.; Coccurello, R.; Cuomo, V.; Gaetani, S. The satiety signal oleoylethanolamide stimulates oxytocin neurosecretion from rat hypothalamic neurons. *Peptides* **2013**, *49*, 21–26. [CrossRef] [PubMed]

166. Romano, A.; Karimian Azari, E.; Tempesta, B.; Mansouri, A.; Micioni Di Bonaventura, M.V.; Ramachandran, D.; Lutz, T.A.; Bedse, G.; Langhans, W.; Gaetani, S. High dietary fat intake influences the activation of specific hindbrain and hypothalamic nuclei by the satiety factor oleoylethanolamide. *Physiol. Behav.* **2014**, *136*, 55–62. [CrossRef] [PubMed]

167. Romano, A.; Coccurello, R.; Giacovazzo, G.; Bedse, G.; Moles, A.; Gaetani, S. Oleoylethanolamide: A novel potential pharmacological alternative to cannabinoid antagonists for the control of appetite. *Biomed. Res. Int.* **2014**, *2014*, 203425. [CrossRef] [PubMed]

168. Gaetani, S.; Kaye, W.H.; Cuomo, V.; Piomelli, D. Role of endocannabinoids and their analogues in obesity and eating disorders. *Eat. Weight Disord.* **2008**, *13*, e42–e48. [CrossRef] [PubMed]

169. Fidaleo, M.; Fanelli, F.; Ceru, M.P.; Moreno, S. Neuroprotective properties of peroxisome proliferator-activated receptor alpha (PPARα) and its lipid ligands. *Curr. Med. Chem.* **2014**, *21*, 2803–2821. [CrossRef] [PubMed]

170. Bedse, G.; Romano, A.; Lavecchia, A.M.; Cassano, T.; Gaetani, S. The role of endocannabinoid signaling in the molecular mechanisms of neurodegeneration in Alzheimer's disease. *J. Alzheimer Dis.* **2015**, *43*, 1115–1136. [CrossRef] [PubMed]

171. Scuderi, C.; Bronzuoli, M.R.; Facchinetti, R.; Pace, L.; Ferraro, L.; Broad, K.D.; Serviddio, G.; Bellanti, F.; Palombelli, G.; Carpinelli, G.; et al. Ultramicronized palmitoylethanolamide rescues learning and memory impairments in a triple transgenic mouse model of Alzheimer's disease by exerting anti-inflammatory and neuroprotective effects. *Transl. Psychiatry* **2018**, *8*, 32. [CrossRef] [PubMed]

172. Bronzuoli, M.R.; Facchinetti, R.; Steardo, L., Jr.; Romano, A.; Stecca, C.; Passarella, S.; Steardo, L.; Cassano, T.; Scuderi, C. Palmitoylethanolamide Dampens Reactive Astrogliosis and Improves Neuronal Trophic Support in a Triple Transgenic Model of Alzheimer's Disease: In Vitro and In Vivo Evidence. *Oxid. Med. Cell. Longev.* **2018**, *2018*, 4720532. [CrossRef] [PubMed]

173. Hanus, L.; Abu-Lafi, S.; Fride, E.; Breuer, A.; Vogel, Z.; Shalev, D.E.; Kustanovich, I.; Mechoulam, R. 2-arachidonyl glyceryl ether, an endogenous agonist of the cannabinoid CB1 receptor. *Proc. Natl. Acad. Sci. USA* **2001**, *98*, 3662–3665. [CrossRef] [PubMed]

174. Porter, A.C.; Sauer, J.M.; Knierman, M.D.; Becker, G.W.; Berna, M.J.; Bao, J.; Nomikos, G.G.; Carter, P.; Bymaster, F.P.; Leese, A.B.; et al. Characterization of a novel endocannabinoid, virodhamine, with antagonist activity at the CB1 receptor. *J. Pharmacol. Exp. Ther.* **2002**, *301*, 1020–1024. [CrossRef] [PubMed]

175. Sharir, H.; Console-Bram, L.; Mundy, C.; Popoff, S.N.; Kapur, A.; Abood, M.E. The Endocannabinoids Anandamide and Virodhamine Modulate the Activity of the Candidate Cannabinoid Receptor GPR55. *J. Neuroimmune Pharmacol.* **2012**, *7*, 856–865. [CrossRef] [PubMed]

176. Kohno, M.; Hasegawa, H.; Inoue, A.; Muraoka, M.; Miyazaki, T.; Oka, K.; Yasukawa, M. Identification of *N*-arachidonylglycine as the endogenous ligand for orphan G-protein-coupled receptor GPR18. *Biochem. Biophys. Res. Commun.* **2006**, *347*, 827–832. [CrossRef] [PubMed]

177. Lipina, C.; Hundal, H.S. Modulation of cellular redox homeostasis by the endocannabinoid system. *Open Biol.* **2016**, *6*, 150276. [CrossRef] [PubMed]

178. Horváth, B.; Mukhopadhyay, P.; Kechrid, M.; Patel, V.; Tanchian, G.; Wink, D.A.; Gertsch, J.; Pacher, P. β-Caryophyllene ameliorates cisplatin-induced nephrotoxicity in a cannabinoid 2 receptor-dependent manner. *Free Radic. Biol. Med.* **2012**, *52*, 1325–1333. [CrossRef] [PubMed]

179. Mukhopadhyay, P.; Pan, H.; Rajesh, M.; Batkai, S.; Patel, V.; Harvey-White, J.; Mukhopadhyay, B.; Hasko, G.; Gao, B.; Mackie, K.; et al. CB1 cannabinoid receptors promote oxidative/nitrosative stress, inflammation and cell death in a murine nephropathy model. *Br. J. Pharmacol.* **2010**, *160*, 657–668. [CrossRef] [PubMed]

180. Mukhopadhyay, P.; Rajesh, M.; Pan, H.; Patel, V.; Mukhopadhyay, B.; Bátkai, S.; Gao, B.; Haskó, G.; Pacher, P. Cannabinoid-2 receptor limits inflammation, oxidative/nitrosative stress, and cell death in nephropathy. *Free Radic. Biol. Med.* **2010**, *48*, 457–467. [CrossRef] [PubMed]

181. Mukhopadhyay, P.; Baggelaar, M.; Erdelyi, K.; Cao, Z.; Cinar, R.; Fezza, F.; Ignatowska-Janlowska, B.; Wilkerson, J.; van Gils, N.; Hansen, T.; et al. The novel, orally available and peripherally restricted selective cannabinoid CB2 receptor agonist LEI-101 prevents cisplatin-induced nephrotoxicity. *Br. J. Pharmacol.* **2016**, *173*, 446–458. [CrossRef] [PubMed]

182. Bedse, G.; Di Domenico, F.; Serviddio, G.; Cassano, T. Aberrant insulin signaling in Alzheimer's disease: Current knowledge. *Front. Neurosci.* **2015**, *9*, 204. [CrossRef] [PubMed]

183. Barone, E.; Di Domenico, F.; Cassano, T.; Arena, A.; Tramutola, A.; Lavecchia, M.A.; Coccia, R.; Butterfield, D.A.; Perluigi, M. Impairment of biliverdin reductase-A promotes brain insulin resistance in Alzheimer disease: A new paradigm. *Free Radic. Biol. Med.* **2016**, *91*, 127–142. [CrossRef] [PubMed]

184. Pardeshi, R.; Bolshette, N.; Gadhave, K.; Ahire, A.; Ahmed, S.; Cassano, T.; Gupta, V.B.; Lahkar, M. Insulin signaling: An opportunistic target to minify the risk of Alzheimer's disease. *Psychoneuroendocrinology* **2017**, *83*, 159–171. [CrossRef] [PubMed]

185. Gruden, G.; Barutta, F.; Kunos, G.; Pacher, P. Role of the endocannabinoid system in diabetes and diabetic complications. *Br. J. Pharmacol.* **2016**, *173*, 1116–1127. [CrossRef] [PubMed]

186. Pacher, P.; Hasko, G. Endocannabinoids and cannabinoid receptors in ischaemia-reperfusion injury and preconditioning. *Br. J. Pharmacol.* **2008**, *153*, 252–262. [CrossRef] [PubMed]

187. Silvestri, C.; Ligresti, A.; Di Marzo, V. Peripheral effects of the endocannabinoid system in energy homeostasis: Adipose tissue, liver and skeletal muscle. *Rev. Endocr. Metab. Disord.* **2011**, *12*, 153–162. [CrossRef] [PubMed]

188. Muriel, P. Role of free radicals in liver diseases. *Hepatol. Int.* **2009**, *3*, 526–536. [CrossRef] [PubMed]

189. Mukhopadhyay, P.; Horváth, B.; Rajesh, M.; Matsumoto, S.; Saito, K.; Bátkai, S.; Patel, V.; Tanchian, G.; Gao, R.Y.; Cravatt, B.F.; et al. Fatty acid amide hydrolase is a key regulator of endocannabinoid-induced myocardial tissue injury. *Free Radic. Biol. Med.* **2011**, *50*, 179–195. [CrossRef] [PubMed]

190. Rajesh, M.; Mukhopadhyay, P.; Haskó, G.; Liaudet, L.; Mackie, K.; Pacher, P. Cannabinoid-1 receptor activation induces reactive oxygen species-dependent and -independent mitogen-activated protein kinase activation and cell death in human coronary artery endothelial cells. *Br. J. Pharmacol.* **2010**, *160*, 688–700. [CrossRef] [PubMed]

191. Bátkai, S.; Osei-Hyiaman, D.; Pan, H.; El-Assal, O.; Rajesh, M.; Mukhopadhyay, P.; Hong, F.; Harvey-White, J.; Jafri, A.; Haskó, G.; et al. Cannabinoid-2 receptor mediates protection against hepatic ischemia/reperfusion injury. *FASEB J.* **2007**, *21*, 1788–1800. [CrossRef] [PubMed]

192. Rajesh, M.; Pan, H.; Mukhopadhyay, P.; Batkai, S.; Osei-Hyiaman, D.; Hasko, G.; Liaudet, L.; Gao, B.; Pacher, P. Cannabinoid-2 receptor agonist HU-308 protects against hepatic ischemia/reperfusion injury by attenuating oxidative stress, inflammatory response, and apoptosis. *J. Leukoc. Biol.* **2007**, *82*, 1382–1389. [CrossRef] [PubMed]

193. Montecucco, F.; Lenglet, S.; Braunersreuther, V.; Burger, F.; Pelli, G.; Bertolotto, M.; Mach, F.; Steffens, S. CB$_2$ cannabinoid receptor activation is cardioprotective in a mouse model of ischemia/reperfusion. *J. Mol. Cell. Cardiol.* **2009**, *46*, 612–620. [CrossRef] [PubMed]

194. Zhang, M.; Adler, M.W.; Abood, M.E.; Ganea, D.; Jallo, J.; Tuma, R.F. CB$_2$ receptor activation attenuates microcirculatory dysfunction during cerebral ischemic/reperfusion injury. *Microvasc. Res.* **2009**, *78*, 86–94. [CrossRef] [PubMed]

195. Murikinati, S.; Juttler, E.; Keinert, T.; Ridder, D.A.; Muhammad, S.; Waibler, Z.; Ledent, C.; Zimmer, A.; Kalinke, U.; Schwaninger, M. Activation of cannabinoid 2 receptors protects against cerebral ischemia by inhibiting neutrophil recruitment. *FASEB J.* **2009**. [CrossRef] [PubMed]

196. Steffens, S.; Veillard, N.R.; Arnaud, C.; Pelli, G.; Burger, F.; Staub, C.; Karsak, M.; Zimmer, A.; Frossard, J.L.; Mach, F. Low dose oral cannabinoid therapy reduces progression of atherosclerosis in mice. *Nature* **2005**, *434*, 782–786. [CrossRef] [PubMed]

197. Rajesh, M.; Mukhopadhyay, P.; Batkai, S.; Hasko, G.; Liaudet, L.; Huffman, J.W.; Csiszar, A.; Ungvari, Z.; Mackie, K.; Chatterjee, S.; et al. CB$_2$-receptor stimulation attenuates TNF-alpha-induced human endothelial cell activation, transendothelial migration of monocytes, and monocyte–endothelial adhesion. *Am. J. Physiol. Heart Circ. Physiol.* **2007**, *293*, H2210–H2218. [CrossRef] [PubMed]

198. Pacher, P.; Mechoulam, R. Is lipid signaling through cannabinoid 2 receptors part of a protective system? *Prog. Lipid Res.* **2011**, *50*, 193–211. [CrossRef] [PubMed]

199. Matthews, A.T.; Lee, J.H.; Borazjani, A.; Mangum, L.C.; Hou, X.; Ross, M.K. Oxyradical stress increases the biosynthesis of 2-arachidonoylglycerol: Involvement of NADPH oxidase. *Am. J. Physiol. Cell Physiol.* **2016**, *311*, C960–C974. [CrossRef] [PubMed]

200. Hoyer, F.F.; Steinmetz, M.; Zimmer, S.; Becker, A.; Lütjohann, D.; Buchalla, R.; Zimmer, A.; Nickenig, G. Atheroprotection via cannabinoid receptor-2 is mediated by circulating and vascular cells in vivo. *J. Mol. Cell. Cardiol.* **2011**, *51*, 1007–1014. [CrossRef] [PubMed]

201. Tiyerili, V.; Zimmer, S.; Jung, S.; Wassmann, K.; Naehle, C.P.; Lütjohann, D.; Zimmer, A.; Nickenig, G.; Wassmann, S. CB$_1$ receptor inhibition leads to decreased vascular AT1 receptor expression, inhibition of oxidative stress and improved endothelial function. *Basic Res. Cardiol.* **2010**, *105*, 465–477. [CrossRef] [PubMed]

202. Zolese, G.; Bacchetti, T.; Masciangelo, S.; Ragni, L.; Ambrosi, S.; Ambrosini, A.; Marini, M.; Ferretti, G. Effect of acylethanolamides on lipid peroxidation and paraoxonase activity. *Biofactors* **2008**, *33*, 201–209. [CrossRef] [PubMed]

203. Gulaya, N.M.; Kuzmenko, A.I.; Margitich, V.M.; Govseeva, N.M.; Melnichuk, S.D.; Goridko, T.M.; Zhukov, A.D. Long-chain *N*-acylethanolamines inhibit lipid peroxidation in rat liver mitochondria under acute hypoxic hypoxia. *Chem. Phys. Lipids* **1998**, *97*, 49–54. [CrossRef]

204. Poli, G.; Albano, E.; Dianzani, M.U. The role of lipid peroxidation in liver damage. *Chem. Phys. Lipids* **1987**, *45*, 117–142. [CrossRef]

205. Emerit, J.; Chaudiere, J. *Free Radicals and Lipid Peroxidation in Cell Biology*; Handbook of Free Radicals and Antioxidants in Biomedicine; CRC Press: Boca Raton, FL, USA, 1989; pp. 177–185.

206. Gulaya, N.M.; Melnik, A.A.; Balkov, D.I.; Volkov, G.L.; Vysotskiy, M.V.; Vaskovsky, V.E. The effect of long-chain *N*-acylethanolamines on some membrane-associated functions of neuroblastoma C1300 N18 cells. *Biochim. Biophys. Acta* **1993**, *1152*, 280–288. [CrossRef]

207. Parinandi, N.L.; Schmid, H.H. Effects of long-chain *N*-acylethanolamines on lipid peroxidation in cardiac mitochondria. *FEBS Lett.* **1988**, *237*, 49–52. [CrossRef]

208. Zolese, G.; Bacchetti, T.; Ambrosini, A.; Wozniak, M.; Bertoli, E.; Ferretti, G. Increased plasma concentrations of palmitoylethanolamide, an endogenous fatty acid amide, affect oxidative damage of human low-density lipoproteins: An in vitro study. *Atherosclerosis* **2005**, *182*, 47–55. [CrossRef] [PubMed]

209. Biernacki, M.; Łuczaj, W.; Gęgotek, A.; Toczek, M.; Bielawska, K.; Skrzydlewska, E. Crosstalk between liver antioxidant and the endocannabinoid systems after chronic administration of the FAAH inhibitor, URB597, to hypertensive rats. *Toxicol. Appl. Pharmacol.* **2016**, *301*, 31–41. [CrossRef] [PubMed]

210. Di Marzo, V.; Maccarrone, M. FAAH and anandamide: Is 2-AG really the odd one out? *Trends Pharmacol. Sci.* **2008**, *29*, 229–233. [CrossRef] [PubMed]

211. Basu, P.P.; Aloysius, M.M.; Shah, N.J.; Brown, R.S., Jr. Review article: The endocannabinoid system in liver disease, a potential therapeutic target. *Aliment. Pharmacol. Ther.* **2014**, *39*, 790–801. [CrossRef] [PubMed]

212. DeLeve, L.D.; Wang, X.; Kanel, G.C.; Atkinson, R.D.; McCuskey, R.S. Prevention of hepatic fibrosis in a murine model of metabolic syndrome with nonalcoholic steatohepatitis. *Am. J. Pathol.* **2008**, *173*, 993–1001. [CrossRef] [PubMed]

213. Mallat, A.; Teixeira-Clerc, F.; Lotersztajn, S. Cannabinoid signaling and liver therapeutics. *J. Hepatol.* **2013**, *59*, 891–896. [CrossRef] [PubMed]

214. Simonian, N.A.; Coyle, J.T. Oxidative stress in neurodegenerative diseases. *Annu. Rev. Pharmacol. Toxicol.* **1996**, *36*, 83–106. [CrossRef] [PubMed]

215. Behl, C. Alzheimer's disease and oxidative stress: Implications for novel therapeutic approaches. *Prog. Neurobiol.* **1999**, *57*, 301–323. [CrossRef]

216. Bedse, G.; Romano, A.; Cianci, S.; Lavecchia, A.M.; Lorenzo, P.; Elphick, M.R.; Laferla, F.M.; Vendemiale, G.; Grillo, C.; Altieri, F.; et al. Altered expression of the CB1 cannabinoid receptor in the triple transgenic mouse model of Alzheimer's disease. *J. Alzheimer Dis.* **2014**, *40*, 701–712. [CrossRef] [PubMed]

217. Gatta, E.; Lefebvre, T.; Gaetani, S.; dos Santos, M.; Marrocco, J.; Mir, A.M.; Cassano, T.; Maccari, S.; Nicoletti, F.; Mairesse, J. Evidence for an imbalance between tau O-GlcNAcylation and phosphorylation in the hippocampus of a mouse model of Alzheimer's disease. *Pharmacol. Res.* **2016**, *105*, 186–197. [CrossRef] [PubMed]

218. Milton, N.G. Role of hydrogen peroxide in the aetiology of Alzheimer's disease: Implications for treatment. *Drugs Aging* **2004**, *21*, 81–100. [CrossRef] [PubMed]

219. Ano, Y.; Sakudo, A.; Kimata, T.; Uraki, R.; Sugiura, K.; Onodera, T. Oxidative damage to neurons caused by the induction of microglial NADPH oxidase in encephalomyocarditis virus infection. *Neurosci. Lett.* **2010**, *469*, 39–43. [CrossRef] [PubMed]

220. Ye, Q.; Huang, B.; Zhang, X.; Zhu, Y.; Chen, X. Astaxanthin protects against MPP+-induced oxidative stress in PC12 cells via the HO-1/NOX2 axis. *BMC Neurosci.* **2012**, *13*, 156. [CrossRef] [PubMed]

221. Jia, J.; Ma, L.; Wu, M.; Zhang, L.; Zhang, X.; Zhai, Q.; Jiang, T.; Wang, Q.; Xiong, L. Anandamide protects HT22 cells exposed to hydrogen peroxide by inhibiting CB1 receptor-mediated type 2 NADPH oxidase. *Oxid. Med. Cell. Longev.* **2014**, *2014*, 893516. [CrossRef] [PubMed]

222. Chung, Y.C.; Bok, E.; Huh, S.H.; Park, J.Y.; Yoon, S.H.; Kim, S.R.; Kim, Y.S.; Maeng, S.; Park, S.H.; Jin, B.K. Cannabinoid receptor type 1 protects nigrostriatal dopaminergic neurons against MPTP neurotoxicity by inhibiting microglial activation. *J. Immunol.* **2011**, *187*, 6508–6517. [CrossRef] [PubMed]

223. Cassano, T.; Calcagnini, S.; Pace, L.; De Marco, F.; Romano, A.; Gaetani, S. Cannabinoid Receptor 2 Signaling in Neurodegenerative Disorders: From Pathogenesis to a Promising Therapeutic Target. *Front. Neurosci.* **2017**, *11*, 30. [CrossRef] [PubMed]

224. Jayant, S.; Sharma, B.M.; Bansal, R.; Sharma, B. Pharmacological benefits of selective modulation of cannabinoid receptor type 2 (CB2) in experimental Alzheimer's disease. *Pharmacol. Biochem. Behav.* **2016**, *140*, 39–50. [CrossRef] [PubMed]

225. Koppel, J.; Vingtdeux, V.; Marambaud, P.; d'Abramo, C.; Jimenez, H.; Stauber, M.; Friedman, R.; Davies, P. CB2 receptor deficiency increases amyloid pathology and alters tau processing in a transgenic mouse model of Alzheimer's disease. *Mol. Med.* **2014**, *20*, 29–36. [CrossRef] [PubMed]

226. Chen, R.; Zhang, J.; Wu, Y.; Wang, D.; Feng, G.; Tang, Y.P.; Teng, Z.; Chen, C. Monoacylglycerol lipase is a therapeutic target for Alzheimer's disease. *Cell Rep.* **2012**, *2*, 1329–1339. [CrossRef] [PubMed]

227. Paloczi, J.; Varga, Z.V.; Hasko, G.; Pacher, P. Neuroprotection in Oxidative Stress-Related Neurodegenerative Diseases: Role of Endocannabinoid System Modulation. *Antioxid. Redox Signal.* **2018**, *29*, 75–108. [CrossRef] [PubMed]

228. Pihlaja, R.; Takkinen, J.; Eskola, O.; Vasara, J.; López-Picón, F.R.; Haaparanta-Solin, M.; Rinne, J.O. Monoacylglycerol lipase inhibitor JZL184 reduces neuroinflammatory response in APdE9 mice and in adult mouse glial cells. *J. Neuroinflamm.* **2015**, *12*, 81. [CrossRef] [PubMed]

229. Kessiova, M.; Alexandrova, A.; Georgieva, A.; Kirkova, M.; Todorov, S. In vitro effects of CB1 receptor ligands on lipid peroxidation and antioxidant defense systems in the rat brain. *Pharmacol. Rep.* **2006**, *58*, 870–875. [PubMed]

230. Sun, H.J.; Lu, Y.; Wang, H.W.; Zhang, H.; Wang, S.R.; Xu, W.Y.; Fu, H.L.; Yao, X.Y.; Yang, F.; Yuan, H.B. Activation of Endocannabinoid Receptor 2 as a Mechanism of Propofol Pretreatment-Induced Cardioprotection against Ischemia-Reperfusion Injury in Rats. *Oxid. Med. Cell. Longev.* **2017**, *2017*, 2186383. [CrossRef] [PubMed]

231. Hayn, M.H.; Ballesteros, I.; de Miguel, F.; Coyle, C.H.; Tyagi, S.; Yoshimura, N.; Chancellor, M.B.; Tyagi, P. Functional and immunohistochemical characterization of CB1 and CB2 receptors in rat bladder. *Urology* **2008**, *72*, 1174–1178. [CrossRef] [PubMed]

232. Wang, Z.Y.; Wang, P.; Bjorling, D.E. Activation of cannabinoid receptor 2 inhibits experimental cystitis. *Am. J. Physiol. Regul. Integr. Comp. Physiol.* **2013**, *304*, R846–R853. [CrossRef] [PubMed]

233. Hermanson, D.J.; Marnett, L.J. Cannabinoids endocannabinoids, and cancer. *Cancer Metastasis Rev.* **2011**, *30*, 599–612. [CrossRef] [PubMed]

234. Ravi, J.; Sneh, A.; Shilo, K.; Nasser, M.W.; Ganju, R.K. FAAH inhibition enhances anandamide mediated anti-tumorigenic effects in non-small cell lung cancer by downregulating the EGF/EGFR pathway. *Oncotarget* **2014**, *5*, 2475–2486. [CrossRef] [PubMed]

235. Clapham, D.E.; Runnels, L.W.; Strübing, C. The TRP ion channel family. *Nat. Rev. Neurosci.* **2001**, *2*, 387–396. [CrossRef] [PubMed]

236. Harteneck, C.; Plant, T.D.; Schultz, G. From worm to man: Three subfamilies of TRP channels. *Trends Neurosci.* **2000**, *23*, 159–166. [CrossRef]

237. Wu, L.J.; Sweet, T.B.; Clapham, D.E. International Union of Basic and Clinical Pharmacology. LXXVI. Current progress in the mammalian TRP ion channel family. *Pharmacol. Rev.* **2010**, *62*, 381–404. [CrossRef] [PubMed]

238. Venkatachalam, K.; Montell, C. TRP channels. *Annu. Rev. Biochem.* **2007**, *76*, 387–417. [CrossRef] [PubMed]

239. Moran, M.M.; Xu, H.; Clapham, D.E. TRP ion channels in the nervous system. *Curr. Opin. Neurobiol.* **2004**, *14*, 362–369. [CrossRef] [PubMed]

240. Desai, B.N.; Clapham, D.E. TRP channels and mice deficient in TRP channels. *Pflugers Arch.* **2005**, *451*, 11–18. [CrossRef] [PubMed]

241. Vriens, J.; Appendino, G.; Nilius, B. Pharmacology of vanilloid transient receptor potential cation channels. *Mol. Pharmacol.* **2009**, *75*, 1262–1279. [CrossRef] [PubMed]

242. Cavanaugh, D.J.; Chesler, A.T.; Jackson, A.C.; Sigal, Y.M.; Yamanaka, H.; Grant, R.; O'Donnell, D.; Nicoll, R.A.; Shah, N.M.; Julius, D.; et al. *Trpv1* reporter mice reveal highly restricted brain distribution and functional expression in arteriolar smooth muscle cells. *J. Neurosci.* **2011**, *31*, 5067–5077. [CrossRef] [PubMed]

243. Caterina, M.J.; Schumacher, M.A.; Tominaga, M.; Rosen, T.A.; Levine, J.D.; Julius, D. The capsaicin receptor: A heat-activated ion channel in the pain pathway. *Nature* **1997**, *389*, 816–824. [CrossRef] [PubMed]

244. Tominaga, M.; Caterina, M.J.; Malmberg, A.B.; Rosen, T.A.; Gilbert, H.; Skinner, K.; Raumann, B.E.; Basbaum, A.I.; Julius, D. The cloned capsaicin receptor integrates multiple pain-producing stimuli. *Neuron* **1998**, *21*, 531–543. [CrossRef]

245. Jordt, S.E.; Tominaga, M.; Julius, D. Acid potentiation of the capsaicin receptor determined by a key extracellular site. *Proc. Natl. Acad. Sci. USA* **2000**, *97*, 8134–8139. [CrossRef] [PubMed]

246. Iida, T.; Moriyama, T.; Kobata, K.; Morita, A.; Murayama, N.; Hashizume, S.; Fushiki, T.; Yazawa, S.; Watanabe, T.; Tominaga, M. TRPV1 activation and induction of nociceptive response by a non-pungent capsaicin-like compound, capsiate. *Neuropharmacology* **2003**, *44*, 958–967. [CrossRef]

247. Blednov, Y.A.; Harris, R.A. Deletion of vanilloid receptor (TRPV1) in mice alters behavioral effects of ethanol. *Neuropharmacology* **2009**, *56*, 814–820. [CrossRef] [PubMed]

248. Ellingson, J.M.; Silbaugh, B.C.; Brasser, S.M. Reduced oral ethanol avoidance in mice lacking transient receptor potential channel vanilloid receptor 1. *Behav. Genet.* **2009**, *39*, 62–72. [CrossRef] [PubMed]

249. Ahern, G.P. Activation of TRPV1 by the satiety factor oleoylethanolamide. *J. Biol. Chem.* **2003**, *278*, 30429–30434. [CrossRef] [PubMed]

250. Huang, S.M.; Bisogno, T.; Trevisani, M.; Al-Hayani, A.; De Petrocellis, L.; Fezza, F.; Tognetto, M.; Petros, T.J.; Krey, J.F.; Chu, C.J.; et al. An endogenous capsaicin-like substance with high potency at recombinant and native vanilloid VR1 receptors. *Proc. Natl. Acad. Sci. USA* **2002**, *99*, 8400–8405. [CrossRef] [PubMed]

251. Chu, C.J.; Huang, S.M.; De Petrocellis, L.; Bisogno, T.; Ewing, S.A.; Miller, J.D.; Zipkin, R.E.; Daddario, N.; Appendino, G.; Di Marzo, V.; et al. *N*-oleoyldopamine, a novel endogenous capsaicin-like lipid that produces hyperalgesia. *J. Biol. Chem.* **2003**, *278*, 13633–13639. [CrossRef] [PubMed]

252. Hwang, S.W.; Cho, H.; Kwak, J.; Lee, S.Y.; Kang, C.J.; Jung, J.; Cho, S.; Min, K.H.; Suh, Y.G.; Kim, D.; et al. Direct activation of capsaicin receptors by products of lipoxygenases: Endogenous capsaicin-like substances. *Proc. Natl. Acad. Sci. USA* **2000**, *97*, 6155–6160. [CrossRef] [PubMed]

253. Numazaki, M.; Tominaga, T.; Takeuchi, K.; Murayama, N.; Toyooka, H.; Tominaga, M. Structural determinant of TRPV1 desensitization interacts with calmodulin. *Proc. Natl. Acad. Sci. USA* **2003**, *100*, 8002–8006. [CrossRef] [PubMed]

254. Rosenbaum, T.; Gordon-Shaag, A.; Munari, M.; Gordon, S.E. Ca^{2+}/calmodulin modulates TRPV1 activation by capsaicin. *J. Gen. Physiol.* **2004**, *123*, 53–62. [CrossRef] [PubMed]

255. Lishko, P.V.; Procko, E.; Jin, X.; Phelps, C.B.; Gaudet, R. The ankyrin repeats of TRPV1 bind multiple ligands and modulate channel sensitivity. *Neuron* **2007**, *54*, 905–918. [CrossRef] [PubMed]

256. Kwon, Y.; Hofmann, T.; Montell, C. Integration of phosphoinositide- and calmodulin-mediated regulation of TRPC6. *Mol. Cell* **2007**, *25*, 491–503. [CrossRef] [PubMed]

257. Premkumar, L.S.; Ahern, G.P. Induction of vanilloid receptor channel activity by protein kinase C. *Nature* **2000**, *408*, 985–990. [CrossRef] [PubMed]

258. De Petrocellis, L.; Harrison, S.; Bisogno, T.; Tognetto, M.; Brandi, I.; Smith, G.D.; Creminon, C.; Davis, J.B.; Geppetti, P.; Di Marzo, V. The vanilloid receptor (VR1)-mediated effects of anandamide are potently enhanced by the cAMP-dependent protein kinase. *J. Neurochem.* **2001**, *77*, 1660–1663. [CrossRef] [PubMed]

259. Docherty, R.J.; Yeats, J.C.; Bevan, S.; Boddeke, H.W. Inhibition of calcineurin inhibits the desensitization of capsaicin-evoked currents in cultured dorsal root ganglion neurones from adult rats. *Pflugers Arch.* **1996**, *431*, 828–837. [CrossRef] [PubMed]

260. Birder, L.A.; Nakamura, Y.; Kiss, S.; Nealen, M.L.; Barrick, S.; Kanai, A.J.; Wang, E.; Ruiz, G.; De Groat, W.C.; Apodaca, G.; et al. Altered urinary bladder function in mice lacking the vanilloid receptor TRPV1. *Nat. Neurosci.* **2002**, *5*, 856–860. [CrossRef] [PubMed]

261. Rong, W.; Hillsley, K.; Davis, J.B.; Hicks, G.; Winchester, W.J.; Grundy, D. Jejunal afferent nerve sensitivity in wild-type and TRPV1 knockout mice. *J. Physiol.* **2004**, *560*, 867–881. [CrossRef] [PubMed]

262. Treesukosol, Y.; Lyall, V.; Heck, G.L.; DeSimone, J.A.; Spector, A.C. A psychophysical and electrophysiological analysis of salt taste in *Trpv1* null mice. *Am. J. Physiol. Regul. Integr. Comp. Physiol.* **2007**, *292*, R1799–R1809. [CrossRef] [PubMed]

263. Cagiano, R.; Cassano, T.; Coluccia, A.; Gaetani, S.; Giustino, A.; Steardo, L.; Tattoli, M.; Trabace, L.; Cuomo, V. Genetic factors involved in the effects of developmental low-level alcohol induced behavioral alterations in rats. *Neuropsychopharmacology* **2002**, *26*, 191–203. [CrossRef]

264. Geppetti, P.; Materazzi, S.; Nicoletti, P. The transient receptor potential vanilloid 1: Role in airway inflammation and disease. *Eur. J. Pharmacol.* **2006**, *533*, 207–214. [CrossRef] [PubMed]

265. Gupta, S.; Sharma, B.; Singh, P.; Sharma, B.M. Modulation of transient receptor potential vanilloid subtype 1 (TRPV1) and norepinephrine transporters (NET) protect against oxidative stress, cellular injury, and vascular dementia. *Curr. Neurovasc. Res.* **2014**, *11*, 94–106. [CrossRef] [PubMed]

266. Gupta, S.; Sharma, B. Pharmacological benefits of agomelatine and vanillin in experimental model of Huntington's disease. *Pharmacol. Biochem. Behav.* **2014**, *122*, 122–135. [CrossRef] [PubMed]

267. Cao, Z.; Balasubramanian, A.; Marrelli, S.P. Pharmacologically induced hypothermia via TRPV1 channel agonism provides neuroprotection following ischemic stroke when initiated 90 min after reperfusion. *Am. J. Physiol. Regul. Integr. Comp. Physiol.* **2014**, *306*, R149–R156. [CrossRef] [PubMed]

268. Neeper, M.P.; Liu, Y.; Hutchinson, T.L.; Wang, Y.; Flores, C.M.; Qin, N. Activation properties of heterologously expressed mammalian TRPV2: Evidence for species dependence. *J. Biol. Chem.* **2007**, *282*, 15894–15902. [CrossRef] [PubMed]

269. Caterina, M.J.; Rosen, T.A.; Tominaga, M.; Brake, A.J.; Julius, D. A capsaicin-receptor homologue with a high threshold for noxious heat. *Nature* **1999**, *398*, 436–441. [CrossRef] [PubMed]

270. Szöllősi, A.G.; Oláh, A.; Tóth, I.B.; Papp, F.; Czifra, G.; Panyi, G.; Bíró, T. Transient receptor potential vanilloid-2 mediates the effects of transient heat shock on endocytosis of human monocyte-derived dendritic cells. *FEBS Lett.* **2013**, *587*, 1440–1445. [CrossRef] [PubMed]

271. Saito, M.; Hanson, P.I.; Schlesinger, P. Luminal chloride-dependent activation of endosome calcium channels: Patch clamp study of enlarged endosomes. *J. Biol. Chem.* **2007**, *282*, 27327–27333. [CrossRef] [PubMed]

272. Abe, K.; Puertollano, R. Role of TRP channels in the regulation of the endosomal pathway. *Physiology* **2011**, *26*, 14–22. [CrossRef] [PubMed]

273. Lévêque, M.; Penna, A.; Le Trionnaire, S.; Belleguic, C.; Desrues, B.; Brinchault, G.; Jouneau, S.; Lagadic-Gossmann, D.; Martin-Chouly, C. Phagocytosis depends on TRPV2-mediated calcium influx and requires TRPV2 in lipids rafts: Alteration in macrophages from patients with cystic fibrosis. *Sci. Rep.* **2018**, *8*, 4310. [CrossRef] [PubMed]

274. Link, T.M.; Park, U.; Vonakis, B.M.; Raben, D.M.; Soloski, M.J.; Caterina, M.J. TRPV2 has a pivotal role in macrophage particle binding and phagocytosis. *Nat. Immunol.* **2010**, *11*, 232–239. [CrossRef] [PubMed]

275. Peier, A.M.; Reeve, A.J.; Andersson, D.A.; Moqrich, A.; Earley, T.J.; Hergarden, A.C.; Story, G.M.; Colley, S.; Hogenesch, J.B.; McIntyre, P.; et al. A heat-sensitive TRP channel expressed in keratinocytes. *Science* **2002**, *296*, 2046–2049. [CrossRef] [PubMed]

276. Smith, G.D.; Gunthorpe, M.J.; Kelsell, R.E.; Hayes, P.D.; Reilly, P.; Facer, P.; Wright, J.E.; Jerman, J.C.; Walhin, J.P.; Ooi, L.; Egerton, J.; et al. TRPV3 is a temperature-sensitive vanilloid receptor-like protein. *Nature* **2002**, *418*, 186–190. [CrossRef] [PubMed]

277. Moqrich, A.; Hwang, S.W.; Earley, T.J.; Petrus, M.J.; Murray, A.N.; Spencer, K.S.; Andahazy, M.; Story, G.M.; Patapoutian, A. Impaired thermosensation in mice lacking TRPV3, a heat and camphor sensor in the skin. *Science* **2005**, *307*, 1468–1472. [CrossRef] [PubMed]

278. Xu, H.; Delling, M.; Jun, J.C.; Clapham, D.E. Oregano, thyme and clove-derived flavors and skin sensitizers activate specific TRP channels. *Nat. Neurosci.* **2006**, *9*, 628–635. [CrossRef] [PubMed]

279. Phelps, C.B.; Wang, R.R.; Choo, S.S.; Gaudet, R. Differential regulation of TRPV1, TRPV3, and TRPV4 sensitivity through a conserved binding site on the ankyrin repeat domain. *J. Biol. Chem.* **2010**, *285*, 731–740. [CrossRef] [PubMed]

280. Mandadi, S.; Sokabe, T.; Shibasaki, K.; Katanosaka, K.; Mizuno, A.; Moqrich, A.; Patapoutian, A.; Fukumi-Tominaga, T.; Mizumura, K.; Tominaga, M. TRPV3 in keratinocytes transmits temperature information to sensory neurons via ATP. *Pflugers Arch.* **2009**, *458*, 1093–1102. [CrossRef] [PubMed]

281. Huang, S.M.; Lee, H.; Chung, M.K.; Park, U.; Yu, Y.Y.; Bradshaw, H.B.; Coulombe, P.A.; Walker, J.M.; Caterina, M.J. Overexpressed transient receptor potential vanilloid 3 ion channels in skin keratinocytes modulate pain sensitivity via prostaglandin E2. *J. Neurosci.* **2008**, *28*, 13727–13737. [CrossRef] [PubMed]

282. Chung, M.K.; Lee, H.; Mizuno, A.; Suzuki, M.; Caterina, M.J. TRPV3 and TRPV4 mediate warmth-evoked currents in primary mouse keratinocytes. *J. Biol. Chem.* **2004**, *279*, 21569–21575. [CrossRef] [PubMed]

283. Liedtke, W.; Choe, Y.; Martí-Renom, M.A.; Bell, A.M.; Denis, C.S.; Sali, A.; Hudspeth, A.J.; Friedman, J.M.; Heller, S. Vanilloid receptor-related osmotically activated channel (VR-OAC), a candidate vertebrate osmoreceptor. *Cell* **2000**, *103*, 525–535. [CrossRef]

284. Güler, A.D.; Lee, H.; Iida, T.; Shimizu, I.; Tominaga, M.; Caterina, M. Heat-evoked activation of the ion channel, TRPV4. *J. Neurosci.* **2002**, *22*, 6408–6414. [CrossRef] [PubMed]

285. Watanabe, H.; Vriens, J.; Prenen, J.; Droogmans, G.; Voets, T.; Nilius, B. Anandamide and arachidonic acid use epoxyeicosatrienoic acids to activate TRPV4 channels. *Nature* **2003**, *424*, 434–438. [CrossRef] [PubMed]

286. Vriens, J.; Owsianik, G.; Fisslthaler, B.; Suzuki, M.; Janssens, A.; Voets, T.; Morisseau, C.; Hammock, B.D.; Fleming, I.; Busse, R.; et al. Modulation of the Ca^2 permeable cation channel TRPV4 by cytochrome P450 epoxygenases in vascular endothelium. *Circ. Res.* **2005**, *97*, 908–915. [CrossRef] [PubMed]

287. Strotmann, R.; Semtner, M.; Kepura, F.; Plant, T.D.; Schöneberg, T. Interdomain interactions control Ca^{2+}-dependent potentiation in the cation channel TRPV4. *PLoS ONE* **2010**, *5*, e10580. [CrossRef] [PubMed]

288. White, J.P.; Cibelli, M.; Urban, L.; Nilius, B.; McGeown, J.G.; Nagy, I. TRPV4: Molecular Conductor of a Diverse Orchestra. *Physiol. Rev.* **2016**, *96*, 911–973. [CrossRef] [PubMed]

289. Takahashi, N.; Hamada-Nakahara, S.; Itoh, Y.; Takemura, K.; Shimada, A.; Ueda, Y.; Kitamata, M.; Matsuoka, R.; Hanawa-Suetsugu, K.; Senju, Y.; et al. TRPV4 channel activity is modulated by direct interaction of the ankyrin domain to PI(4,5)P$_2$. *Nat. Commun.* **2014**, *5*, 4994. [CrossRef] [PubMed]

290. Gao, X.; Wu, L.; O'Neil, R.G. Temperature-modulated diversity of TRPV4 channel gating: Activation by physical stresses and phorbol ester derivatives through protein kinase C-dependent and -independent pathways. *J. Biol. Chem.* **2003**, *278*, 27129–27137. [CrossRef] [PubMed]

291. Fan, H.C.; Zhang, X.; McNaughton, P.A. Activation of the TRPV4 ion channel is enhanced by phosphorylation. *J. Biol. Chem.* **2009**, *284*, 27884–27891. [CrossRef] [PubMed]

292. Wegierski, T.; Lewandrowski, U.; Müller, B.; Sickmann, A.; Walz, G. Tyrosine phosphorylation modulates the activity of TRPV4 in response to defined stimuli. *J. Biol. Chem.* **2009**, *284*, 2923–2933. [CrossRef] [PubMed]

293. Lee, E.J.; Shin, S.H.; Chun, J.; Hyun, S.; Kim, Y.; Kang, S.S. The modulation of TRPV4 channel activity through its Ser 824 residue phosphorylation by SGK1. *Anim. Cells Syst.* **2010**, *14*, 99–114. [CrossRef]

294. Delany, N.S.; Hurle, M.; Facer, P.; Alnadaf, T.; Plumpton, C.; Kinghorn, I.; See, C.G.; Costigan, M.; Anand, P.; Woolf, C.J.; et al. Identification and characterization of a novel human vanilloid receptor-like protein, VRL-2. *Physiol. Genom.* **2001**, *4*, 165–174. [CrossRef] [PubMed]

295. Schumacher, M.A.; Jong, B.E.; Frey, S.L.; Sudanagunta, S.P.; Capra, N.F.; Levine, J.D. The stretch-inactivated channel, a vanilloid receptor variant, is expressed in small-diameter sensory neurons in the rat. *Neurosci. Lett.* **2000**, *287*, 215–218. [CrossRef]

296. Suzuki, M.; Mizuno, A.; Kodaira, K.; Imai, M. Impaired pressure sensation in mice lacking TRPV4. *J. Biol. Chem.* **2003**, *278*, 22664–22668. [CrossRef] [PubMed]

297. Birder, L.; Kullmann, F.A.; Lee, H.; Barrick, S.; de Groat, W.; Kanai, A.; Caterina, M. Activation of urothelial transient receptor potential vanilloid 4 by 4alpha-phorbol 12,13-didecanoate contributes to altered bladder reflexes in the rat. *J. Pharmacol. Exp. Ther.* **2007**, *323*, 227–235. [CrossRef] [PubMed]

298. Gevaert, T.; Vriens, J.; Segal, A.; Everaerts, W.; Roskams, T.; Talavera, K.; Owsianik, G.; Liedtke, W.; Daelemans, D.; Dewachter, I.; et al. Deletion of the transient receptor potential cation channel TRPV4 impairs murine bladder voiding. *J. Clin. Investig.* **2007**, *117*, 3453–3462. [CrossRef] [PubMed]

299. Alvarez, D.F.; King, J.A.; Weber, D.; Addison, E.; Liedtke, W.; Townsley, M.I. Transient receptor potential vanilloid 4-mediated disruption of the alveolar septal barrier: A novel mechanism of acute lung injury. *Circ. Res.* **2006**, *99*, 988–995. [CrossRef] [PubMed]

300. Hamanaka, K.; Jian, M.Y.; Weber, D.S.; Alvarez, D.F.; Townsley, M.I.; Al-Mehdi, A.B.; King, J.A.; Liedtke, W.; Parker, J.C. TRPV4 initiates the acute calcium-dependent permeability increase during ventilator-induced lung injury in isolated mouse lungs. *Am. J. Physiol. Lung Cell. Mol. Physiol.* **2007**, *293*, L923–L932. [CrossRef] [PubMed]

301. Alessandri-Haber, N.; Dina, O.A.; Joseph, E.K.; Reichling, D.; Levine, J.D. A transient receptor potential vanilloid 4-dependent mechanism of hyperalgesia is engaged by concerted action of inflammatory mediators. *J. Neurosci.* **2006**, *26*, 3864–3874. [CrossRef] [PubMed]

302. Vennekens, R.; Hoenderop, J.G.; Prenen, J.; Stuiver, M.; Willems, P.H.; Droogmans, G.; Nilius, B.; Bindels, R.J. Permeation and gating properties of the novel epithelial Ca^{2+} channel. *J. Biol. Chem.* **2000**, *275*, 3963–3969. [CrossRef] [PubMed]

303. Yue, L.; Peng, J.B.; Hediger, M.A.; Clapham, D.E. CaT1 manifests the pore properties of the calcium-release-activated calcium channel. *Nature* **2001**, *410*, 705–709. [CrossRef] [PubMed]

304. Clapham, D.E. TRP channels as cellular sensors. *Nature* **2003**, *426*, 517–524. [CrossRef] [PubMed]

305. Hoenderop, J.G.; Vennekens, R.; Müller, D.; Prenen, J.; Droogmans, G.; Bindels, R.J.; Nilius, B. Function and expression of the epithelial Ca^{2+} channel family: Comparison of mammalian ECaC1 and 2. *J. Physiol.* **2001**, *537*, 747–761. [CrossRef] [PubMed]

306. Lambers, T.T.; Weidema, A.F.; Nilius, B.; Hoenderop, J.G.; Bindels, R.J. Regulation of the mouse epithelial Ca^{2+} channel TRPV6 by the Ca^{2+}-sensor calmodulin. *J. Biol. Chem.* **2004**, *279*, 28855–28861. [CrossRef] [PubMed]

307. Niemeyer, B.A.; Bergs, C.; Wissenbach, U.; Flockerzi, V.; Trost, C. Competitive regulation of CaT-like-mediated Ca^{2+} entry by protein kinase C and calmodulin. *Proc. Natl. Acad. Sci. USA* **2001**, *98*, 3600–3605. [CrossRef] [PubMed]

308. Nilius, B.; Vennekens, R.; Prenen, J.; Hoenderop, J.G.; Bindels, R.J.; Droogmans, G. Whole-cell and single channel monovalent cation currents through the novel rabbit epithelial Ca^{2+} channel ECaC. *J. Physiol.* **2000**, *527 Pt 2*, 239–248. [CrossRef] [PubMed]

309. Voets, T.; Janssens, A.; Prenen, J.; Droogmans, G.; Nilius, B. Mg^{2+}-dependent gating and strong inward rectification of the cation channel TRPV6. *J. Gen. Physiol.* **2003**, *121*, 245–260. [CrossRef] [PubMed]

310. Lee, J.; Cha, S.K.; Sun, T.J.; Huang, C.L. PIP2 activates TRPV5 and releases its inhibition by intracellular Mg^{2+}. *J. Gen. Physiol.* **2005**, *126*, 439–451. [CrossRef] [PubMed]

311. Rohács, T.; Lopes, C.M.; Michailidis, I.; Logothetis, D.E. PI(4,5)P2 regulates the activation and desensitization of TRPM8 channels through the TRP domain. *Nat. Neurosci.* **2005**, *8*, 626–634. [CrossRef] [PubMed]

312. Thyagarajan, B.; Lukacs, V.; Rohacs, T. Hydrolysis of phosphatidylinositol 4,5-bisphosphate mediates calcium-induced inactivation of TRPV6 channels. *J. Biol. Chem.* **2008**, *283*, 14980–14987. [CrossRef] [PubMed]

313. Thyagarajan, B.; Benn, B.S.; Christakos, S.; Rohacs, T. Phospholipase C-mediated regulation of transient receptor potential vanilloid 6 channels: Implications in active intestinal Ca^{2+} transport. *Mol. Pharmacol.* **2009**, *75*, 608–616. [CrossRef] [PubMed]

314. Hoenderop, J.G.; van der Kemp, A.W.; Hartog, A.; van de Graaf, S.F.; van Os, C.H.; Willems, P.H.; Bindels, R.J. Molecular identification of the apical Ca^{2+} channel in 1, 25-dihydroxyvitamin D3-responsive epithelia. *J. Biol. Chem.* **1999**, *274*, 8375–8378. [CrossRef] [PubMed]

315. Hoenderop, J.G.; van Leeuwen, J.P.; van der Eerden, B.C.; Kersten, F.F.; van der Kemp, A.W.; Mérillat, A.M.; Waarsing, J.H.; Rossier, B.C.; Vallon, V.; Hummler, E.; et al. Renal Ca^{2+} wasting, hyperabsorption, and reduced bone thickness in mice lacking TRPV5. *J. Clin. Investig.* **2003**, *112*, 1906–1914. [CrossRef] [PubMed]

316. Van der Eerden, B.C.; Hoenderop, J.G.; de Vries, T.J.; Schoenmaker, T.; Buurman, C.J.; Uitterlinden, A.G.; Pols, H.A.; Bindels, R.J.; van Leeuwen, J.P. The epithelial Ca^{2+} channel TRPV5 is essential for proper osteoclastic bone resorption. *Proc. Natl. Acad. Sci. USA* **2005**, *102*, 17507–17512. [CrossRef] [PubMed]

317. Peng, J.B.; Chen, X.Z.; Berger, U.V.; Weremowicz, S.; Morton, C.C.; Vassilev, P.M.; Brown, E.M.; Hediger, M.A. Human calcium transport protein CaT1. *Biochem. Biophys. Res. Commun.* **2000**, *278*, 326–332. [CrossRef] [PubMed]

318. Hirnet, D.; Olausson, J.; Fecher-Trost, C.; Bödding, M.; Nastainczyk, W.; Wissenbach, U.; Flockerzi, V.; Freichel, M. The TRPV6 gene, cDNA and protein. *Cell Calcium* **2003**, *33*, 509–518. [CrossRef]

319. Peng, J.B.; Chen, X.Z.; Berger, U.V.; Vassilev, P.M.; Tsukaguchi, H.; Brown, E.M.; Hediger, M.A. Molecular cloning and characterization of a channel-like transporter mediating intestinal calcium absorption. *J. Biol. Chem.* **1999**, *274*, 22739–22746. [CrossRef] [PubMed]

320. Zhuang, L.; Peng, J.B.; Tou, L.; Takanaga, H.; Adam, R.M.; Hediger, M.A.; Freeman, M.R. Calcium-selective ion channel, CaT1, is apically localized in gastrointestinal tract epithelia and is aberrantly expressed in human malignancies. *Lab. Investig.* **2002**, *82*, 1755–1764. [CrossRef] [PubMed]

321. Nijenhuis, T.; Hoenderop, J.G.; van der Kemp, A.W.; Bindels, R.J. Localization and regulation of the epithelial Ca^{2+} channel TRPV6 in the kidney. *J. Am. Soc. Nephrol.* **2003**, *14*, 2731–2740. [CrossRef] [PubMed]

322. Suzuki, Y.; Kovacs, C.S.; Takanaga, H.; Peng, J.B.; Landowski, C.P.; Hediger, M.A. Calcium channel TRPV6 is involved in murine maternal-fetal calcium transport. *J. Bone Min. Res.* **2008**, *23*, 1249–1256. [CrossRef] [PubMed]

323. Fernandes, E.S.; Vong, C.T.; Quek, S.; Cheong, J.; Awal, S.; Gentry, C.; Aubdool, A.A.; Liang, L.; Bodkin, J.V.; Bevan, S.; et al. Superoxide generation and leukocyte accumulation: Key elements in the mediation of leukotriene B$_4$-induced itch by transient receptor potential ankyrin 1 and transient receptor potential vanilloid 1. *FASEB J.* **2013**, *27*, 1664–1673. [CrossRef] [PubMed]

324. Sisignano, M.; Park, C.K.; Angioni, C.; Zhang, D.D.; von Hehn, C.; Cobos, E.J.; Ghasemlou, N.; Xu, Z.Z.; Kumaran, V.; Lu, R.; et al. 5,6-EET is released upon neuronal activity and induces mechanical pain hypersensitivity via TRPA1 on central afferent terminals. *J. Neurosci.* **2012**, *32*, 6364–6372. [CrossRef] [PubMed]

325. Ross, R.A.; Craib, S.J.; Stevenson, L.A.; Pertwee, R.G.; Henderson, A.; Toole, J.; Ellington, H.C. Pharmacological characterization of the anandamide cyclooxygenase metabolite: Prostaglandin E2 ethanolamide. *J. Pharmacol. Exp. Ther.* **2002**, *301*, 900–907. [CrossRef] [PubMed]

326. Yu, M.; Ives, D.; Ramesha, C.S. Synthesis of prostaglandin E2 ethanolamide from anandamide by cyclooxygenase-2. *J. Biol. Chem.* **1997**, *272*, 21181–21186. [CrossRef] [PubMed]

327. Ueda, N.; Yamamoto, K.; Yamamoto, S.; Tokunaga, T.; Shirakawa, E.; Shinkai, H.; Ogawa, M.; Sato, T.; Kudo, I.; Inoue, K.; et al. Lipoxygenase-catalyzed oxygenation of arachidonylethanolamide, a cannabinoid receptor agonist. *Biochim. Biophys. Acta* **1995**, *1254*, 127–134. [CrossRef]

328. Ueda, N.; Kurahashi, Y.; Yamamoto, K.; Yamamoto, S.; Tokunaga, T. Enzymes for anandamide biosynthesis and metabolism. *J. Lipid Mediat. Cell Signal.* **1996**, *14*, 57–61. [CrossRef]

329. Craib, S.J.; Ellington, H.C.; Pertwee, R.G.; Ross, R.A. A possible role of lipoxygenases in the activation of vanilloid receptors by anandamide in the guinea-pig bronchus. *Br. J. Pharmacol.* **2001**, *134*, 30–37. [CrossRef] [PubMed]

330. Smart, D.; Gunthorpe, M.J.; Jerman, J.C.; Nasir, S.; Gray, J.; Muir, A.I.; Chambers, J.K.; Randall, A.D.; Davis, J.B. The endogenous lipid anandamide is a full agonist at the human vanilloid receptor (hVR1). *Br. J. Pharmacol.* **2000**, *129*, 227–230. [CrossRef] [PubMed]

331. Jacobsson, S.O.; Wallin, T.; Fowler, C.J. Inhibition of rat C6 glioma cell proliferation by endogenous and synthetic cannabinoids. Relative involvement of cannabinoid and vanilloid receptors. *J. Pharmacol. Exp. Ther.* **2001**, *299*, 951–959. [PubMed]

332. Sarker, K.P.; Obara, S.; Nakata, M.; Kitajima, I.; Maruyama, I. Anandamide induces apoptosis of PC-12 cells: Involvement of superoxide and caspase-3. *FEBS Lett.* **2000**, *472*, 39–44. [CrossRef]

333. Maccarrone, M.; Lorenzon, T.; Bari, M.; Melino, G.; Finazzi-Agro, A. Anandamide induces apoptosis in human cells via vanilloid receptors. Evidence for a protective role of cannabinoid receptors. *J. Biol. Chem.* **2000**, *275*, 31938–31945. [CrossRef] [PubMed]

334. Yang, Z.H.; Wang, X.H.; Wang, H.P.; Hu, L.Q.; Zheng, X.M.; Li, S.W. Capsaicin mediates cell death in bladder cancer T24 cells through reactive oxygen species production and mitochondrial depolarization. *Urology* **2010**, *75*, 735–741. [CrossRef] [PubMed]

335. Ma, F.; Zhang, L.; Westlund, K.N. Reactive oxygen species mediate TNFR1 increase after TRPV1 activation in mouse DRG neurons. *Mol. Pain* **2009**, *5*, 31. [CrossRef] [PubMed]

336. Talbot, S.; Dias, J.P.; Lahjouji, K.; Bogo, M.R.; Campos, M.M.; Gaudreau, P.; Couture, R. Activation of TRPV1 by capsaicin induces functional kinin B(1) receptor in rat spinal cord microglia. *J. Neuroinflamm.* **2012**, *9*, 16. [CrossRef] [PubMed]

337. Adam-Vizi, V.; Starkov, A.A. Calcium and mitochondrial reactive oxygen species generation: How to read the facts. *J. Alzheimer Dis.* **2010**, *20* (Suppl. 2), S413–S426. [CrossRef] [PubMed]

338. Nishio, S.; Teshima, Y.; Takahashi, N.; Thuc, L.C.; Saito, S.; Fukui, A.; Kume, O.; Fukunaga, N.; Hara, M.; Nakagawa, M.; et al. Activation of CaMKII as a key regulator of reactive oxygen species production in diabetic rat heart. *J. Mol. Cell. Cardiol.* **2012**, *52*, 1103–1111. [CrossRef] [PubMed]

339. Pandey, D.; Gratton, J.P.; Rafikov, R.; Black, S.M.; Fulton, D.J. Calcium/calmodulin-dependent kinase II mediates the phosphorylation and activation of NADPH oxidase 5. *Mol. Pharmacol.* **2011**, *80*, 407–415. [CrossRef] [PubMed]

340. Kishimoto, E.; Naito, Y.; Handa, O.; Okada, H.; Mizushima, K.; Hirai, Y.; Nakabe, N.; Uchiyama, K.; Ishikawa, T.; Takagi, T.; et al. Oxidative stress-induced posttranslational modification of TRPV1 expressed in esophageal epithelial cells. *Am. J. Physiol. Gastrointest. Liver Physiol.* **2011**, *301*, G230–G238. [CrossRef] [PubMed]

341. Yoshida, T.; Inoue, R.; Morii, T.; Takahashi, N.; Yamamoto, S.; Hara, Y.; Tominaga, M.; Shimizu, S.; Sato, Y.; Mori, Y. Nitric oxide activates TRP channels by cysteine S-nitrosylation. *Nat. Chem. Biol.* **2006**, *2*, 596–607. [CrossRef] [PubMed]

342. Takahashi, N.; Mori, Y. TRP Channels as Sensors and Signal Integrators of Redox Status Changes. *Front. Pharmacol.* **2011**, *2*, 58. [CrossRef] [PubMed]

343. Susankova, K.; Tousova, K.; Vyklicky, L.; Teisinger, J.; Vlachova, V. Reducing and oxidizing agents sensitize heat-activated vanilloid receptor (TRPV1) current. *Mol. Pharmacol.* **2006**, *70*, 383–394. [CrossRef] [PubMed]

344. Taylor-Clark, T.E.; McAlexander, M.A.; Nassenstein, C.; Sheardown, S.A.; Wilson, S.; Thornton, J.; Carr, M.J.; Undem, B.J. Relative contributions of TRPA1 and TRPV1 channels in the activation of vagal bronchopulmonary C-fibres by the endogenous autacoid 4-oxononenal. *J. Physiol.* **2008**, *586*, 347–359. [CrossRef] [PubMed]

345. Pei, Z.; Zhuang, Z.; Sang, H.; Wu, Z.; Meng, R.; He, E.Y.; Scott, G.I.; Maris, J.R.; Li, R.; Ren, J. α,β-Unsaturated aldehyde crotonaldehyde triggers cardiomyocyte contractile dysfunction: Role of TRPV1 and mitochondrial function. *Pharmacol. Res.* **2014**, *82*, 40–50. [CrossRef] [PubMed]

346. Inoue, I.; Goto, S.; Matsunaga, T.; Nakajima, T.; Awata, T.; Hokari, S.; Komoda, T.; Katayama, S. The ligands/activators for peroxisome proliferator-activated receptor alpha (PPARalpha) and PPARgamma increase Cu^{2+},Zn^{2+}-superoxide dismutase and decrease p22phox message expressions in primary endothelial cells. *Metabolism* **2001**, *50*, 3–11. [CrossRef] [PubMed]

347. Girnun, G.D.; Domann, F.E.; Moore, S.A.; Robbins, M.E. Identification of a functional peroxisome proliferator-activated receptor response element in the rat catalase promoter. *Mol. Endocrinol.* **2002**, *16*, 2793–2801. [CrossRef] [PubMed]

348. Diep, Q.N.; Amiri, F.; Touyz, R.M.; Cohn, J.S.; Endemann, D.; Neves, M.F.; Schiffrin, E.L. PPARalpha activator effects on Ang II-induced vascular oxidative stress and inflammation. *Hypertension* **2002**, *40*, 866–871. [CrossRef] [PubMed]

349. Landmesser, U.; Cai, H.; Dikalov, S.; McCann, L.; Hwang, J.; Jo, H.; Holland, S.M.; Harrison, D.G. Role of p47 in vascular oxidative stress and hypertension caused by angiotensin II. *Hypertension* **2002**, *40*, 511–515. [CrossRef] [PubMed]

350. Martinez, A.A.; Morgese, M.G.; Pisanu, A.; Macheda, T.; Paquette, M.A.; Seillier, A.; Cassano, T.; Carta, A.R.; Giuffrida, A. Activation of PPAR gamma receptors reduces levodopa-induced dyskinesias in 6-OHDA-lesioned rats. *Neurobiol. Dis.* **2015**, *74*, 295–304. [CrossRef] [PubMed]

351. Impellizzeri, D.; Esposito, E.; Attley, J.; Cuzzocrea, S. Targeting inflammation: New therapeutic approaches in chronic kidney disease (CKD). *Pharmacol. Res.* **2014**, *81*, 91–102. [CrossRef] [PubMed]

352. Di Paola, R.; Impellizzeri, D.; Mondello, P.; Velardi, E.; Aloisi, C.; Cappellani, A.; Esposito, E.; Cuzzocrea, S. Palmitoylethanolamide reduces early renal dysfunction and injury caused by experimental ischemia and reperfusion in mice. *Shock* **2012**, *38*, 356–366. [CrossRef] [PubMed]

353. Moreno, S.; Mugnaini, E.; Ceru, M.P. Immunocytochemical localization of catalase in the central nervous system of the rat. *J. HistoChem. Cytochem.* **1995**, *43*, 1253–1267. [CrossRef] [PubMed]

354. Moreno, S.; Nardacci, R.; Ceru, M.P. Regional and ultrastructural immunolocalization of copper-zinc superoxide dismutase in rat central nervous system. *J. Histochem. Cytochem.* **1997**, *45*, 1611–1622. [CrossRef] [PubMed]

355. Farioli-Vecchioli, S.; Moreno, S.; Ceru, M.P. Immunocytochemical localization of acyl-CoA oxidase in the rat central nervous system. *J. Neurocytol.* **2001**, *30*, 21–33. [CrossRef] [PubMed]

356. Poynter, M.E.; Daynes, R.A. Peroxisome proliferator-activated receptor alpha activation modulates cellular redox status, represses nuclear factor-kappaB signaling, and reduces inflammatory cytokine production in aging. *J. Biol. Chem.* **1998**, *273*, 32833–32841. [CrossRef] [PubMed]

357. Cimini, A.; Benedetti, E.; Cristiano, L.; Sebastiani, P.; D'Amico, M.A.; D'Angelo, B.; Di Loreto, S. Expression of peroxisome proliferator-activated receptors (PPARs) and retinoic acid receptors (RXRs) in rat cortical neurons. *Neuroscience* **2005**, *130*, 325–337. [CrossRef] [PubMed]

358. Sayre, L.M.; Perry, G.; Smith, M.A. Oxidative Stress and Neurotoxicity. *Chem. Res. Toxicol.* **2008**, *21*, 172–188. [CrossRef] [PubMed]

359. Sultana, R.; Butterfield, D.A. Role of oxidative stress in the progression of Alzheimer's disease. *J. Alzheimer Dis.* **2010**, *19*, 341–353. [CrossRef] [PubMed]

360. Fanelli, F.; Sepe, S.; D'Amelio, M.; Bernardi, C.; Cristiano, L.; Cimini, A.; Cecconi, F.; Ceru', M.P.; Moreno, S. Age-dependent roles of peroxisomes in the hippocampus of a transgenic mouse model of Alzheimer's disease. *Mol. Neurodegener.* **2013**, *8*, 8. [CrossRef] [PubMed]

361. Duncan, R.S.; Chapman, K.D.; Koulen, P. The neuroprotective properties of palmitoylethanolamine against oxidative stress in a neuronal cell line. *Mol. Neurodegener.* **2009**, *4*, 50. [CrossRef] [PubMed]

362. Raso, G.M.; Esposito, E.; Vitiello, S.; Iacono, A.; Santoro, A.; D'Agostino, G.; Sasso, O.; Russo, R.; Piazza, P.V.; Calignano, A.; et al. Palmitoylethanolamide stimulation induces allopregnanolone synthesis in C6 Cells and primary astrocytes: Involvement of peroxisome-proliferator activated receptor-a. *J. Neuroendocrinol.* **2011**, *23*, 591–600. [CrossRef] [PubMed]

363. Avagliano, C.; Russo, R.; De Caro, C.; Cristiano, C.; La Rana, G.; Piegari, G.; Paciello, O.; Citraro, R.; Russo, E.; De Sarro, G.; et al. Palmitoylethanolamide protects mice against 6-OHDA-induced neurotoxicity and endoplasmic reticulum stress: In vivo and in vitro evidence. *Pharmacol. Res.* **2016**, *113*, 276–289. [CrossRef] [PubMed]

364. Manea, A.; Manea, S.A.; Todirita, A.; Albulescu, I.C.; Raicu, M.; Sasson, S.; Simionescu, M. High-glucose-increased expression and activation of NADPH oxidase in human vascular smooth muscle cells is mediated by 4-hydroxynonenal-activated PPARα and PPARβ/δ. *Cell Tissue Res.* **2015**, *361*, 593–604. [CrossRef] [PubMed]

365. Irving, A.; Abdulrazzaq, G.; Chan, S.L.F.; Penman, J.; Harvey, J.; Alexander, S.P.H. Cannabinoid Receptor-Related Orphan G Protein-Coupled Receptors. *Adv. Pharmacol.* **2017**, *80*, 223–247. [CrossRef] [PubMed]

366. Gantz, I.; Muraoka, A.; Yang, Y.K.; Samuelson, L.C.; Zimmerman, E.M.; Cook, H.; Yamada, T. Cloning and chromosomal localization of a gene (GPR18) encoding a novel seven transmembrane receptor highly expressed in spleen and testis. *Genomics* **1997**, *42*, 462–466. [CrossRef] [PubMed]

367. Vassilatis, D.K.; Hohmann, J.G.; Zeng, H.; Li, F.; Ranchalis, J.E.; Mortrud, M.T.; Brown, A.; Rodriguez, S.S.; Weller, J.R.; Wright, A.C.; et al. The G protein-coupled receptor repertoires of human and mouse. *Proc. Natl. Acad. Sci. USA* **2003**, *100*, 4903–4908. [CrossRef] [PubMed]

368. Lu, V.B.; Puhl, H.L., 3rd; Ikeda, S.R. *N*-Arachidonyl glycine does not activate G protein-coupled receptor 18 signaling via canonical pathways. *Mol. Pharmacol.* **2013**, *83*, 267–282. [CrossRef] [PubMed]

369. Finlay, D.B.; Joseph, W.R.; Grimsey, N.L.; Glass, M. GPR18 undergoes a high degree of constitutive trafficking but is unresponsive to *N*-Arachidonoyl Glycine. *PeerJ* **2016**, *4*, e1835. [CrossRef] [PubMed]

370. Penumarti, A.; Abdel-Rahman, A.A. The novel endocannabinoid receptor GPR18 is expressed in the rostral ventrolateral medulla and exerts tonic restraining influence on blood pressure. *J. Pharmacol. Exp. Ther.* **2014**, *349*, 29–38. [CrossRef] [PubMed]

371. Matouk, A.I.; Taye, A.; El-Moselhy, M.A.; Heeba, G.H.; Abdel-Rahman, A.A. The Effect of Chronic Activation of the Novel Endocannabinoid Receptor GPR18 on Myocardial Function and Blood Pressure in Conscious Rats. *J. Cardiovasc. Pharmacol.* **2017**, *69*, 23–33. [CrossRef] [PubMed]

372. Sawzdargo, M.; Nguyen, T.; Lee, D.K.; Lynch, K.R.; Cheng, R.; Heng, H.H.; George, S.R.; O'Dowd, B.F. Identification and cloning of three novel human G protein-coupled receptor genes GPR52, PsiGPR53 and GPR55: GPR55 is extensively expressed in human brain. *Brain Res. Mol. Brain Res.* **1999**, *64*, 193–198. [CrossRef]

373. Ryberg, E.; Larsson, N.; Sjögren, S.; Hjorth, S.; Hermansson, N.O.; Leonova, J.; Elebring, T.; Nilsson, K.; Drmota, T.; Greasley, P.J. The orphan receptor GPR55 is a novel cannabinoid receptor. *Br. J. Pharmacol.* **2007**, *152*, 1092–1101. [CrossRef] [PubMed]

374. Romero-Zerbo, S.Y.; Rafacho, A.; Díaz-Arteaga, A.; Suárez, J.; Quesada, I.; Imbernon, M.; Ross, R.A.; Dieguez, C.; Rodríguez de Fonseca, F.; Nogueiras, R.; et al. A role for the putative cannabinoid receptor GPR55 in the islets of Langerhans. *J. Endocrinol.* **2011**, *211*, 177–185. [CrossRef] [PubMed]

375. Whyte, L.S.; Ryberg, E.; Sims, N.A.; Ridge, S.A.; Mackie, K.; Greasley, P.J.; Ross, R.A.; Rogers, M.J. The putative cannabinoid receptor GPR55 affects osteoclast function in vitro and bone mass in vivo. *Proc. Natl. Acad. Sci. USA* **2009**, *106*, 16511–16516. [CrossRef] [PubMed]

376. Pietr, M.; Kozela, E.; Levy, R.; Rimmerman, N.; Lin, Y.H.; Stella, N.; Vogel, Z.; Juknat, A. Differential changes in GPR55 during microglial cell activation. *FEBS Lett.* **2009**, *583*, 2071–2076. [CrossRef] [PubMed]

377. Waldeck-Weiermair, M.; Zoratti, C.; Osibow, K.; Balenga, N.; Goessnitzer, E.; Waldhoer, M.; Malli, R.; Graier, W.F. Integrin clustering enables anandamide-induced Ca^{2+} signaling in endothelial cells via GPR55 by protection against CB1-receptor-triggered repression. *J. Cell Sci.* **2008**, *121*, 1704–1717. [CrossRef] [PubMed]

378. Kapur, A.; Zhao, P.; Sharir, H.; Bai, Y.; Caron, M.G.; Barak, L.S.; Abood, M.E. Atypical responsiveness of the orphan receptor GPR55 to cannabinoid ligands. *J. Biol. Chem.* **2009**, *284*, 29817–29827. [CrossRef] [PubMed]

379. Yin, H.; Chu, A.; Li, W.; Wang, B.; Shelton, F.; Otero, F.; Nguyen, D.G.; Caldwell, J.S.; Chen, Y.A. Lipid G protein-coupled receptor ligand identification using beta-arrestin PathHunter assay. *J. Biol. Chem.* **2009**, *284*, 12328–12338. [CrossRef] [PubMed]

380. Henstridge, C.M.; Balenga, N.A.; Ford, L.A.; Ross, R.A.; Waldhoer, M.; Irving, A.J. The GPR55 ligand L-alpha-lysophosphatidylinositol promotes RhoA-dependent Ca^{2+} signaling and NFAT activation. *FASEB J.* **2009**, *23*, 183–193. [CrossRef] [PubMed]

381. Oka, S.; Toshida, T.; Maruyama, K.; Nakajima, K.; Yamashita, A.; Sugiura, T. 2-Arachidonoyl-sn-glycero-3-phosphoinositol: A possible natural ligand for GPR55. *J. Biochem.* **2009**, *145*, 13–20. [CrossRef] [PubMed]

382. Oka, S.; Nakajima, K.; Yamashita, A.; Kishimoto, S.; Sugiura, T. Identification of GPR55 as a lysophosphatidylinositol receptor. *Biochem. Biophys. Res. Commun.* **2007**, *362*, 928–934. [CrossRef] [PubMed]

383. Bondarenko, A.; Waldeck-Weiermair, M.; Naghdi, S.; Poteser, M.; Malli, R.; Graier, W.F. GPR55-dependent and -independent ion signalling in response to lysophosphatidylinositol in endothelial cells. *Br. J. Pharmacol.* **2010**, *161*, 308–320. [CrossRef] [PubMed]

384. Moreno, E.; Andradas, C.; Medrano, M.; Caffarel, M.M.; Pérez-Gómez, E.; Blasco-Benito, S.; Gómez-Cañas, M.; Pazos, M.R.; Irving, A.J.; Lluís, C.; et al. Targeting CB2-GPR55 receptor heteromers modulates cancer cell signaling. *J. Biol. Chem.* **2014**, *289*, 21960–21972. [CrossRef] [PubMed]

385. Fredriksson, R.; Höglund, P.J.; Gloriam, D.E.; Lagerström, M.C.; Schiöth, H.B. Seven evolutionarily conserved human rhodopsin G protein-coupled receptors lacking close relatives. *FEBS Lett.* **2003**, *554*, 381–388. [CrossRef]

386. Soga, T.; Ohishi, T.; Matsui, T.; Saito, T.; Matsumoto, M.; Takasaki, J.; Matsumoto, S.; Kamohara, M.; Hiyama, H.; Yoshida, S.; et al. Lysophosphatidylcholine enhances glucose-dependent insulin secretion via an orphan G-protein-coupled receptor. *Biochem. Biophys. Res. Commun.* **2005**, *326*, 744–751. [CrossRef] [PubMed]

387. Sakamoto, Y.; Inoue, H.; Kawakami, S.; Miyawaki, K.; Miyamoto, T.; Mizuta, K.; Itakura, M. Expression and distribution of Gpr119 in the pancreatic islets of mice and rats: Predominant localization in pancreatic polypeptide-secreting PP-cells. *Biochem. Biophys. Res. Commun.* **2006**, *351*, 474–480. [CrossRef] [PubMed]

388. Chu, Z.L.; Carroll, C.; Alfonso, J.; Gutierrez, V.; He, H.; Lucman, A.; Pedraza, M.; Mondala, H.; Gao, H.; Bagnol, D.; et al. A role for intestinal endocrine cell-expressed g protein-coupled receptor 119 in glycemic control by enhancing glucagon-like Peptide-1 and glucose-dependent insulinotropic Peptide release. *Endocrinology* **2008**, *149*, 2038–2047. [CrossRef] [PubMed]

389. Lauffer, L.M.; Iakoubov, R.; Brubaker, P.L. GPR119 is essential for oleoylethanolamide-induced glucagon-like peptide-1 secretion from the intestinal enteroendocrine L-cell. *Diabetes* **2009**, *58*, 1058–1066. [CrossRef] [PubMed]

390. Yang, J.W.; Kim, H.S.; Im, J.H.; Kim, J.W.; Jun, D.W.; Lim, S.C.; Lee, K.; Choi, J.M.; Kim, S.K.; Kang, K.W. GPR119: A promising target for nonalcoholic fatty liver disease. *FASEB J.* **2016**, *30*, 324–335. [CrossRef] [PubMed]

391. Cvijanovic, N.; Isaacs, N.J.; Rayner, C.K.; Feinle-Bisset, C.; Young, R.L.; Little, T.J. Duodenal fatty acid sensor and transporter expression following acute fat exposure in healthy lean humans. *Clin. Nutr.* **2017**, *36*, 564–569. [CrossRef] [PubMed]

392. Overton, H.A.; Babbs, A.J.; Doel, S.M.; Fyfe, M.C.; Gardner, L.S.; Griffin, G.; Jackson, H.C.; Procter, M.J.; Rasamison, C.M.; Tang-Christensen, M.; et al. Deorphanization of a G protein-coupled receptor for oleoylethanolamide and its use in the discovery of small-molecule hypophagic agents. *Cell Metab.* **2006**, *3*, 167–175. [CrossRef] [PubMed]

393. Chu, Z.L.; Carroll, C.; Chen, R.; Alfonso, J.; Gutierrez, V.; He, H.; Lucman, A.; Xing, C.; Sebring, K.; Zhou, J.; et al. *N*-oleoyldopamine enhances glucose homeostasis through the activation of GPR119. *Mol. Endocrinol.* **2010**, *24*, 161–170. [CrossRef] [PubMed]

394. Hansen, K.B.; Rosenkilde, M.M.; Knop, F.K.; Wellner, N.; Diep, T.A.; Rehfeld, J.F.; Andersen, U.B.; Holst, J.J.; Hansen, H.S. 2-Oleoyl glycerol is a GPR119 agonist and signals GLP-1 release in humans. *J. Clin. Endocrinol. Metab.* **2011**, *96*, E1409–E1417. [CrossRef] [PubMed]

395. Balenga, N.A.; Aflaki, E.; Kargl, J.; Platzer, W.; Schröder, R.; Blättermann, S.; Kostenis, E.; Brown, A.J.; Heinemann, A.; Waldhoer, M. GPR55 regulates cannabinoid 2 receptor-mediated responses in human neutrophils. *Cell Res.* **2011**, *21*, 1452–1469. [CrossRef] [PubMed]

396. Chiurchiù, V.; Lanuti, M.; De Bardi, M.; Battistini, L.; Maccarrone, M. The differential characterization of GPR55 receptor in human peripheral blood reveals a distinctive expression in monocytes and NK cells and a proinflammatory role in these innate cells. *Int. Immunol.* **2015**, *27*, 153–160. [CrossRef] [PubMed]

397. He, L.; He, T.; Farrar, S.; Ji, L.; Liu, T.; Ma, X. Antioxidants Maintain Cellular Redox Homeostasis by Elimination of Reactive Oxygen Species. *Cell. Physiol. Biochem.* **2017**, *44*, 532–553. [CrossRef] [PubMed]

398. Chelikani, P.; Fita, I.; Loewen, P.C. Diversity of structures and properties among catalases. *Cell. Mol. Life Sci.* **2004**, *61*, 192–208. [CrossRef] [PubMed]

399. Bannister, J.V.; Bannister, W.H.; Rotilio, G. Aspects of the structure, function, and applications of superoxide dismutase. *CRC Crit. Rev. Biochem.* **1987**, *22*, 111–180. [CrossRef] [PubMed]

400. Zelko, I.N.; Mariani, T.J.; Folz, R.J. Superoxide dismutase multigene family: A comparison of the CuZn-SOD (SOD1), Mn-SOD (SOD2), and EC-SOD (SOD3) gene structures, evolution, and expression. *Free Radic. Biol. Med.* **2002**, *33*, 337–349. [CrossRef]

401. Brigelius-Flohé, R. Tissue-specific functions of individual glutathione peroxidases. *Free Radic. Biol. Med.* **1999**, *27*, 951–965. [CrossRef]

402. Arnér, E.S.; Holmgren, A. Physiological functions of thioredoxin and thioredoxin reductase. *Eur. J. Biochem.* **2000**, *267*, 6102–6109. [CrossRef] [PubMed]

403. Meister, A.; Anderson, M.E. Glutathione. *Annu. Rev. Biochem.* **1983**, *52*, 711–760. [CrossRef] [PubMed]

404. Palace, V.P.; Khaper, N.; Qin, Q.; Singal, P.K. Antioxidant potentials of vitamin A and carotenoids and their relevance to heart disease. *Free Radic. Biol. Med.* **1999**, *26*, 746–761. [CrossRef]

405. Rice, M.E. Ascorbate regulation and its neuroprotective role in the brain. *Trends Neurosci.* **2000**, *23*, 209–216. [CrossRef]

406. McCay, P.B. Vitamin E: Interactions with free radicals and ascorbate. *Annu. Rev. Nutr.* **1985**, *5*, 323–340. [CrossRef] [PubMed]

407. Turunen, M.; Olsson, J.; Dallner, G. Metabolism and function of coenzyme Q. *Biochim. Biophys. Acta* **2004**, *1660*, 171–199. [CrossRef] [PubMed]

408. Paiva, S.A.; Russell, R.M. Beta-carotene and other carotenoids as antioxidants. *J. Am. Coll. Nutr.* **1999**, *18*, 426–433. [CrossRef] [PubMed]

409. Giudetti, A.M.; Salzet, M.; Cassano, T. Oxidative Stress in Aging Brain: Nutritional and Pharmacological Interventions for Neurodegenerative Disorders. *Oxid. Med. Cell. Longev.* **2018**, *2018*, 3416028. [CrossRef] [PubMed]

410. Heim, K.E.; Tagliaferro, A.R.; Bobilya, D.J. Flavonoid antioxidants: Chemistry, metabolism and structure-activity relationships. *J. Nutr. Biochem.* **2002**, *13*, 572–584. [CrossRef]

411. Sandoval-Acuña, C.; Ferreira, J.; Speisky, H. Polyphenols and mitochondria: An update on their increasingly emerging ROS-scavenging independent actions. *Arch. Biochem. Biophys.* **2014**, *559*, 75–90. [CrossRef] [PubMed]

412. Tabassum, A.; Bristow, R.G.; Venkateswaran, V. Ingestion of selenium and other antioxidants during prostate cancer radiotherapy: A good thing? *Cancer Treat. Rev.* **2010**, *36*, 230–234. [CrossRef] [PubMed]

413. Prasad, A.S.; Bao, B.; Beck, F.W.; Kucuk, O.; Sarkar, F.H. Antioxidant effect of zinc in humans. *Free Radic. Biol. Med.* **2004**, *37*, 1182–1190. [CrossRef] [PubMed]

414. Rizzo, A.M.; Berselli, P.; Zava, S.; Montorfano, G.; Negroni, M.; Corsetto, P.; Berra, B. Endogenous antioxidants and radical scavengers. *Adv. Exp. Med. Biol.* **2010**, *698*, 52–67. [CrossRef] [PubMed]

415. Reiter, R.J.; Tan, D.X.; Poeggeler, B.; Menendez-Pelaez, A.; Chen, L.D.; Saarela, S. Melatonin as a free radical scavenger: Implications for aging and age-related diseases. *Ann. N. Y. Acad. Sci.* **1994**, *719*, 1–12. [CrossRef] [PubMed]

416. Burton, G.W.; Traber, M.G. Vitamin E: Antioxidant activity, biokinetics, and bioavailability. *Annu. Rev. Nutr.* **1990**, *10*, 357–382. [CrossRef] [PubMed]

417. Bowman, G.L.; Shannon, J.; Frei, B.; Kaye, J.A.; Quinn, J.F. Uric acid as a CNS antioxidant. *J. Alzheimer Dis.* **2010**, *19*, 1331–1336. [CrossRef] [PubMed]

418. Cotelle, N. Role of flavonoids in oxidative stress. *Curr. Top. Med. Chem.* **2001**, *1*, 569–590. [CrossRef] [PubMed]

419. Hussain, T.; Tan, B.; Yin, Y.; Blachier, F.; Tossou, M.C.; Rahu, N. Oxidative Stress and Inflammation: What Polyphenols Can Do for Us? *Oxid. Med. Cell. Longev.* **2016**, *2016*, 7432797. [CrossRef] [PubMed]

420. Martinez, J.; Moreno, J.J. Role of Ca^{2+}-Independent Phospholipase A_2 on Arachidonic Acid Release Induced by Reactive Oxygen Species. *Arch. Biochem. Biophys.* **2001**, *392*, 257–262. [CrossRef] [PubMed]

421. Bátkai, S.; Rajesh, M.; Mukhopadhyay, P.; Haskó, G.; Liaudet, L.; Cravatt, B.F.; Csiszár, A.; Ungvári, Z.; Pacher, P. Decreased age-related cardiac dysfunction, myocardial nitrative stress, inflammatory gene expression, and apoptosis in mice lacking fatty acid amide hydrolase. *Am. J. Physiol. Heart Circ. Physiol.* **2007**, *293*, H909–H918. [CrossRef] [PubMed]

422. Wei, Y.; Wang, X.; Wang, L. Presence and regulation of cannabinoid receptors in human retinal pigment epithelial cells. *Mol. Vis.* **2009**, *15*, 1243–1251. [PubMed]

423. Wang, M.; Abais, J.M.; Meng, N.; Zhang, Y.; Ritter, J.K.; Li, P.L.; Tang, W.X. Upregulation of cannabinoid receptor-1 and fibrotic activation of mouse hepatic stellate cells during Schistosoma J. infection: Role of NADPH oxidase. *Free Radic. Biol. Med.* **2014**, *71*, 109–120. [CrossRef] [PubMed]

8

Glutathione: Antioxidant Properties Dedicated to Nanotechnologies

Caroline Gaucher * [iD], Ariane Boudier, Justine Bonetti, Igor Clarot, Pierre Leroy and Marianne Parent [iD]

Université de Lorraine, CITHEFOR, F-54000 Nancy, France; ariane.boudier@univ-lorraine.fr (A.B.); justine.bonetti@univ-lorraine.fr (J.B.); igor.clarot@univ-lorraine.fr (I.C.); pierre.leroy@univ-lorraine.fr (P.L.); marianne.parent@univ-lorraine.fr (M.P.)

* Correspondence: caroline.gaucher@univ-lorraine.fr

Abstract: Which scientist has never heard of glutathione (GSH)? This well-known low-molecular-weight tripeptide is perhaps the most famous natural antioxidant. However, the interest in GSH should not be restricted to its redox properties. This multidisciplinary review aims to bring out some lesser-known aspects of GSH, for example, as an emerging tool in nanotechnologies to achieve targeted drug delivery. After recalling the biochemistry of GSH, including its metabolism pathways and redox properties, its involvement in cellular redox homeostasis and signaling is described. Analytical methods for the dosage and localization of GSH or glutathiolated proteins are also covered. Finally, the various therapeutic strategies to replenish GSH stocks are discussed, in parallel with its use as an addressing molecule in drug delivery.

Keywords: glutathione; antioxidant; redox signaling; nanotechnologies; repletion; targeted drug delivery

---

1. Introduction: Biochemical Implication of Glutathione in Redox Homeostasis

Reduced glutathione (GSH; Figure 1) is the main low-molecular-weight thiol-containing peptide present in most living cells from bacteria to mammals (except some bacteria and amoebae) [1]. Since its discovery 130 years ago in baker's yeast (*Saccharomyces cerevisiae*) by J. de Rey Pailhade, who named it "philothion", many works have tried to establish and have elucidated its pivotal role in aerobic life. Its structure and redox role were established by Sir Frederick Gowland Hopkins in 1922 [2]. Glutathione was first claimed to be a dipeptide, and then a tripeptide, that is, γ-L-glutamyl-L-cysteinylglycine [3].

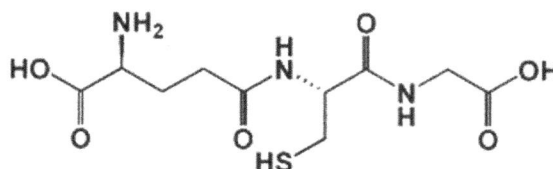

Figure 1. Condensed structural chemical formula of glutathione (IUPAC name: (2S)-2-amino-4-{[(1R)-1-[(carboxymethyl)carbamoyl]-2-sulfanylethyl] carbamoyl}butanoic acid).

In the 1970s, the cellular glutathione cycle, involving two ATP-dependent enzymatically catalyzed steps for its synthesis, was established by Meister (Figure 2) [4,5]. The first enzyme, the γ-glutamylcysteinyl ligase (EC 6.3.2.3; GCL), is a heterodimeric rate-limiting enzyme. In animals and humans, the transcription of the GCL gene is regulated by nuclear factor erythroid-derived 2-like 2 (NFE2L2), which is sensitive to oxidative stress. Indeed, NFE2L2 activates the transcription of genes under the control of the antioxidant responsive element in various cell types [6]. The second enzyme, the glutathione synthase (EC 6.3.2.2; GS), catalyzes the formation of the covalent bond between the glycine residue and the γ-glutamyl-cysteine dipeptide. The rate of GSH synthesis is controlled by the cell content of L-cysteine [5] and ATP, and the ratio between the two subunits of the GCL [7], as well as its feedback inhibition by GSH [8] and oxidative stimulation of GCL enzymatic activity [9]. Although all cell types synthesize GSH, the main GSH source in the body remains the liver [10,11].

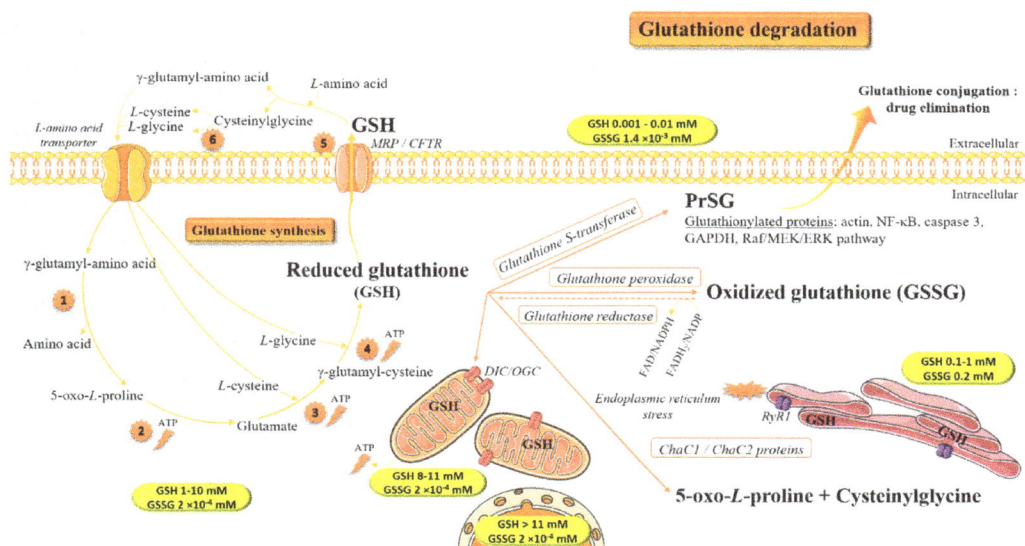

Figure 2. The homeostasis of reduced (GSH) and oxidized/disulfide (GSSG) glutathione within cells [12–17].

The synthesis of GSH is controlled by enzymes of Meister's cycle: **1.** γ-Glutamyl cyclotransferase. **2.** 5-Oxoprolinase. **3.** γ-Glutamyl-cysteine ligase. **4.** GS; **5.** γ-Glutamyl transferase. **6.** Dipeptidase. These last two enzymes contribute to extracellular GSH catabolism, whereas glutathione-specific γ-glutamylcyclotransferases, the ChaC1 and ChaC2 proteins (EC 4.3.2.7) handle its intracellular catabolism. After synthesis, GSH is distributed between intracellular organelles by transporters such as the dicarboxylate carrier (DIC) and the oxoglutarate carrier (OGC) on the mitochondria and the ryanodine receptor type 1 (RyR1) on the endoplasmic reticulum. The multidrug resistance-associated proteins (MRPs) and the cystic fibrosis transmembrane conductance regulator (CFTR) are in charge of GSH cell efflux.

The γ-bond between the two amino acids, glutamic acid and cysteine, provides peculiar characteristics, such as insusceptibility to proteolysis. Moreover, the thiol-containing cysteine residue confers redox catalytic properties. Glutathione indeed resists hydrolysis of most of the proteases and peptidases, except γ-glutamyltransferase (EC 2.3.2.2; GGT) and the enzymes from the ChaC family. GGT, an exofacial plasmic membrane, is able to transfer the γ-glutamyl residue of glutathione to an acceptor (e.g., peptides) and release the dipeptide cysteinylglycine. It is the only known enzyme able to catabolize both GSH and GSH adducts (e.g., oxidized glutathione, glutathione *S*-conjugates and glutathione complexes) [18,19]. The glutathione catabolism is controlled by GGT, and the released cysteinylglycine is next degraded by a dipeptidase; then resulting free amino acids enter the cell to permit the de novo GSH synthesis. GGT is a glycosylated glycoprotein that shows multiple sites of *N*-glycosylation depending on the species and localization of the enzyme. For example, seven *N*-glycosylation sites have been identified in human GGT [20]. Furthermore, GGT is redox-regulated at the transcriptional and translational levels as well as in its enzymatic activity [20,21]. Other cytosolic enzymes from the ChaC family have recently been reported to catalyze the cleavage of glutathione. The ChaC enzymes, ChaC1 and ChaC2, are cytosolic glutathione-specific γ-glutamylcyclotransferases, cleaving the amide bond via transamidation using the α-amine of the L-glutamyl residue, releasing it as cyclic 5-oxo-L-proline and cysteinylglycine dipeptide. The ChaC1 and ChaC2 enzymes show around 50% of sequence homology and specifically degrade glutathione but no other γ-glutamyl peptides or oxidized glutathione [22,23]. The ChaC2 proteins are characterized by a lower catalytic efficiency than ChaC1 and are constitutively expressed [23]. ChaC1 is a proapoptotic enzyme under the regulation of CHOP (C/EBP homologue protein) transcription factor during the unfolding protein response of endoplasmic reticulum stress [24].

Therefore, the intracellular and extracellular GSH concentrations are determined by the balance between its synthesis and catabolism, as well as by its transport between the cytosol and the different organelles or the extracellular space. The mechanisms of GSH transport into the mitochondria and the endoplasmic reticulum have not been established. However, the DIC and the OGC seem to contribute to the transport of GSH across the mitochondrial inner membrane [25], and RyR1 participates in the accumulation of GSH in the endoplasmic reticulum [26,27]. Although some of the GSH synthesized within cells is delivered to intracellular compartments, much of it is exported across the plasma membrane into the extracellular spaces, especially under oxidative stress [28]. Plasma membrane proteins such as MRPs and the CFTR are implicated in the GSH export from cells essentially under oxidative stress [29,30]. The ability to export both GSH and oxidized derivatives of GSH endows these transporters with the capacity to directly regulate the cellular thiol-redox status and therefore the ability to influence many key signaling and biochemical pathways.

The physiological functions of glutathione range from (i) the maintenance of cysteine under a reduced state within proteins; (ii) the formation of a cysteine pool; (iii) the metabolism of oestrogens, leukotrienes, and prostaglandins and the production of deoxyribonucleotides; (v) the maturation of iron–sulfur clusters in proteins; and (vi) the transduction of redox signals to the cell transcription machinery; to (vii) the maintenance of the cell redox potential [31]. Indeed, as a result of its ability to exist in different redox states, GSH is implicated in processes of the maintenance and regulation of the thiol-redox status [32].

2. Glutathione and Antioxidant/Pro-Oxidant Properties

Even if the glutathione reducing power was described early on by reacting with the redox probe methylene blue [2], its redox role corresponding to a Nernstian response was clearly established in this century [33]. From a thermodynamic point of view (Gibbs free energy of redox reactions at the equilibrium, excluding enzyme activity in the redox buffering), two molecules of GSH simultaneously exchange two electrons and two protons with its disulfide form (GSSG). Taking into account the high concentration of glutathione in cells (in the millimolar range) and the high proportion of its reduced form (more than 98% in healthy cells), the GSSG/2 GSH redox couple is considered as the main cellular redox buffer. The standard potential value $E°$ of the couple GSSG/2 GSH is equal to +197 mV, and because of its pH dependence according to the Nernst equation (Equation (1)), its apparent potential $E°'$ at the physiological pH is equal to −240 mV.

$$E°' = E° - 0.059 \times pH \times \log \frac{[GSH]^2}{[GSSG]} \tag{1}$$

The redox metabolism of the cells depends also on redox enzymes working under steady-state conditions instead of the equilibrium defining thermodynamic systems. From this point of view, the enzymes' reaction rate and kinetic constants (k_{cat} and K_m values), as well as GSH concentration and localization, are fundamental to highlight kinetic competition and to completely understand the GSH metabolism [17,34].

Therefore, the concentration of GSH as well as the [GSH]/[GSSG] ratio is a marker of oxidative stress and of the cell redox homeostasis. Regarding GSH reducing properties, it plays the role of an antioxidant as a scavenger of electrophilic and oxidant species either in a direct way or through enzymatic catalysis: (i) it directly quenches reactive hydroxyl free radicals, other oxygen-centered free radicals, and radical centers on DNA as well as on other biomolecules such as methylglyoxal and 4-hydroxynonenal; and (ii) GSH is the co-substrate of glutathione peroxidase (EC 1.11.1.9; GPx), permitting the reduction of peroxides (hydrogen and lipid peroxides) and producing GSSG. In turn, GSSG is reduced to 2 GSH by using NADPH reducing equivalents and glutathione disulfide reductase (EC 1.6.4.2; GR) catalysis. Electrophilic endogenous compounds and xenobiotics (drugs, pollutants and their phase I metabolites) are conjugated with GSH through activation by glutathione-S-transferases (EC 2.5.1.18; GSTs). The resulting conjugates are substrates of GGT, which initiates the mercapturic acid pathway and facilitates toxic elimination.

The overall cellular redox homeostasis is aimed at maintaining harmful reactive oxygen and nitrogen species and GSSG at very low levels and GSH at a high level. However, GSH can play a pro-oxidant role, which occurs to a lesser extent than its antioxidant role. This process has been reported during the GSH catabolism via GGT catalysis (Figure 3) [35,36]. The mechanism relies upon a shift of pKa of the SH group in the cysteine residue between GSH (pKa of 8.7) and its breakdown product cysteinylglycine (pKa of 6.4). Consequently, the proportion of the more reactive thiolate form is higher in cysteinylglycine than in GSH at the physiological pH value: the reduction rate of ferric ions to ferrous ions is higher, and the production of hydroxyl radicals and superoxide anions through Fenton and Haber–Weiss reactions is more abundant. The GSH pro-oxidant effect occurs, at least initially, on the outer side of the plasma membrane inducing lipid peroxidation, which destabilizes the cell membrane structure. Then, pro-oxidant effects, which are not stopped by the antioxidant defense systems [36], are propagated inside the cell through a signaling process. The pro-oxidant action of GGT is linked to the presence of redox active metals in the extracellular space. The reactivity of free redox active metals is strongly prevented in vivo by complexation with ferritin, transferrin or ceruloplasmin, for example. In this regard, the GGT activity can be postulated as able to reduce and to promote the release of iron ions from transferrin [37,38] as well as copper ions from ceruloplasmin [39]. An excess production of reactive oxygen species through GSH catabolism will produce DNA damages [40,41] or trigger the lipid peroxidation, already documented in vitro for linoleic acid [42] and for low-density lipoproteins (LDLs). Indeed, LDLs' oxidation process catalyzed during the reduction of iron (Fe^{3+} to Fe^{2+}) is known to play a central role in atherogenesis and vascular damage. Moreover, thiol-containing residues such as cysteine and homocysteine are known to reduce Fe^{3+} and promote Fe^{2+}-dependent LDL oxidation [43]. The γ-glutamate residue of GSH decreases the interactions between the thiol function of the cysteine residue and iron, precluding Fe^{3+} reduction and hence LDL oxidation [44,45]. The catabolism of GSH by GGT removing the γ-glutamate residue from the cysteine residue increases the iron reduction and LDL oxidation remarkably [38].

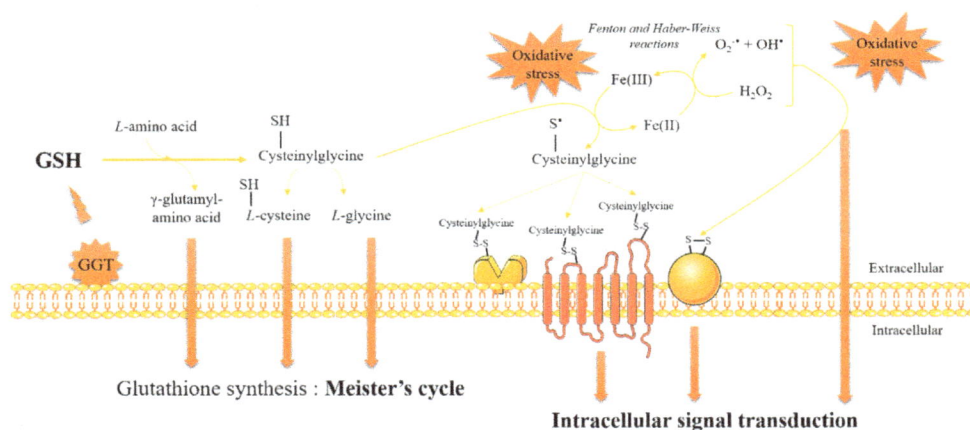

Figure 3. The pro-oxidant activity of γ-glutamyltransferase (GGT) adapted from [35].

3. Glutathione and Redox Signaling

Glutathione plays a crucial role in cell signaling via two pathways: (i) the modification of the redox potential toward oxidative values linked to the GSH concentration decrease and/or GSSG increase can activate transcription factors, which provokes gene activation and the synthesis of proteins with antioxidant properties; and (ii) the formation of the disulfide bond between protein thiol groups (PSHs) and GSH generates mixed (protein/non-protein) disulfides, that is, S-glutathiolated proteins (PSSGs).

Three main redox systems, the GSSG/2 GSH couple, the NADP+/NADPH couple and the thioredoxin system, regulate the intracellular redox potential [33]. However, as the intracellular concentration of GSH is very high, the ratio of the concentration of GSSG and GSH is fundamental for signal transductions, such as in the cell-cycle regulation [33]. Depending on the conditions, the in vivo redox potential of the GSSG/2 GSH couple ranges from −260 to −150 mV [46]. In fact, shifting the GSSG/2 GSH ratio toward the oxidizing state (redox potential of up to −150 mV) reduces cell proliferation and increases apoptosis through the activation of several signaling pathways, including calcineurin, NF-κB, protein kinase B, c-Jun N-terminal kinase, apoptosis signal-regulated kinase 1, and mitogen-activated protein kinase [47]. Furthermore, the cellular redox environment fluctuates during the cell cycle. Indeed, the cellular GSH content is significantly higher in the G2 and M phases compared with G1, while cells in the S-phase show an intermediate redox state [48]. Pharmacologic and genetic manipulations of the cellular redox environment perturb normal cell-cycle progression [49,50].

The process S-glutathiolation, a reversible post-translational modification of proteins, may have a role in the protection of PSHs from irreversible oxidation and in the redox regulation of the protein function, serving for cell signaling [51]. Indeed, if the modified cysteine is critical for the protein function, the S-glutathiolation will also either inactivate the protein or compromise cellular functions. Several S-glutathiolation mechanisms have been proposed: the direct reaction of GSH with partially oxidized reactive PSHs (thiyl radicals or sulfenic acids), thiol–disulfide exchange between PSHs and GSSG or between PSHs and oxidized GSH (sulfenic acid (GSOH)), nucleophilic attack of a protein thiolate on S-nitrosoglutathione (GSNO), and finally, PSHs' S-nitrosation followed by S-glutathiolation by GSH to yield the rate of mixed disulfides' formation. Protein S-glutathiolation can also change the protein activity and have a role in redox signaling. Under normal physiological conditions, the glutathiolation status of some proteins is important for many vital functions such as actin polymerization, transcription factor activation, and apoptosis [51]. Glutaredoxin, whose major isoforms in mammals are Grx1, Grx2, and Grx5, as well as thioredoxin, catalyzes S-glutathiolation and deglutathiolation of proteins to protect SH-groups from oxidation and restore functionally active thiols [52].

4. Methodologies for Dosage of Glutathione/Glutathiolated Proteins

As glutathione plays a fundamental role in cellular homeostasis, the changes in the GSH/GSSG ratio and concentrations are especially important in the evaluation and diagnosis of many redox-related pathologies, such as cancers [53], neurodegenerative diseases [54] or stroke [55], and cardiovascular diseases [56]. Glutathione in biological fluids (e.g., plasma) is known to demonstrate great instability, with a half-life of about 20 min [57]. The methodology used for GSH or GSSG quantification is therefore essential to achieve (i) the specificity required to discriminate between the various forms of glutathione and other endogenous thiols present in the biological matrices (cells, tissues, fluids, etc.), as well as (ii) the mandatory selectivity to separate the reduced and oxidized glutathione forms. Another important methodological criterion is sensitivity. For GSH, this parameter is often not critical because of its high concentration in cells (from 1 to 10 mM) and plasma (from 1 to 6 μM [58]). This will often be a problem for GSSG, which is present at low concentrations under physiological conditions, at around 1% of intracellular GSH levels.

At present, there are many methods for evaluating GSH and GSSG in biological samples, from the classical enzymo-colorimetric method developed by Tietze in 1969 [59], to spectrophotometric [60] or spectrofluorimetric [61] methods. The lack of chromophores and fluorophores in the glutathione family has led to the development of numerous derivatization methods (e.g., *N*-pyrenemaleimide or *O*-phthalaldehyde (OPA) [62–66]) or the use of electrochemical methods [67], mass spectrometry [68], chemiluminescence [69], nuclear magnetic resonance [70] or surface-enhanced Raman scattering [71]. Separation methods are also in full extension for this type of application, using chromatographic techniques (ultra-performance liquid chromatography [72], high-performance liquid chromatography [73], and gas chromatography [74]) or electrophoretic techniques [75], such as, for example, the quality control of GSH produced by microorganisms for pharmaceutical use [76].

The different methodologies mentioned above can be very effective but require specific equipment and an important analysis time, as well as peculiar sample processing or treatment. In this context, the use of nanotechnologies (essentially gold and silver metallic nanoparticles (NPs)) appears to be an interesting solution to quantify glutathiolated species. Gold and other metallic species are indeed characterized by an important avidity to bind sulfhydryl compounds [77–79]. In an organism, these atoms, including those under a NP state, form a bond with the thiol function of glutathione, even if the sulfur–metal interfacial chemistry remains controversial in the literature [77,80]. Over the past years, quantification on the basis of NPs has been largely developed to evaluate GSH in intracellular and/or extracellular concentrations in various biological matrices such as plasma, urine or saliva. Many colorimetric methods using gold NPs (AuNPs) (sensor or probes) [81] have been developed on the basis of their high molar absorbance coefficient associated with a specific plasmonic resonance-band shift (the maximum wavelength moves from a dispersed to an aggregated state or vice versa; see, e.g., [82]). The development of such nanosystems is very interesting but can lead to many problems of interference as a result, in particular, of chemical structures close to glutathione in large quantities in the body, such as cysteine or homocysteine [83]. Current methods make it possible to reach nanomolar concentrations, such as capillary electrophoresis coupled laser-induced fluorescence, as described by Shen et al. [84]. To a lesser extent, silver NPs are also used to evaluate glutathione in a biological medium with the same advantages as AuNPs described previously [85,86]. Other, more marginal examples of NPs developed specifically to quantify GSH or GSSG, such as NPs of alumina or zinc, can be found in the literature [87,88].

All the examples mentioned above show that nanotechnology is the future of the determination of many biological molecules, glutathione clearly being a part of it.

5. Repletion of Glutathione: Therapeutic Opportunities and Challenges

In cancer therapy, the depletion of glutathione has emerged as a valuable strategy to increase the sensitivity of cancer cells to radiations and toxic drugs, especially for aggressive and/or metastatic cancers [89–91]. However, a great majority of diseases (diabetes [92], cardiovascular diseases [56], HIV/AIDS [93], sepsis [94], cystic fibrosis [95], stroke [55], and brain disorders such as Alzheimer's and Parkinson's diseases or schizophrenia [96–98]), are associated with a decrease in GSH, combined with various oxidative stress states. Similarly, it has been demonstrated that the GSH antioxidant defenses of the body decrease linearly with age (oxidation of the GSSG/2 GSH couple in plasma: +0.7 mV/year after 45 years of age [99]), leaving us vulnerable to many age-related diseases. As a result, therapeutic strategies to restore the GSH pool are needed, ideally through oral administration for such chronic conditions. This is especially challenging because of the physicochemical properties of GSH (low partition coefficient; PubChem's calculated log P = -4.5) and its high degradation rate in the gastrointestinal tract through bacterial and epithelial GGT catalysis [100]. Two complementary approaches might increase GSH bioavailability: one is based on chemistry and the other is based on drug delivery technology (Figure 4a).

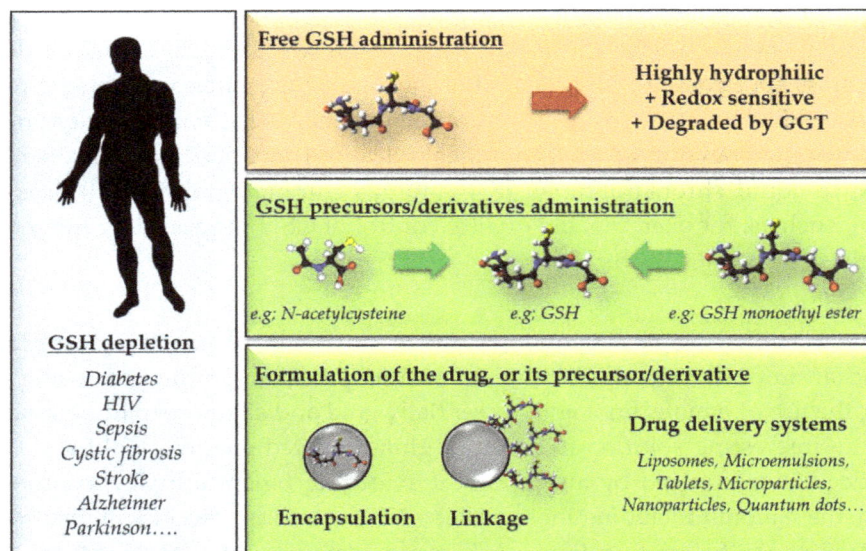

(a)

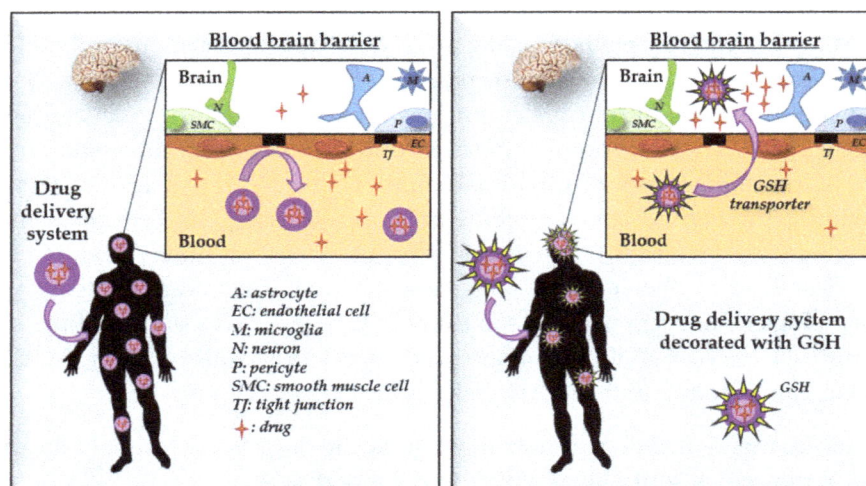

(b)

Figure 4. Schematic representations of the links between nanotechnologies and glutathione. (a) How nanotechnologies can help to reconstitute the glutathione pool? (b) How GSH can help nanotechnologies to reach their target? The example of Brain delivery.

The administration of prodrugs of GSH (or GSH precursors such as cysteine) is a first option. However, cysteine cannot be administered directly because of its toxicity and instability [101]; therefore precursors of cysteine, for example, the well-known *N*-acetylcysteine (NAC), are used. NAC is a potent antioxidant and an established antidote for acetaminophen overdose (which depletes hepatic GSH). Both parenteral and oral administrations are approved by the Food and Drug Administration for this indication, with different therapeutic schemes: loading dose followed by 17 additional doses over 72 h for oral NAC versus loading dose and 2 additional doses over 21 h for parenteral NAC [102]. Although several human clinical trials have investigated the potential of oral NAC to replenish GSH in chronic depletions (e.g., in HIV patients), all have failed to give sufficient benefits to gain regulatory approval, even at high doses (up to 2 g/day) [103]. These results can be explained by different mechanisms of GSH depletion between acute and chronic conditions and/or by the low NAC bioavailability when given per os (6–10% [104]). To improve tissue distribution, lipophilic derivatives of NAC were prepared: they gave encouraging results in cells (NAC amide [105]) or after peritoneal (NAC amide [106]) or oral administration in rats (NAC ethyl ester [107]). This strategy was also extended to GSH, creating more lipophilic derivatives through esterification. Glutathione esters (mainly mono- and di-methylesters) have been investigated as potential oral delivery compounds because they present a higher hydrophobicity and less sensitivity toward GGT degradation [108–111], but no conclusive data on their ability to restore the GSH pool in humans are currently reported in the literature. Furthermore, other cysteine or glutathione precursors have been evaluated with varying results: L-methionine; S-adenosylmethionine (SAMe) [112]; L-2-oxothiazolidine-4-carboxylate (OTC, procysteine), which is enzymatically converted to cysteine within liver cells [113]; 2-(RS)-n-propylthiazolidine-4(R)-carboxylic-acid (PTCA); D-ribose-L-cysteine; L-cysteine-glutathione mixed disulphide [114]; and γ-glutamylcysteine [115].

The second option for improving the bioavailability of GSH (or its derivatives) is to use a drug delivery system. In the literature, GSH has been encapsulated into various galenic forms for oral administration: liposomes [116], water-in-oil microemulsions [117], pellets of montmorillonite and glutathione [118], polymeric NPs and microparticles prepared with natural or synthetic polymers [119–121], hydrogels [122], and mucoadhesive films for sublingual delivery [123], as well as orobuccal tablets in combination with L-cystine, vitamin C and selenium [124]. Only this latter form has been tested per os in humans, with promising results: the GSH blood level increased significantly with time after administration of this tablet containing 250 mg of GSH to 15 healthy volunteers (both sexes, 20–40 years old) [124]. Aside from improving bioavailability, an additional benefit of formulations is to increase patient compliance while hiding the undesirable organoleptic (odor and flavor) properties of the thiol drugs.

The GSH can also be chemically linked to the carrier surface (instead of being passively encapsulated into the carrier). The main problem encountered with GSH conjugation on molecules remains the preservation of the thiol function, that is, to avoid formation of a disulfide. Many works use GSH as a stabilizer for metallic (mainly gold or silver) NPs [125–127] or nanoclusters [128] by the interaction between sulfur and metallic atoms, as previously explained. However, this prevents their use for the peptide repletion event if these particles seem to be well-tolerated by cells and the organism [129]. Only few works have reported the synthesis of GSH conjugates with a preservation of its antioxidant property. Two main strategies were led, grafting GSH either to polymers used as raw material for NP preparation, or to preformed NPs. First, GSH was covalently linked to chitosan [130] and polyethylene glycol [131]. Yields of grafting were 99% for polyethylene glycol–GSH oligomers [131] and 111 µmol GSH/g of functionalized chitosan [130]. In an in vitro model of oxidative stress (human brain neuroblastoma cells' SH-SY5Y cell line; exposed to H_2O_2 for 24 h), cells pre-treated by oligomers (polyethylene glycol conjugated to GSH) were protected from oxidative damage [131]. Second, GSH was anchored to core shell (CdSe/ZnS) quantum dots (up to 40 GSH moieties per quantum dot [132]. These quantum dots were tested in an in vivo model using *Hydra vulgaris* [132]. The authors showed the localization of GSH binding proteins inside the animals after internalization, as a result of the fluorescent properties of the quantum dots. GSH was also conjugated to gold NPs (AuNPs) via a linker (lipoic acid), which was previously shown to passivate the NP surface [133,134], and which limited the access of the thiol function to the gold core [135]. In this work, the authors report the possible oligomerization of GSH during the process, which could explain the high grafting density (ca. 7500 GSH moieties per AuNP) on AuNPs. The preservation of GSH properties was demonstrated using classical redox tests. Compared to non-conjugated GSH AuNPs, an activity enhanced by factors of 10,000 and 36,000 was reported for AuNPs functionalized by GSH using 2,2′-azino-bis(3-éthylbenzothiazoline-6-sulphonic) acid (ABTS) and ferric reducing antioxidant power (FRAP), respectively [135].

To conclude, very few of these works have moved from research into clinic applications (apart from precursors/prodrugs of GSH such as NAC, and one GSH-containing orobuccal tablet), especially for oral GSH supplementation. The collaboration between the chemical and galenic approaches seems nevertheless to offer promising opportunities in the future.

6. GSH Decoration as a Tool for Targeted Drug Delivery Systems

Glutathione is now also being investigated as a molecular tool in the hand of chemists and pharmacists to specifically deliver drugs to the brain (Figure 4b) or to obtain controlled drug release in the intracellular compartment. These two aspects are discussed in this section.

6.1. Brain-Targeted Drug Delivery

Drug delivery to the central nervous system represents one of the major pharmaceutical challenges, as the passage of macromolecules as well as 98% of small molecules is prevented by the blood–brain barrier under physiological conditions [136]. However, brain drug delivery can be achieved by taking advantage of the numerous endogenous specialized transport systems of this biological barrier. In the last years, GSH has emerged as a potential candidate to facilitate the receptor-mediated transcytosis of nanocarriers. The sodium-dependent (active) glutathione transporter is indeed present in all mammalian species, with a preferential expression in the central nervous system and the blood–brain barrier [137–139]. The conjugation of GSH on several pharmaceutical forms safely enhanced the delivery of various encapsulated drugs and nucleic acids to the brain. The story of G-technology, a liposomal system with a polyethylene glycol (PEG) coating modified with GSH, is developed as an example of the successful transfer from the pre-clinic to the clinic. Rip et al. evaluated the uptake of GSH-coated–PEGylated liposomes encapsulating carboxyfluorescein (an autoquenched fluorescent tracer) by brain endothelial cells, as well as their pharmacokinetic behavior and brain distribution after intraperitoneal or intravenous administration to rats [140]. The results demonstrated a temperature-dependent uptake of liposomes by the endothelial cells (about 2 times higher for GSH–PEG liposomes compared to uncoated liposomes). In rats, both administration routes gave comparable circulating levels and tissue distribution, and the brain levels of the fluorescent tracer were increased 4-fold by the GSH coating. This technology was used to deliver amyloid-targeting antibody fragments to the brain in a mouse model of Alzheimer's disease after intravenous bolus [141]. The liposomes were prepared by the ethanol injection method, with cholesterol, mPEG-2000-1,2-distearoyl-sn-glycero-3-phosphoethanolamine, and different lipids: the brain accumulation was higher for egg-yolk phosphatidylcholine liposomes than 1,2-dimyristoyl-sn-glycero-3-phosphocholine liposomes. Maussang et al. studied the mechanisms of increased in vivo brain delivery of the model drug ribavirin when encapsulated into PEGylated liposomes conjugated with GSH, intravenously administered to rats [142]. They demonstrated that this brain-specific uptake was positively correlated with increasing amounts of GSH coating and involved a receptor-mediated mechanism. These GSH–PEG liposomes (G-technology) have also demonstrated brain targeting as well as therapeutic efficacy in murine models of brain cancer (2B3-101; drug: doxorubicin [143,144]) and neuroinflammation (2B3-201; drug: methylprednisolone [145]). As an example, the major results obtained with 2B3-101 in cells and animals are presented in Figure 5. The 2B3-201 product has recently completed a phase I trial in healthy volunteers [146], while the 2B3-101 product has completed a phase I/IIa trial in patients with various forms of brain cancer (ClinicalTrials.gov Identifier: NCT01386580 [147,148]) and is currently being tested in a phase II trial in patients with breast cancer and leptomeningeal metastases (ClinicalTrials.gov Identifier: NCT01818713).

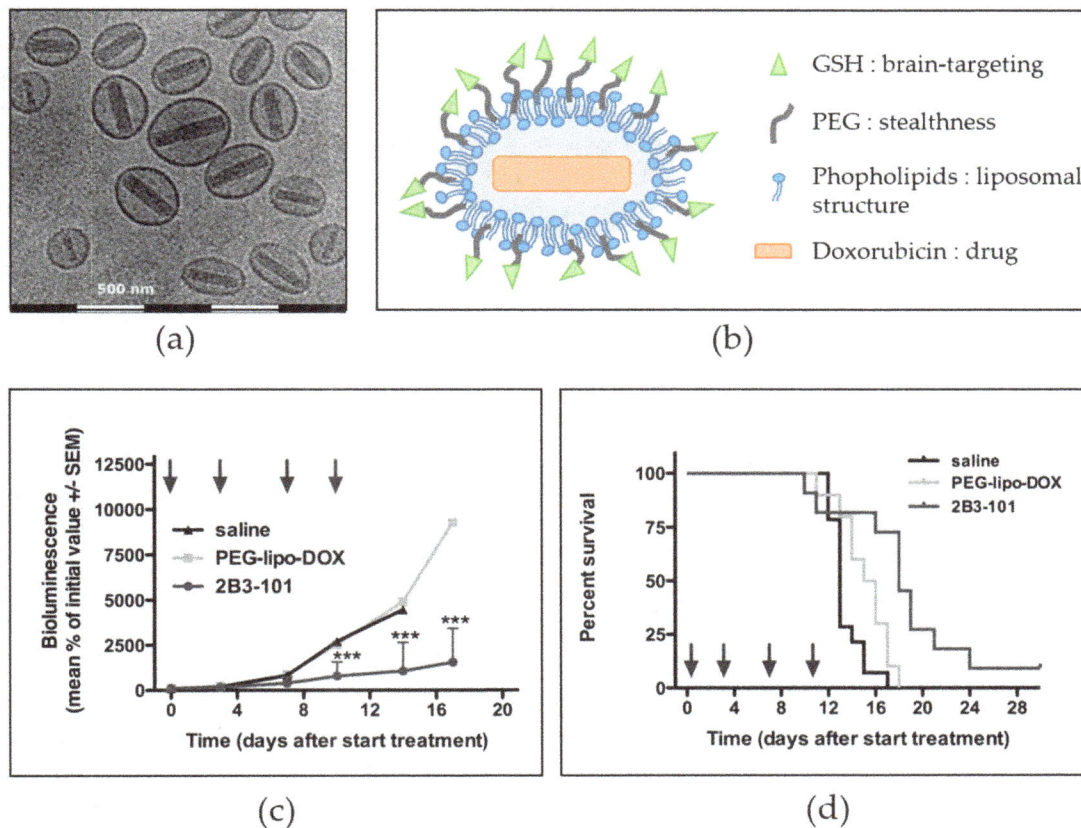

Figure 5. Brain targeting with reduced glutathione (GSH) decoration: example of the 2B3-101 product (GSH-coated–polyethylene glycol (PEG)ylated liposome containing doxorubicin). (**a**) Cryo-electron microscopy image of 2B3-101; (**b**) schematic representation of the liposomal structure; (**c**) inhibition of brain tumor growth in mice with experimental brain tumors; (**d**) increased survival of mice with experimental brain tumors. Animals received twice-weekly IV administrations (arrows on the graph) of saline ($n = 14$), 2B3-101 ($n = 10$) or PEGylated liposomal doxorubicin (PEG-lipo-DOX; $n = 10$), all at 5 mg/kg doxorubicin equivalents. *** $p < 0.001$, 2B3-101 vs saline and PEG-lipo-DOX; (**a**,**c**,**d**) are reproduced with permission from [144].

GSH-coating is also under investigation to obtain the brain delivery of drugs encapsulated into NPs. Veszelka et al. have, for example, demonstrated on cells that GSH coating leads to a higher cell uptake of polystyrene NPs than biotin coating [149]. GSH-coated poly(lactic-*co*-glycolic acid) (PLGA)–PEG NPs containing docetaxel [150], doxorubicin [151] or paclitaxel [152] have also been developed and characterized for drug release, cytotoxicity and blood–brain barrier permeation. In animals, bovine serum albumin (BSA) NPs with a GSH ligand led to 10-fold higher brain concentrations of a neuroprotective agent than the drug solution, 5 h after intravenous injection [153]. In another study, a hydrophilic model drug was 3 times more concentrated in the brain after intravenous injection of GSH-coated BSA NPs, compared to the same uncoated NPs [154]. Finally, in a middle cerebral artery occlusion model of stroke, GSH-coated PLGA–PEG NPs containing the thyroid T3 hormone showed better therapeutic efficacy than T3 solution or uncoated NPs, on both tissue infarction (reduction of 58%, 34%, and 51%, respectively) and brain edema (reduction of 75%, 59% and 68%, respectively) [155]. Although these GSH-coated NPs are not already in use in clinical trials, they highlight that GSH-mediated brain targeting can be used with different galenic forms, for various drugs. Recently, this strategy has also been proved to be successful in vitro for gene delivery to brain endothelial cells [156], thus opening another wide field of applications.

6.2. Intracellular-Targeted Drug Delivery

Because of the difference in GSH concentrations between plasma and cytosol (0.001 mM vs. 1 to 10 mM), the intracellular compartment is a more reductive environment than plasma. As a result, the difference in redox potential has been exploited by researchers to create stimuli-sensitive NPs. Using this strategy, a drug is not only protected in the blood flow but is also released specifically in this reductive environment, thus achieving intracellular targeting. Other external stimuli have been described on the basis of physical (light and electromagnetic field), chemical (pH and temperature) or even biochemical (enzyme) signals. To go further, there is growing research to develop sequential or simultaneous multi-stimuli responsive delivery systems. Interesting reviews on this topic can be found in the literature (e.g., [157–159]). As far as the redox stimulus is concerned, two main strategies are usually described, based either on the reduction of disulfide bounds structuring the NPs or on ligand exchange at the surface of inorganic NPs. An extensive literature deals with the design of new bio-reducible polymers (such as poly(ethylenimine), poly(amido amine) or polymers based on peptide or nucleic acid derivatives) [159,160]. In these works, the authors use the reduction of disulfide bounds (introduced into the polymer structure) by intracellular GSH to trigger the drug release through NP disorganization or disassembly. Another approach focuses on di-selenide or carbon–selenide bonds, which are more sensitive to the GSH concentration than disulfide bonds [161]. Chemical and pre-clinical proofs of concept have been brought forward for applications in gene silencing and imaging [162], as well as in the delivery of genes [160], proteins and anti-proliferative drugs [159,162]. None of these objects has nevertheless reached the clinical level so far.

Apart from disulfide reduction by GSH, another strategy using ligand exchange at the surface of AuNPs has been described (Figure 6). As previously explained, there is a strong avidity of AuNPs towards the thiol function of GSH. After internalization of AuNPs into the cellular cytoplasm, the drug grafted on the surface of the gold core is progressively released and replaced by GSH through thiol–gold binding. This was used to deliver the drug (e.g., paclitaxel) or for cell imaging [162,163]. However, intracellular GSH may be depleted, which could lead to oxidative stress in addition to other redox side-effects that may be induced by AuNPs [164].

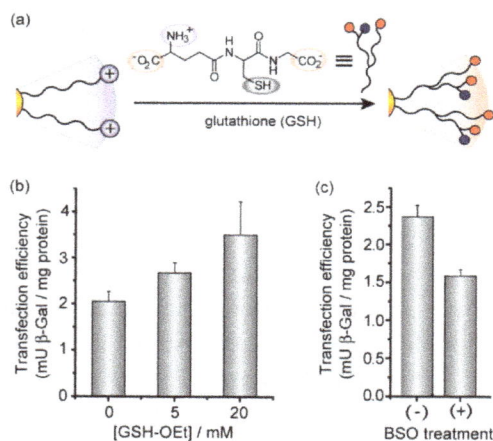

Figure 6. Example of ligand exchange strategy involving reduced glutathione (GSH) for targeted intracellular gene delivery. (**a**) Scheme of the ligand exchange reaction between native cationic ligands and cellular glutathione on gold nanoparticles' surface. (**b**) Elevation in transfection level depending on dose of glutathione monoester (GSH–Oet). Monkey kidney cells were preincubated with GSH–Oet for 1 h then washed prior to transfection, to transiently increase the GSH level. (**c**) Decrease in transfection efficiency upon L-buthionine-[S,R]-sulfoximine (BSO) treatment. Cells were plated in BSO-containing (2 mM) media and incubated for 24 h. BSO is an inhibitor of γ-glutamylcysteine synthetase and thus suppresses baseline GSH production. Reprinted with permission from [163].

7. Conclusions

Since its discovery, GSH has been shown to play ubiquitous roles in most living cells, from prokaryotic to eukaryotic organisms. GSH was defined as the intracellular redox buffer, and its major function, either free or associated to proteins, is tightly connected to redox reactions, mainly acting as a reductant versus oxygen and its derived reactive species. From physico-chemical and biochemical points of view, GSH redox properties are well defined and act in cell signaling through post-translational modifications. Disturbance of redox homeostasis related to the depletion of GSH has been shown more and more to be implicated in many pathophysiological states, opening a means for its use as a drug. Glutathione has clearly penetrated fields other than biology, such as therapeutics, with associated nanotechnology approaches for improving its bioavailability and targeting ability. Indeed, growing research considers GSH not only as a drug, but also as a tool for stimuli responsive in drug delivery systems.

Acknowledgments: The authors acknowledge support of EA 3452 CITHEFOR by the "Impact Biomolecules" project of the "Lorraine Université d'Excellence" (Investissements d'avenir—ANR).

Conflicts of Interest: The authors declare no conflict of interest.

Abbreviations

ABTS	2,2′-Azino-bis(3-éthylbenzothiazoline-6-sulphonic) acid
AuNP	Gold nanoparticle
BSA	Bovine serum albumin
BSO	L-Buthionine-[S,R]-sulfoximine
CFTR	Cystic fibrosis transmembrane conductance regulator
DIC	Dicarboxylate carrier
FRAP	Ferric reducing antioxidant power
GCL	γ-Glutamylcysteinyl ligase
GGT	γ-Glutamyltransferase
GPx	Glutathione peroxidase
GR	Glutathione disulfide reductase
GS	Glutathione synthase
GSH	Reduced glutathione
GSH-Oet	Glutathione monoester
GSNO	S-Nitrosoglutathione
GSOH	Glutathione sulfenic acid
GSSG	Disulfide glutathione
GSTs	Glutathione-S-transferases
LDL	Low-density lipoprotein
MRP	Multidrug resistance-associated protein
NAC	N-Acetylcysteine
NFE2L2	Nuclear factor erythroid-derived 2-like 2
NP	Nanoparticle
OGC	Oxoglutarate carrier
OPA	O-Phthalaldehyde
OTC	L-2-Oxothiazolidine-4-carboxylate
PEG	Poly(ethylene)glycol
PLGA	Poly(lactic-co-glycolic acid)
PSHs	Protein thiol groups
PSSGs	S-Glutathiolated proteins
PTCA	2-(RS)-n-Propylthiazolidine-4(R)-carboxylic-acid
RyR1	Ryanodine receptor type 1
SAMe	S-Adenosylmethionine

References

1. Hamilton, C.J.; Arbach, M.; Groom, M. Beyond Glutathione: Different Low Molecular Weight Thiols as Mediators of Redox Regulation and Other Metabolic Functions in Lower Organisms. In *Recent Advances in Redox Active Plant and Microbial Products*; Jacob, C., Kirsch, G., Slusarenko, A., Winyard, P., Burkholz, T., Eds.; Springer: Dordrecht, The Netherlands, 2014; ISBN 978-94-017-8925-3.

2. Gowland Hopkins, F.; Dixon, M. On glutathione. II. A thermostable oxidation-reduction system. *J. Biol. Chem.* **1922**, *54*, 527–563.

3. Hunter, G.; Eagles, B.A. Glutathione: A critical study. *J. Biol. Chem.* **1927**, *72*, 147–166.

4. Meister, A.; Tate, S.S. Glutathione and related gamma-glutamyl compounds: Biosynthesis and utilization. *Annu. Rev. Biochem.* **1976**, *45*, 559–604. [CrossRef] [PubMed]

5. Meister, A.; Anderson, M.E. Glutathione. *Annu. Rev. Biochem.* **1983**, *52*, 711–760. [CrossRef] [PubMed]

6. Baldelli, S.; Aquilano, K.; Ciriolo, M.R. Punctum on two different transcription factors regulated by PGC-1α: Nuclear factor erythroid-derived 2-like 2 and nuclear respiratory factor 2. *Biochim. Biophys. Acta* **2013**, *1830*, 4137–4146. [CrossRef] [PubMed]

7. Chen, Y.; Shertzer, H.G.; Schneider, S.N.; Nebert, D.W.; Dalton, T.P. Glutamate cysteine ligase catalysis: Dependence on ATP and modifier subunit for regulation of tissue glutathione levels. *J. Biol. Chem.* **2005**, *280*, 33766–33774. [CrossRef] [PubMed]

8. Taylor, C.G.; Nagy, L.E.; Bray, T.M. Nutritional and hormonal regulation of glutathione homeostasis. *Curr. Top. Cell. Regul.* **1996**, *34*, 189–208. [PubMed]

9. Krejsa, C.M.; Franklin, C.C.; White, C.C.; Ledbetter, J.A.; Schieven, G.L.; Kavanagh, T.J. Rapid Activation of Glutamate Cysteine Ligase following Oxidative Stress. *J. Biol. Chem.* **2010**, *285*, 16116–16124. [CrossRef] [PubMed]

10. Lauterburg, B.H.; Adams, J.D.; Mitchell, J.R. Hepatic glutathione homeostasis in the rat: Efflux accounts for glutathione turnover. *Hepatology* **1984**, *4*, 586–590. [CrossRef] [PubMed]

11. DeLeve, L.D.; Kaplowitz, N. Glutathione metabolism and its role in hepatotoxicity. *Pharmacol. Ther.* **1991**, *52*, 287–305. [CrossRef]

12. Cooper, A.J.; Pinto, J.T.; Callery, P.S. Reversible and irreversible protein glutathionylation: Biological and Clinical aspects. *Expert Opin. Drug Metab. Toxicol.* **2011**, *7*, 891–910. [CrossRef] [PubMed]

13. Pineda-Molina, E.; Klatt, P.; Vázquez, J.; Marina, A.; García de Lacoba, M.; Pérez-Sala, D.; Lamas, S. Glutathionylation of the p50 subunit of NF-kappaB: A mechanism for redox-induced inhibition of DNA binding. *Biochemistry* **2001**, *40*, 14134–14142. [CrossRef] [PubMed]

14. Huang, Z.; Pinto, J.T.; Deng, H.; Richie, J.P. Inhibition of caspase-3 activity and activation by protein glutathionylation. *Biochem. Pharmacol.* **2008**, *75*, 2234–2244. [CrossRef] [PubMed]

15. Pastore, A.; Piemonte, F. Protein glutathionylation in cardiovascular diseases. *Int. J. Mol. Sci.* **2013**, *14*, 20845–20876. [CrossRef] [PubMed]

16. Circu, M.L.; Aw, T.Y. Glutathione and modulation of cell apoptosis. *Biochim. Biophys. Acta* **2012**, *1823*, 1767–1777. [CrossRef] [PubMed]

17. Deponte, M. The Incomplete Glutathione Puzzle: Just Guessing at Numbers and Figures? *Antioxid. Redox Signal.* **2017**, *27*, 1130–1161. [CrossRef] [PubMed]

18. Taniguchi, N.; Ikeda, Y. Gamma-glutamyl transpeptidase: Catalytic mechanism and gene expression. *Adv. Enzymol. Relat. Areas Mol. Biol.* **1998**, *72*, 239–278. [PubMed]

19. Ohkama-Ohtsu, N.; Radwan, S.; Peterson, A.; Zhao, P.; Badr, A.F.; Xiang, C.; Oliver, D.J. Characterization of the extracellular gamma-glutamyl transpeptidases, GGT1 and GGT2, in Arabidposis. *Plant J.* **2007**, *49*, 865–877. [CrossRef] [PubMed]

20. Hanigan, M.H. Gamma-glutamyl transpeptidase: Redox regulation and drug resistance. *Adv. Cancer Res.* **2014**, *122*, 103–141. [CrossRef] [PubMed]

21. Zhang, H.; Forman, H.J. Redox regulation of gamma-glutamyl transpeptidase. *Am. J. Respir. Cell Mol. Biol.* **2009**, *41*, 509–515. [CrossRef] [PubMed]

22. Kumar, A.; Tikoo, S.; Maity, S.; Sengupta, S.; Sengupta, S.; Kaur, A.; Bachhawat, A.K. Mammalian proapoptotic factor ChaC1 and its homologues function as γ-glutamyl cyclotransferases acting specifically on glutathione. *EMBO Rep.* **2012**, *13*, 1095–1101. [CrossRef] [PubMed]

23. Kaur, A.; Gautam, R.; Srivastava, R.; Chandel, A.; Kumar, A.; Karthikeyan, S.; Bachhawat, A.K. ChaC2, an Enzyme for Slow Turnover of Cytosolic Glutathione. *J. Biol. Chem.* **2017**, *292*, 638–651. [CrossRef] [PubMed]

24. Mungrue, I.N.; Pagnon, J.; Kohannim, O.; Gargalovic, P.S.; Lusis, A.J. CHAC1/MGC4504 is a novel proapoptotic component of the unfolded protein response, downstream of the ATF4-ATF3-CHOP cascade. *J. Immunol.* **2009**, *182*, 466–476. [CrossRef] [PubMed]

25. Lash, L.H. Mitochondrial glutathione transport: Physiological, pathological and toxicological implications. *Chem. Biol. Interact.* **2006**, *163*, 54–67. [CrossRef] [PubMed]

26. Bánhegyi, G.; Csala, M.; Nagy, G.; Sorrentino, V.; Fulceri, R.; Benedetti, A. Evidence for the transport of glutathione through ryanodine receptor channel type 1. *Biochem. J.* **2003**, *376*, 807–812. [CrossRef] [PubMed]

27. Csala, M.; Fulceri, R.; Mandl, J.; Benedetti, A.; Bánhegyi, G. Ryanodine receptor channel-dependent glutathione transport in the sarcoplasmic reticulum of skeletal muscle. *Biochem. Biophys. Res. Commun.* **2001**, *287*, 696–700. [CrossRef] [PubMed]

28. Belcastro, E.; Wu, W.; Fries-Raeth, I.; Corti, A.; Pompella, A.; Leroy, P.; Lartaud, I.; Gaucher, C. Oxidative stress enhances and modulates protein S-nitrosation in smooth muscle cells exposed to S-nitrosoglutathione. *Nitric Oxide Biol. Chem.* **2017**, *69*, 10–21. [CrossRef] [PubMed]

29. Ballatori, N.; Krance, S.M.; Marchan, R.; Hammond, C.L. Plasma membrane glutathione transporters and their roles in cell physiology and pathophysiology. *Mol. Asp. Med.* **2009**, *30*, 13–28. [CrossRef] [PubMed]

30. Muanprasat, C.; Wongborisuth, C.; Pathomthongtaweechai, N.; Satitsri, S.; Hongeng, S. Protection against oxidative stress in beta thalassemia/hemoglobin E erythrocytes by inhibitors of glutathione efflux transporters. *PLoS ONE* **2013**, *8*, e55685. [CrossRef] [PubMed]

31. Dickinson, D.A.; Forman, H.J. Cellular glutathione and thiols metabolism. *Biochem. Pharmacol.* **2002**, *64*, 1019–1026. [CrossRef]

32. Forman, H.J.; Zhang, H.; Rinna, A. Glutathione: Overview of its protective roles, measurement, and biosynthesis. *Mol. Asp. Med.* **2009**, *30*, 1–12. [CrossRef] [PubMed]

33. Schafer, F.Q.; Buettner, G.R. Redox environment of the cell as viewed through the redox state of the glutathione disulfide/glutathione couple. *Free Radic. Biol. Med.* **2001**, *30*, 1191–1212. [CrossRef]

34. Nagy, P. Kinetics and mechanisms of thiol-disulfide exchange covering direct substitution and thiol-oxidation pathways. *Antioxid. Redox Signal.* **2013**, *18*, 1623–1641. [CrossRef] [PubMed]

35. Paolicchi, A.; Dominici, S.; Pieri, L.; Maellaro, E.; Pompella, A. Glutathione catabolism as a signaling mechanism. *Biochem. Pharmacol.* **2002**, *64*, 1027–1035. [CrossRef]

36. Dominici, S.; Paolicchi, A.; Corti, A.; Maellaro, E.; Pompella, A. Prooxidant reactions promoted by soluble and cell-bound gamma-glutamyltransferase activity. *Methods Enzymol.* **2005**, *401*, 484–501. [CrossRef] [PubMed]

37. Drozdz, R.; Parmentier, C.; Hachad, H.; Leroy, P.; Siest, G.; Wellman, M. gamma-Glutamyltransferase dependent generation of reactive oxygen species from a glutathione/transferrin system. *Free Radic. Biol. Med.* **1998**, *25*, 786–792. [CrossRef]

38. Dominici, S.; Pieri, L.; Comporti, M.; Pompella, A. Possible role of membrane gamma-glutamyltransferase activity in the facilitation of transferrin-dependent and -independent iron uptake by cancer cells. *Cancer Cell Int.* **2003**, *3*, 7. [CrossRef] [PubMed]

39. Glass, G.A.; Stark, A.A. Promotion of glutathione-gamma-glutamyl transpeptidase-dependent lipid peroxidation by copper and ceruloplasmin: The requirement for iron and the effects of antioxidants and antioxidant enzymes. *Environ. Mol. Mutagen.* **1997**, *29*, 73–80. [CrossRef]

40. Schmidt, A.M.; Hori, O.; Brett, J.; Yan, S.D.; Wautier, J.L.; Stern, D. Cellular receptors for advanced glycation end products. Implications for induction of oxidant stress and cellular dysfunction in the pathogenesis of vascular lesions. *Arterioscler. Thromb. J. Vasc. Biol.* **1994**, *14*, 1521–1528. [CrossRef]

41. Gimbrone, M.A. Vascular endothelium: An integrator of pathophysiologic stimuli in atherosclerosis. *Am. J. Cardiol.* **1995**, *75*, 67B–70B. [CrossRef]

42. Ross, R. The pathogenesis of atherosclerosis: A perspective for the 1990s. *Nature* **1993**, *362*, 801–809. [CrossRef] [PubMed]

43. Bradley, J.R. TNF-mediated inflammatory disease. *J. Pathol.* **2008**, *214*, 149–160. [CrossRef] [PubMed]

44. Paolicchi, A.; Minotti, G.; Tonarelli, P.; Tongiani, R.; De Cesare, D.; Mezzetti, A.; Dominici, S.; Comporti, M.; Pompella, A. Gamma-glutamyl transpeptidase-dependent iron reduction and LDL oxidation—A potential mechanism in atherosclerosis. *J. Investig. Med.* **1999**, *47*, 151–160. [PubMed]

45. Berliner, J.A.; Heinecke, J.W. The role of oxidized lipoproteins in atherogenesis. *Free Radic. Biol. Med.* **1996**, *20*, 707–727. [CrossRef]

46. Jones, D.P. Redox potential of GSH/GSSG couple: Assay and biological significance. *Methods Enzymol.* **2002**, *348*, 93–112. [PubMed]

47. Sen, C.K. Cellular thiols and redox-regulated signal transduction. *Curr. Top. Cell. Regul.* **2000**, *36*, 1–30. [PubMed]

48. Conour, J.E.; Graham, W.V.; Gaskins, H.R. A combined in vitro/bioinformatic investigation of redox regulatory mechanisms governing cell cycle progression. *Physiol. Genom.* **2004**, *18*, 196–205. [CrossRef] [PubMed]

49. Menon, S.G.; Sarsour, E.H.; Spitz, D.R.; Higashikubo, R.; Sturm, M.; Zhang, H.; Goswami, P.C. Redox regulation of the G1 to S phase transition in the mouse embryo fibroblast cell cycle. *Cancer Res.* **2003**, *63*, 2109–2117. [PubMed]

50. Menon, S.G.; Sarsour, E.H.; Kalen, A.L.; Venkataraman, S.; Hitchler, M.J.; Domann, F.E.; Oberley, L.W.; Goswami, P.C. Superoxide signaling mediates N-acetyl-L-cysteine-induced G1 arrest: Regulatory role of cyclin D1 and manganese superoxide dismutase. *Cancer Res.* **2007**, *67*, 6392–6399. [CrossRef] [PubMed]

51. Belcastro, E.; Gaucher, C.; Corti, A.; Leroy, P.; Lartaud, I.; Pompella, A. Regulation of protein function by S-nitrosation and S-glutathionylation: Processes and targets in cardiovascular pathophysiology. *Biol. Chem.* **2017**, *398*, 1267–1293. [CrossRef] [PubMed]

52. Holmgren, A. Redox regulation by thioredoxin and thioredoxin reductase. *BioFactors* **2000**, *11*, 63–64. [CrossRef] [PubMed]

53. Pastore, A.; Federici, G.; Bertini, E.; Piemonte, F. Analysis of glutathione: Implication in redox and detoxification. *Clin. Chim. Acta* **2003**, *333*, 19–39. [CrossRef]

54. Schulz, J.B.; Lindenau, J.; Seyfried, J.; Dichgans, J. Glutathione, oxidative stress and neurodegeneration. *Eur. J. Biochem.* **2000**, *267*, 4904–4911. [CrossRef] [PubMed]

55. Anderson, M.F.; Nilsson, M.; Eriksson, P.S.; Sims, N.R. Glutathione monoethyl ester provides neuroprotection in a rat model of stroke. *Neurosci. Lett.* **2004**, *354*, 163–165. [CrossRef] [PubMed]

56. Vargas, F.; Rodríguez-Gómez, I.; Pérez-Abud, R.; Vargas Tendero, P.; Baca, Y.; Wangensteen, R. Cardiovascular and renal manifestations of glutathione depletion induced by buthionine sulfoximine. *Am. J. Hypertens.* **2012**, *25*, 629–635. [CrossRef] [PubMed]

57. Beutler, E.; Duron, O.; Kelly, B.M. Improved method for the determination of blood glutathione. *J. Lab. Clin. Med.* **1963**, *61*, 882–888. [PubMed]

58. Mansoor, M.A.; Svardal, A.M.; Ueland, P.M. Determination of the in vivo redox status of cysteine, cysteinylglycine, homocysteine, and glutathione in human plasma. *Anal. Biochem.* **1992**, *200*, 218–229. [CrossRef]

59. Tietze, F. Enzymic method for quantitative determination of nanogram amounts of total and oxidized glutathione: Applications to mammalian blood and other tissues. *Anal. Biochem.* **1969**, *27*, 502–522. [CrossRef]

60. Chen, Z.; Wang, Z.; Chen, J.; Wang, S.; Huang, X. Sensitive and selective detection of glutathione based on resonance light scattering using sensitive gold nanoparticles as colorimetric probes. *Analyst* **2012**, *137*, 3132–3137. [CrossRef] [PubMed]

61. Xu, H.; Hepel, M. "Molecular beacon"—Based fluorescent assay for selective detection of glutathione and cysteine. *Anal. Chem.* **2011**, *83*, 813–819. [CrossRef] [PubMed]

62. Piccoli, G.; Fiorani, M.; Biagiarelli, B.; Palma, F.; Potenza, L.; Amicucci, A.; Stocchi, V. Simultaneous high-performance capillary electrophoretic determination of reduced and oxidized glutathione in red blood cells in the femtomole range. *J. Chromatogr. A* **1994**, *676*, 239–246. [CrossRef]

63. Park, S.K.; Boulton, R.B.; Noble, A.C. Automated HPLC analysis of glutathione and thiol-containing compounds in grape juice and wine using pre-column derivatization with fluorescence detection. *Food Chem.* **2000**, *68*, 475–480. [CrossRef]

64. Parmentier, C.; Leroy, P.; Wellman, M.; Nicolas, A. Determination of cellular thiols and glutathione-related enzyme activities: Versatility of high-performance liquid chromatography-spectrofluorimetric detection. *J. Chromatogr. B. Biomed. Sci. Appl.* **1998**, *719*, 37–46. [CrossRef]

65. Parmentier, C.; Wellman, M.; Nicolas, A.; Siest, G.; Leroy, P. Simultaneous measurement of reactive oxygen species and reduced glutathione using capillary electrophoresis and laser-induced fluorescence detection in cultured cell lines. *Electrophoresis* **1999**, *20*, 2938–2944. [CrossRef]

66. Lewicki, K.; Marchand, S.; Matoub, L.; Lulek, J.; Coulon, J.; Leroy, P. Development of a fluorescence-based microtiter plate method for the measurement of glutathione in yeast. *Talanta* **2006**, *70*, 876–882. [CrossRef] [PubMed]

67. Rezaei, B.; Khosropour, H.; Ensafi, A.A.; Hadadzadeh, H.; Farrokhpour, H. A Differential Pulse Voltammetric Sensor for Determination of Glutathione in Real Samples Using a Trichloro(terpyridine)ruthenium(III)/Multiwall Carbon Nanotubes Modified Paste Electrode. *IEEE Sens. J.* **2015**, *15*, 483–490. [CrossRef]

68. Burford, N.; Eelman, M.D.; Mahony, D.E.; Morash, M. Definitive identification of cysteine and glutathione complexes of bismuth by mass spectrometry: Assessing the biochemical fate of bismuth pharmaceutical agents. *Chem. Commun.* **2003**, *1*, 146–147. [CrossRef]

69. Han, H.-Y.; He, Z.-K.; Zeng, Y.-E. Chemiluminescence method for the determination of glutathione in human serum using the $Ru(phen)_3^{2+}$-$KMnO_4$ system. *Microchim. Acta* **2006**, *155*, 431–434. [CrossRef]

70. Mandal, P.K.; Tripathi, M.; Sugunan, S. Brain oxidative stress: Detection and mapping of anti-oxidant marker "Glutathione" in different brain regions of healthy male/female, MCI and Alzheimer patients using non-invasive magnetic resonance spectroscopy. *Biochem. Biophys. Res. Commun.* **2012**, *417*, 43–48. [CrossRef] [PubMed]

71. Huang, G.G.; Hossain, M.K.; Han, X.X.; Ozaki, Y. A novel reversed reporting agent method for surface-enhanced Raman scattering; highly sensitive detection of glutathione in aqueous solutions. *Analyst* **2009**, *134*, 2468–2474. [CrossRef] [PubMed]

72. Vallverdú-Queralt, A.; Verbaere, A.; Meudec, E.; Cheynier, V.; Sommerer, N. Straightforward method to quantify GSH, GSSG, GRP, and hydroxycinnamic acids in wines by UPLC-MRM-MS. *J. Agric. Food Chem.* **2015**, *63*, 142–149. [CrossRef] [PubMed]

73. Parent, M.; Dahboul, F.; Schneider, R.; Clarot, I.; Maincent, P.; Leroy, P.; Boudier, A. A Complete Physicochemical Identity Card of S-Nitrosoglutathione. Available online: http://www.eurekaselect.com/105996/article (accessed on 22 March 2018).

74. Neuschwander-Tetri, B.A.; Roll, F.J. Glutathione measurement by high-performance liquid chromatography separation and fluorometric detection of the glutathione-orthophthalaldehyde adduct. *Anal. Biochem.* **1989**, *179*, 236–241. [CrossRef]

75. Serru, V.; Baudin, B.; Ziegler, F.; David, J.P.; Cals, M.J.; Vaubourdolle, M.; Mario, N. Quantification of reduced and oxidized glutathione in whole blood samples by capillary electrophoresis. *Clin. Chem.* **2001**, *47*, 1321–1324. [PubMed]

76. European Department for the Quality of Medicines. *Glutathione, Monograph 01/2017: 1670, European Pharmacopoeia*; European Department for the Quality of Medicines: Strasbourg, France, 2018.

77. Pensa, E.; Cortés, E.; Corthey, G.; Carro, P.; Vericat, C.; Fonticelli, M.H.; Benítez, G.; Rubert, A.A.; Salvarezza, R.C. The chemistry of the sulfur-gold interface: In search of a unified model. *Acc. Chem. Res.* **2012**, *45*, 1183–1192. [CrossRef] [PubMed]

78. Lin, Z.; Monteiro-Riviere, N.A.; Riviere, J.E. Pharmacokinetics of metallic nanoparticles. *Wiley Interdiscip. Rev. Nanomed. Nanobiotechnol.* **2015**, *7*, 189–217. [CrossRef] [PubMed]

79. Bhattacharjee, A.; Chakraborty, K.; Shukla, A. Cellular copper homeostasis: Current concepts on its interplay with glutathione homeostasis and its implication in physiology and human diseases. *Metallomics* **2017**, *9*, 1376–1388. [CrossRef] [PubMed]

80. Reimers, J.R.; Ford, M.J.; Marcuccio, S.M.; Ulstrup, J.; Hush, N.S. Competition of van der Waals and chemical forces on gold–sulfur surfaces and nanoparticles. *Nat. Rev. Chem.* **2017**, *1*, 17. [CrossRef]

81. Tsogas, G.Z.; Kappi, F.A.; Vlessidis, A.G.; Giokas, D.L. Recent Advances in Nanomaterial Probes for Optical Biothiol Sensing: A Review. *Anal. Lett.* **2018**, *51*, 443–468. [CrossRef]

82. Li, Z.-J.; Zheng, X.-J.; Zhang, L.; Liang, R.-P.; Li, Z.-M.; Qiu, J.-D. Label-free colorimetric detection of biothiols utilizing SAM and unmodified Au nanoparticles. *Biosens. Bioelectron.* **2015**, *68*, 668–674. [CrossRef] [PubMed]

83. Li, J.-F.; Huang, P.-C.; Wu, F.-Y. Highly selective and sensitive detection of glutathione based on anti-aggregation of gold nanoparticles via pH regulation. *Sens. Actuators B Chem.* **2017**, *240*, 553–559. [CrossRef]

84. Shen, C.-C.; Tseng, W.-L.; Hsieh, M.-M. Selective enrichment of aminothiols using polysorbate 20-capped gold nanoparticles followed by capillary electrophoresis with laser-induced fluorescence. *J. Chromatogr. A* **2009**, *1216*, 288–293. [CrossRef] [PubMed]

85. Shen, L.-M.; Chen, Q.; Sun, Z.-Y.; Chen, X.-W.; Wang, J.-H. Assay of biothiols by regulating the growth of silver nanoparticles with C-dots as reducing agent. *Anal. Chem.* **2014**, *86*, 5002–5008. [CrossRef] [PubMed]

86. Kappi, F.A.; Papadopoulos, G.A.; Tsogas, G.Z.; Giokas, D.L. Low-cost colorimetric assay of biothiols based on the photochemical reduction of silver halides and consumer electronic imaging devices. *Talanta* **2017**, *172*, 15–22. [CrossRef] [PubMed]

87. Dringen, R.; Koehler, Y.; Derr, L.; Tomba, G.; Schmidt, M.M.; Treccani, L.; Colombi Ciacchi, L.; Rezwan, K. Adsorption and reduction of glutathione disulfide on α-Al$_2$O$_3$ nanoparticles: Experiments and modeling. *Langmuir* **2011**, *27*, 9449–9457. [CrossRef] [PubMed]

88. Barman, U.; Mukhopadhyay, G.; Goswami, N.; Ghosh, S.S.; Paily, R.P. Detection of Glutathione by Glutathione-S-Transferase-Nanoconjugate Ensemble Electrochemical Device. *IEEE Trans. Nanobiosci.* **2017**, *16*, 271–279. [CrossRef] [PubMed]

89. Estrela, J.; Obrador, E.; Navarro, J.; Delavega, M.; Pellicer, J. Elimination of Ehrlich Tumors by ATP-Induced Growth-Inhibition, Glutathione Depletion and X-Rays. *Nat. Med.* **1995**, *1*, 84–88. [CrossRef] [PubMed]

90. Mena, S.; Benlloch, M.; Ortega, A.; Carretero, J.; Obrador, E.; Asensi, M.; Petschen, I.; Brown, B.D.; Estrela, J.M. Bcl-2 and glutathione depletion sensitizes B16 melanoma to combination therapy and eliminates metastatic disease. *Clin. Cancer Res.* **2007**, *13*, 2658–2666. [CrossRef] [PubMed]

91. Rocha, C.R.R.; Garcia, C.C.M.; Vieira, D.B.; Quinet, A.; de Andrade-Lima, L.C.; Munford, V.; Belizario, J.E.; Menck, C.F.M. Glutathione depletion sensitizes cisplatin- and temozolomide-resistant glioma cells in vitro and in vivo. *Cell Death Dis.* **2014**, *5*, e1505. [CrossRef] [PubMed]

92. Lagman, M.; Ly, J.; Saing, T.; Kaur Singh, M.; Vera Tudela, E.; Morris, D.; Chi, P.-T.; Ochoa, C.; Sathananthan, A.; Venketaraman, V. Investigating the causes for decreased levels of glutathione in individuals with type II diabetes. *PLoS ONE* **2015**, *10*, e0118436. [CrossRef] [PubMed]

93. Herzenberg, L.A.; DeRosa, S.C.; Dubs, J.G.; Roederer, M.; Anderson, M.T.; Ela, S.W.; Deresinski, S.C.; Herzenberg, L.A. Glutathione deficiency is associated with impaired survival in HIV disease. *Proc. Natl. Acad. Sci. USA* **1997**, *94*, 1967–1972. [CrossRef] [PubMed]

94. Biolo, G.; Antonione, R.; De Cicco, M. Glutathione metabolism in sepsis. *Crit. Care Med.* **2007**, *35*, S591–S595. [CrossRef] [PubMed]

95. Day, B.J. Glutathione—A radical treatment for cystic fibrosis lung disease? *Chest* **2005**, *127*, 12–14. [CrossRef] [PubMed]

96. Martin, H.L.; Teismann, P. Glutathione—A review on its role and significance in Parkinson's disease. *FASEB J.* **2009**, *23*, 3263–3272. [CrossRef] [PubMed]

97. Pocernich, C.B.; Butterfield, D.A. Elevation of glutathione as a therapeutic strategy in Alzheimer disease. *Biochim. Biophys. Acta* **2012**, *1822*, 625–630. [CrossRef] [PubMed]

98. Gu, F.; Chauhan, V.; Chauhan, A. Glutathione redox imbalance in brain disorders. *Curr. Opin. Clin. Nutr. Metab. Care* **2015**, *18*, 89–95. [CrossRef] [PubMed]

99. Jones, D.P.; Mody, V.C.; Carlson, J.L.; Lynn, M.J.; Sternberg, P. Redox analysis of human plasma allows separation of pro-oxidant events of aging from decline in antioxidant defenses. *Free Radic. Biol. Med.* **2002**, *33*, 1290–1300. [CrossRef]

100. Witschi, A.; Reddy, S.; Stofer, B.; Lauterburg, B.H. The systemic availability of oral glutathione. *Eur. J. Clin. Pharmacol.* **1992**, *43*, 667–669. [CrossRef] [PubMed]

101. Shibui, Y.; Sakai, R.; Manabe, Y.; Masuyama, T. Comparisons of l-cysteine and d-cysteine toxicity in 4-week repeated-dose toxicity studies of rats receiving daily oral administration. *J. Toxicol. Pathol.* **2017**, *30*, 217–229. [CrossRef] [PubMed]

102. Greene, S.C.; Noonan, P.K.; Sanabria, C.; Peacock, W.F. Effervescent N-Acetylcysteine Tablets versus Oral Solution N-Acetylcysteine in Fasting Healthy Adults: An Open-Label, Randomized, Single-Dose, Crossover, Relative Bioavailability Study. *Curr. Ther. Res. Clin. Exp.* **2016**, *83*, 1–7. [CrossRef] [PubMed]

103. Dröge, W.; Breitkreutz, R. N-acetyl-cysteine in the therapy of HIV-positive patients. *Curr. Opin. Clin. Nutr. Metab. Care* **1999**, *2*, 493–498. [CrossRef] [PubMed]

104. Borgström, L.; Kågedal, B.; Paulsen, O. Pharmacokinetics of N-acetylcysteine in man. *Eur. J. Clin. Pharmacol.* **1986**, *31*, 217–222. [CrossRef] [PubMed]

105. Grinberg, L.; Fibach, E.; Amer, J.; Atlas, D. N-acetylcysteine amide, a novel cell-permeating thiol, restores cellular glutathione and protects human red blood cells from oxidative stress. *Free Radic. Biol. Med.* **2005**, *38*, 136–145. [CrossRef] [PubMed]

106. Patel, S.P.; Sullivan, P.G.; Pandya, J.D.; Goldstein, G.A.; VanRooyen, J.L.; Yonutas, H.M.; Eldahan, K.C.; Morehouse, J.; Magnuson, D.S.K.; Rabchevsky, A.G. N-acetylcysteine amide preserves mitochondrial bioenergetics and improves functional recovery following spinal trauma. *Exp. Neurol.* **2014**, *257*, 95–105. [CrossRef] [PubMed]

107. Giustarini, D.; Milzani, A.; Dalle-Donne, I.; Tsikas, D.; Rossi, R. N-Acetylcysteine ethyl ester (NACET): A novel lipophilic cell-permeable cysteine derivative with an unusual pharmacokinetic feature and remarkable antioxidant potential. *Biochem. Pharmacol.* **2012**, *84*, 1522–1533. [CrossRef] [PubMed]

108. Anderson, M.E.; Powrie, F.; Puri, R.N.; Meister, A. Glutathione monoethyl ester: Preparation, uptake by tissues, and conversion to glutathione. *Arch. Biochem. Biophys.* **1985**, *239*, 538–548. [CrossRef]

109. Grattagliano, I.; Wieland, P.; Schranz, C.; Lauterburg, B.H. Effect of oral glutathione monoethyl ester and glutathione on circulating and hepatic sulfhydrils in the rat. *Pharmacol. Toxicol.* **1994**, *75*, 343–347. [CrossRef] [PubMed]

110. Minhas, H.S.; Thornalley, P.J. Comparison of the delivery of reduced glutathione into P388D1 cells by reduced glutathione and its mono- and diethyl ester derivatives. *Biochem. Pharmacol.* **1995**, *49*, 1475–1482. [CrossRef]

111. Zampagni, M.; Wright, D.; Cascella, R.; D'Adamio, G.; Casamenti, F.; Evangelisti, E.; Cardona, F.; Goti, A.; Nacmias, B.; Sorbi, S.; et al. Novel S-acyl glutathione derivatives prevent amyloid oxidative stress and cholinergic dysfunction in Alzheimer disease models. *Free Radic. Biol. Med.* **2012**, *52*, 1362–1371. [CrossRef] [PubMed]

112. Lieber, C.S. S-Adenosyl-L-methionine and alcoholic liver disease in animal models: Implications for early intervention in human beings. *Alcohol* **2002**, *27*, 173–177. [CrossRef]

113. Fawcett, J.P.; Schiller, B.; Jiang, R.; Moran, J.; Walker, R.J. Supplementation with L-2-oxothiazolidine-4-carboxylic acid, a cysteine precursor, does not protect against lipid peroxidation in puromycin aminonucleoside-induced nephropathy. *Exp. Nephrol.* **1996**, *4*, 248–252. [PubMed]

114. Oz, H.S.; Chen, T.S.; Nagasawa, H. Comparative efficacies of 2 cysteine prodrugs and a glutathione delivery agent in a colitis model. *Transl. Res. J. Lab. Clin. Med.* **2007**, *150*, 122–129. [CrossRef] [PubMed]

115. Zarka, M.H.; Bridge, W.J. Oral administration of γ-glutamylcysteine increases intracellular glutathione levels above homeostasis in a randomised human trial pilot study. *Redox Biol.* **2017**, *11*, 631–636. [CrossRef] [PubMed]

116. Rosenblat, M.; Volkova, N.; Coleman, R.; Aviram, M. Anti-oxidant and anti-atherogenic properties of liposomal glutathione: Studies in vitro, and in the atherosclerotic apolipoprotein E-deficient mice. *Atherosclerosis* **2007**, *195*, e61–e68. [CrossRef] [PubMed]

117. Wen, J.; Du, Y.; Li, D.; Alany, R. Development of water-in-oil microemulsions with the potential of prolonged release for oral delivery of L-glutathione. *Pharm. Dev. Technol.* **2013**, *18*, 1424–1429. [CrossRef] [PubMed]

118. Baek, M.; Choy, J.-H.; Choi, S.-J. Montmorillonite intercalated with glutathione for antioxidant delivery: Synthesis, characterization, and bioavailability evaluation. *Int. J. Pharm.* **2012**, *425*, 29–34. [CrossRef] [PubMed]

119. Trapani, A.; Laquintana, V.; Denora, N.; Lopedota, A.; Cutrignelli, A.; Franco, M.; Trapani, G.; Liso, G. Eudragit RS 100 microparticles containing 2-hydroxypropyl-β-cyclodextrin and glutathione: Physicochemical characterization, drug release and transport studies. *Eur. J. Pharm. Sci.* **2007**, *30*, 64–74. [CrossRef] [PubMed]

120. Trapani, A.; Lopedota, A.; Franco, M.; Cioffi, N.; Ieva, E.; Garcia-Fuentes, M.; Alonso, M.J. A comparative study of chitosan and chitosan/cyclodextrin nanoparticles as potential carriers for the oral delivery of small peptides. *Eur. J. Pharm. Biopharm.* **2010**, *75*, 26–32. [CrossRef] [PubMed]

121. Naji-Tabasi, S.; Razavi, S.M.A.; Mehditabar, H. Fabrication of basil seed gum nanoparticles as a novel oral delivery system of glutathione. *Carbohydr. Polym.* **2017**, *157*, 1703–1713. [CrossRef] [PubMed]

122. Mandracchia, D.; Denora, N.; Franco, M.; Pitarresi, G.; Giammona, G.; Trapani, G. New Biodegradable Hydrogels Based on Inulin and alpha,beta-Polyaspartylhydrazide Designed for Colonic Drug Delivery: In Vitro Release of Glutathione and Oxytocin. *J. Biomater. Sci. Polym. Ed.* **2011**, *22*, 313–328. [CrossRef] [PubMed]

123. Chen, G.; Bunt, C.; Wen, J. Mucoadhesive polymers-based film as a carrier system for sublingual delivery of glutathione. *J. Pharm. Pharmacol.* **2015**, *67*, 26–34. [CrossRef] [PubMed]

124. Buonocore, D.; Grosini, M.; Giardina, S.; Michelotti, A.; Carrabetta, M.; Seneci, A.; Verri, M.; Dossena, M.; Marzatico, F. Bioavailability Study of an Innovative Orobuccal Formulation of Glutathione. *Oxid. Med. Cell. Longev.* **2016**, *2016*, 3286365. [CrossRef] [PubMed]

125. Beqa, L.; Singh, A.K.; Khan, S.A.; Senapati, D.; Arumugam, S.R.; Ray, P.C. Gold nanoparticle-based simple colorimetric and ultrasensitive dynamic light scattering assay for the selective detection of Pb(II) from paints, plastics, and water samples. *ACS Appl. Mater. Interfaces* **2011**, *3*, 668–673. [CrossRef] [PubMed]

126. Zhang, Z.; Jia, J.; Lai, Y.; Ma, Y.; Weng, J.; Sun, L. Conjugating folic acid to gold nanoparticles through glutathione for targeting and detecting cancer cells. *Bioorg. Med. Chem.* **2010**, *18*, 5528–5534. [CrossRef] [PubMed]

127. Valusová, E.; Svec, P.; Antalík, M. Structural and thermodynamic behavior of cytochrome c assembled with glutathione-covered gold nanoparticles. *J. Biol. Inorg. Chem.* **2009**, *14*, 621–630. [CrossRef] [PubMed]

128. Polavarapu, L.; Manna, M.; Xu, Q.-H. Biocompatible glutathione capped gold clusters as one- and two-photon excitation fluorescence contrast agents for live cells imaging. *Nanoscale* **2011**, *3*, 429–434. [CrossRef] [PubMed]

129. Simpson, C.A.; Salleng, K.J.; Cliffel, D.E.; Feldheim, D.L. In vivo toxicity, biodistribution, and clearance of glutathione-coated gold nanoparticles. *Nanomed. Nanotechnol. Biol. Med.* **2013**, *9*, 257–263. [CrossRef] [PubMed]

130. Koo, S.H.; Lee, J.-S.; Kim, G.-H.; Lee, H.G. Preparation, Characteristics, and Stability of Glutathione-Loaded Nanoparticles. *J. Agric. Food Chem.* **2011**, *59*, 11264–11269. [CrossRef] [PubMed]

131. Williams, S.R.; Lepene, B.S.; Thatcher, C.D.; Long, T.E. Synthesis and characterization of poly(ethylene glycol)-glutathione conjugate self-assembled nanoparticles for antioxidant delivery. *Biomacromolecules* **2009**, *10*, 155–161. [CrossRef] [PubMed]

132. Tortiglione, C.; Quarta, A.; Tino, A.; Manna, L.; Cingolani, R.; Pellegrino, T. Synthesis and biological assay of GSH functionalized fluorescent quantum dots for staining Hydra vulgaris. *Bioconjug. Chem.* **2007**, *18*, 829–835. [CrossRef] [PubMed]

133. Tournebize, J.; Boudier, A.; Sapin-Minet, A.; Maincent, P.; Leroy, P.; Schneider, R. Role of gold nanoparticles capping density on stability and surface reactivity to design drug delivery platforms. *ACS Appl. Mater. Interfaces* **2012**, *4*, 5790–5799. [CrossRef] [PubMed]

134. Tournebize, J.; Boudier, A.; Joubert, O.; Eidi, H.; Bartosz, G.; Maincent, P.; Leroy, P.; Sapin-Minet, A. Impact of gold nanoparticle coating on redox homeostasis. *Int. J. Pharm.* **2012**, *438*, 107–116. [CrossRef] [PubMed]

135. Luo, M.; Boudier, A.; Clarot, I.; Maincent, P.; Schneider, R.; Leroy, P. Gold Nanoparticles Grafted by Reduced Glutathione With Thiol Function Preservation. *Colloid Interface Sci. Commun.* **2016**, *14*, 8–12. [CrossRef]

136. Levin, V.A. Relationship of octanol/water partition coefficient and molecular weight to rat brain capillary permeability. *J. Med. Chem.* **1980**, *23*, 682–684. [CrossRef] [PubMed]

137. Kannan, R.; Kuhlenkamp, J.F.; Jeandidier, E.; Trinh, H.; Ookhtens, M.; Kaplowitz, N. Evidence for carrier-mediated transport of glutathione across the blood-brain barrier in the rat. *J. Clin. Investig.* **1990**, *85*, 2009–2013. [CrossRef] [PubMed]

138. Zlokovic, B.V.; Mackic, J.B.; McComb, J.G.; Weiss, M.H.; Kaplowitz, N.; Kannan, R. Evidence for transcapillary transport of reduced glutathione in vascular perfused guinea-pig brain. *Biochem. Biophys. Res. Commun.* **1994**, *201*, 402–408. [CrossRef] [PubMed]

139. Kannan, R.; Chakrabarti, R.; Tang, D.; Kim, K.J.; Kaplowitz, N. GSH transport in human cerebrovascular endothelial cells and human astrocytes: Evidence for luminal localization of Na+-dependent GSH transport in HCEC. *Brain Res.* **2000**, *852*, 374–382. [CrossRef]

140. Rip, J.; Chen, L.; Hartman, R.; van den Heuvel, A.; Reijerkerk, A.; van Kregten, J.; van der Boom, B.; Appeldoorn, C.; de Boer, M.; Maussang, D.; et al. Glutathione PEGylated liposomes: Pharmacokinetics and delivery of cargo across the blood-brain barrier in rats. *J. Drug Target.* **2014**, *22*, 460–467. [CrossRef] [PubMed]

141. Rotman, M.; Welling, M.M.; Bunschoten, A.; de Backer, M.E.; Rip, J.; Nabuurs, R.J.A.; Gaillard, P.J.; van Buchem, M.A.; van der Maarel, S.M.; van der Weerd, L. Enhanced glutathione PEGylated liposomal brain delivery of an anti-amyloid single domain antibody fragment in a mouse model for Alzheimer's disease. *J. Control. Release* **2015**, *203*, 40–50. [CrossRef] [PubMed]

142. Maussang, D.; Rip, J.; van Kregten, J.; van den Heuvel, A.; van der Pol, S.; van der Boom, B.; Reijerkerk, A.; Chen, L.; de Boer, M.; Gaillard, P.; et al. Glutathione conjugation dose-dependently increases brain-specific liposomal drug delivery in vitro and in vivo. *Drug Discov. Today Technol.* **2016**, *20*, 59–69. [CrossRef] [PubMed]

143. Birngruber, T.; Raml, R.; Gladdines, W.; Gatschelhofer, C.; Gander, E.; Ghosh, A.; Kroath, T.; Gaillard, P.J.; Pieber, T.R.; Sinner, F. Enhanced doxorubicin delivery to the brain administered through glutathione PEGylated liposomal doxorubicin (2B3-101) as compared with generic Caelyx,(®)/Doxil(®)—A cerebral open flow microperfusion pilot study. *J. Pharm. Sci.* **2014**, *103*, 1945–1948. [CrossRef] [PubMed]

144. Gaillard, P.J.; Appeldoorn, C.C.M.; Dorland, R.; van Kregten, J.; Manca, F.; Vugts, D.J.; Windhorst, B.; van Dongen, G.A.M.S.; de Vries, H.E.; Maussang, D.; et al. Pharmacokinetics, brain delivery, and efficacy in brain tumor-bearing mice of glutathione pegylated liposomal doxorubicin (2B3-101). *PLoS ONE* **2014**, *9*, e82331. [CrossRef] [PubMed]

145. Gaillard, P.J.; Appeldoorn, C.C.M.; Rip, J.; Dorland, R.; van der Pol, S.M.A.; Kooij, G.; de Vries, H.E.; Reijerkerk, A. Enhanced brain delivery of liposomal methylprednisolone improved therapeutic efficacy in a model of neuroinflammation. *J. Control. Release* **2012**, *164*, 364–369. [CrossRef] [PubMed]

146. Kanhai, K.M.S.; Zuiker, R.G.J.A.; Stavrakaki, I.; Gladdines, W.; Gaillard, P.J.; Klaassen, E.S.; Groeneveld, G.J. Glutathione-PEGylated liposomal methylprednisolone in comparison to free methylprednisolone: Slow release characteristics and prolonged lymphocyte depression in a first-in-human study. *Br. J. Clin. Pharmacol.* 2018. [CrossRef] [PubMed]

147. Gaillard, P.J.; Kerklaan, B.M.; Aftimos, P.; Altintas, S.; Jager, A.; Gladdines, W.; Lonnqvist, F.; Soetekouw, P.; Verheul, H.; Awada, A.; et al. Abstract CT216: Phase I dose escalating study of 2B3-101, glutathione PEGylated liposomal doxorubicin, in patients with solid tumors and brain metastases or recurrent malignant glioma. *Cancer Res.* **2014**, *74*, CT216. [CrossRef]

148. Brandsma, D.; Kerklaan, B.M.; Diéras, V.; Altintas, S.; Anders, C.K.; Ballester, M.A.; Gelderblom, H.; Soetekouw, P.M.M.B.; Gladdines, W.; Lonnqvist, F.; et al. Phase 1/2a study of glutathione pegylated liposomal doxorubicin (2b3-101) in patients with brain metastases (BM) from solid tumors or recurrent high grade gliomas (HGG). *Ann. Oncol.* **2014**, *25*, iv157–iv158. [CrossRef]

149. Veszelka, S.; Meszaros, M.; Kiss, L.; Kota, Z.; Pali, T.; Hoyk, Z.; Bozso, Z.; Fulop, L.; Toth, A.; Rakhely, G.; et al. Biotin and Glutathione Targeting of Solid Nanoparticles to Cross Human Brain Endothelial Cells. *Curr. Pharm. Des.* **2017**, *23*, 4198–4205. [CrossRef] [PubMed]

150. Grover, A.; Hirani, A.; Pathak, Y.; Sutariya, V. Brain-targeted delivery of docetaxel by glutathione-coated nanoparticles for brain cancer. *AAPS PharmSciTech* **2014**, *15*, 1562–1568. [CrossRef] [PubMed]

151. Geldenhuys, W.; Wehrung, D.; Groshev, A.; Hirani, A.; Sutariya, V. Brain-targeted delivery of doxorubicin using glutathione-coated nanoparticles for brain cancers. *Pharm. Dev. Technol.* **2015**, *20*, 497–506. [CrossRef] [PubMed]

152. Geldenhuys, W.; Mbimba, T.; Bui, T.; Harrison, K.; Sutariya, V. Brain-targeted delivery of paclitaxel using glutathione-coated nanoparticles for brain cancers. *J. Drug Target.* **2011**, *19*, 837–845. [CrossRef] [PubMed]

153. Raval, N.; Mistry, T.; Acharya, N.; Acharya, S. Development of glutathione-conjugated asiatic acid-loaded bovine serum albumin nanoparticles for brain-targeted drug delivery. *J. Pharm. Pharmacol.* **2015**, *67*, 1503–1511. [CrossRef] [PubMed]

154. Patel, P.; Acharya, N.; Acharya, S. Development and characterization of glutathione-conjugated albumin nanoparticles for improved brain delivery of hydrophilic fluorescent marker. *Drug Deliv.* **2013**, *20*, 143–155. [CrossRef] [PubMed]

155. Mdzinarishvili, A.; Sutariya, V.; Talasila, P.K.; Geldenhuys, W.J.; Sadana, P. Engineering triiodothyronine (T3) nanoparticle for use in ischemic brain stroke. *Drug Deliv. Transl. Res.* **2013**, *3*, 309–317. [CrossRef] [PubMed]

156. Englert, C.; Trützschler, A.-K.; Raasch, M.; Bus, T.; Borchers, P.; Mosig, A.S.; Traeger, A.; Schubert, U.S. Crossing the blood-brain barrier: Glutathione-conjugated poly(ethylene imine) for gene delivery. *J. Control. Release* **2016**, *241*, 1–14. [CrossRef] [PubMed]

157. Yin, J.; Chen, Y.; Zhang, Z.-H.; Han, X. Stimuli-Responsive Block Copolymer-Based Assemblies for Cargo Delivery and Theranostic Applications. *Polymers* **2016**, *8*, 268. [CrossRef]

158. Liu, X.; Yang, Y.; Urban, M.W. Stimuli-Responsive Polymeric Nanoparticles. *Macromol. Rapid Commun.* **2017**, *38*, 13. [CrossRef] [PubMed]

159. Cheng, R.; Meng, F.; Deng, C.; Klok, H.-A.; Zhong, Z. Dual and multi-stimuli responsive polymeric nanoparticles for programmed site-specific drug delivery. *Biomaterials* **2013**, *34*, 3647–3657. [CrossRef] [PubMed]

160. Son, S.; Namgung, R.; Kim, J.; Singha, K.; Kim, W.J. Bioreducible polymers for gene silencing and delivery. *Acc. Chem. Res.* **2012**, *45*, 1100–1112. [CrossRef] [PubMed]

161. Ma, N.; Li, Y.; Xu, H.; Wang, Z.; Zhang, X. Dual redox responsive assemblies formed from diselenide block copolymers. *J. Am. Chem. Soc.* **2010**, *132*, 442–443. [CrossRef] [PubMed]

162. Han, L.; Zhang, X.-Y.; Wang, Y.-L.; Li, X.; Yang, X.-H.; Huang, M.; Hu, K.; Li, L.-H.; Wei, Y. Redox-responsive theranostic nanoplatforms based on inorganic nanomaterials. *J. Control. Release* **2017**, *259*, 40–52. [CrossRef] [PubMed]

163. Ghosh, P.S.; Kim, C.-K.; Han, G.; Forbes, N.S.; Rotello, V.M. Efficient Gene Delivery Vectors by Tuning the Surface Charge Density of Amino Acid-Functionalized Gold Nanoparticles. *ACS Nano* **2008**, *2*, 2213–2218. [CrossRef] [PubMed]

164. Tournebize, J.; Sapin-Minet, A.; Bartosz, G.; Leroy, P.; Boudier, A. Pitfalls of assays devoted to evaluation of oxidative stress induced by inorganic nanoparticles. *Talanta* **2013**, *116*, 753–763. [CrossRef] [PubMed]

9

Solvent Extraction of Polyphenolics from the Indigenous African Fruit *Ximenia caffra* and Characterization by LC-HRMS

Dewald Oosthuizen [1], Neill J. Goosen [1,*] (iD), Maria A. Stander [2] (iD), Aliyu D. Ibrahim [3], Mary-Magdalene Pedavoah [4] (iD), Grace O. Usman [5] and Taiwo Aderinola [6] (iD)

[1] Department of Process Engineering, Stellenbosch University, Stellenbosch 7600, South Africa; oosthuizen.dewald@gmail.com

[2] Central Analytical Facility, Stellenbosch University, Stellenbosch 7600, South Africa; lcms@sun.ac.za

[3] Department of Microbiology, Usmanu Danfodiyo University, Sokoto PMB 2346, Nigeria; aid4life@yahoo.com

[4] Department of Applied Chemistry and Biochemistry, University for Development Studies, Navrongo, Ghana; mmpeddy@yahoo.com

[5] Department of Food, Nutrition and Home Sciences, Kogi State University, Anyigba 1008, Nigeria; ojaligu@yahoo.co.uk

[6] Department of Food Science and Technology, The Federal University of Technology, Akure PMB 704, Nigeria; aderinolata@futa.edu.ng

* Correspondence: njgoosen@sun.ac.za

Abstract: Indigenous and non-commercial fruits can be an important source of antioxidant polyphenols; however, the identity and content of polyphenols from non-commercial fruits are often poorly described. The study aimed to extract, identify, and quantify polyphenols from the skin of the indigenous Africa fruit *Ximenia caffra*, using solvent extraction. Three solvents (hexane, acetone, and 70% v/v ethanol) over three extraction times (30, 60 and 120 min) were used in a 3^2 full factorial experimental design to determine effects on polyphenol recovery, and individual polyphenolics were characterised using liquid chromatography high-resolution mass spectrometry (LC-HRMS). Ethanol was the most effective extraction solvent, and extracts had high levels of total phenolics and flavonoids (65 mg gallic and 40 mg catechin equivalents per gram dry sample respectively), and high antioxidant activity (18.2 mg mL^{-1} ascorbic acid equivalents). LC-HRMS positively identified 16 compounds, of which 14 were flavonoids including flavonoid glycosides, and indicated that concentrations of some flavonoids decreased for extraction times beyond 60 min. It was concluded that the fruit of *Ximenia caffra* is rich in natural polyphenolic antioxidants; the present work identified and quantified a number of these, while also establishing suitable solvent extraction conditions for the recovery of these potentially high-value compounds.

Keywords: bioactive phytochemicals; flavonoids; indigenous African fruit; natural antioxidants; polyphenols; solvent extraction

1. Introduction

Fruits of the indigenous African tree *Ximenia caffra* (Sonder) have been shown to contain high amounts of polyphenolic compounds in both the pulp and skins [1]. Natural polyphenols are known for their antioxidant properties, and the evidence linking regular consumption of these natural antioxidants with improved health outcomes is continually growing [2–4]. *Ximenia caffra* has been identified as a promising indigenous African plant for commercialisation due to its variety of commercial, cultural, and medicinal uses [5–7]; it is widely distributed within and indigenous to

Southern and Eastern Africa, including Madagascar [6]. In season, the plant produces edible fruits which are utilised as food by humans and animals, while different parts of the plant including the leaves, bark, and roots are used in traditional medicine to treat a range of diseases and disorders [6,8–10], with reports of antibacterial and antifungal activity of *X. caffra* extracts providing support for the ethnomedicinal uses of the plant [9,11]. Commercial activity around the fruit has thus far mainly revolved around production of jellies and jams, and extraction of the commercially valuable seed oil [6,12], and very little attention has been devoted to studying the high amount of polyphenols in the fruit.

The fruit pulp and skins of *X. caffra* are a potential source from which natural antioxidants could be extracted, especially the skins, which contain higher amounts of polyphenols than the pulp, and which are regularly not consumed due to poor palatability [1,6,13]. Polyphenols from plants are of particular interest due to their potential health benefits, disease prevention, and pharmacological activity [2,14–16]; natural polyphenols are particularly sought after for their antioxidant activity, especially in the large and lucrative food preservative market [2,17,18]. Polyphenols can also find applications as food colourants, and as the raw materials for industrial applications e.g., for the production of paints, cosmetics, and paper [16,19].

Little is known about the specific polyphenols that occur in *X. caffra* fruit, or the extraction methods and conditions which would maximise polyphenol recovery. Extraction conditions like the type of extraction process employed, the physical condition of raw material, the extraction conditions, and type of solvent all affect the efficiency of product recovery from plant material [2,16,20–22], and therefore need to be considered. Different extraction techniques have been demonstrated for polyphenol extraction, including various non-conventional extraction technologies that may improve extraction efficiency and decrease extraction times [23]; yet, organic solvent extraction and supercritical fluid extraction are the most commonly employed commercial extraction techniques [16,20]. Due to the varying polarities of individual polyphenols, each raw material needs to be specifically matched with the most suitable solvent, and might require the use of combinations of solvents, sequential extraction steps, or the use of co-solvents in the case of supercritical fluid extraction, in order to affect optimal extraction efficiency [16,20,24]. A further complication of polyphenol extraction is that severe extraction conditions e.g., elevated temperature or long extraction times could cause polyphenols to degrade or be converted into undesirable by-products [21,25], thereby further emphasizing the need for determining optimal polyphenol extraction conditions.

The study aimed to optimize extraction conditions for the recovery of polyphenols from the fruit of *X. caffra*, to identify specific compounds in the extracts. This was achieved by employing different extraction solvents and extraction times via Soxhlet extraction, and measuring total phenolic and flavonoid contents, as well as antioxidant activity of the extracts, and identifying individual polyphenols using LC-HRMS.

2. Materials and Methods

2.1. Chemicals and Reagents

Extraction solvents were purchased from Kimix Chemical and Lab Supplies, Cape Town South Africa, and had the following purities: hexane 96%, ethanol 99.7%, and acetone 99.0% minimum. Folin-Ciocalteu's phenol reagent and sodium hydroxide were purchased from Merck (Darmstadt, Germany). Sodium carbonate, gallic acid, ±catechin hydrate, sodium nitrite, *N,N*-Dimethyl-*p*-phenylenediamine dihydrochloride (DMPD), iron(iii)chloride, L-ascorbic acid, sodium acetate trihydrate, aluminium chloride and 0.1 M acetic acid were purchased from Sigma-Aldrich (St. Louis, MO, USA). All chemicals were of analytical grade. Phenolic and flavonoid standards were obtained from Sigma (Darmstadt, Germany).

For all high performance liquid chromatography (HPLC) analyses, methanol and acetonitrile were purchased from Merck Millipore (Darmstadt, Germany) and Sigma-Aldrich (St. Louis, MO, USA), respectively, while HPLC-grade water was prepared using tandem Elix and Milli-Q academic (Merck Millipore) water purification systems.

2.2. Raw Material Collection and Preparation

Ripe fruits of X. caffra var. natalensis were collected in the Hoedspruit area, Limpopo Province, South Africa on the 10 January 2015, at the GPS coordinates: 24°25′12″ S 30°47′42″ E. Fruits were positively identified by a local botanist, Mr. Dave Rushworth, and were kept on ice until processed. Processing entailed separating the skin and fleshy portion of the fruit from the seeds through physical means, homogenizing the fruit flesh and skins together in a food processor and filtering the resultant pulp through a cotton cloth. The filtered juice was frozen at $-20\ ^{\circ}C$, and the solid residue remaining after filtration was then dried in a drying oven at 55 °C for approximately 6 h, and crushed by hand using a mortar and pestle until all material passed a mesh size of 2 mm. The dried material was thoroughly mixed by hand in order to ensure homogenous distribution, and stored in airtight containers at room temperature until used for solvent extraction. The juice was utilised for further nutritional evaluation, for which the findings will be reported elsewhere.

2.3. Experimental Design and Extraction Equipment

A 3^2 full factorial design with 5 replicates was employed to investigate the effects of two factors (type of solvent, and extraction time) each at three different levels, on the extraction of polyphenols from the raw material using the Soxhlet extraction method. As certain polyphenolic compounds can degrade when subjected to elevated temperatures for extended times [26], the appropriate extraction time for polyphenolic recovery needs to be determined. The solvents were chosen to represent three different polarities: hexane (non-polar), acetone (intermediate polarity), and a 70 vol % aqueous ethanol solution (polar, although slightly less polar than water, as suggested by Kim and Lee [27]). The extraction times chosen were 30, 60, and 120 min. The solvent substrate ratio was chosen as 10:1 (volume per weight) as per Aspé and Fernández [26], and kept constant for each run.

At the end of the trial, a single extraction using 70% ethanol as a solvent was also done to generate samples within which individual phenolic compounds were identified; experimental conditions and sampling procedures were identical to the other ethanol extraction runs, and samples were taken at 30, 60 and 120 min extraction time.

The extraction apparatus consisted of a standard Soxhlet setup, with glass thimble holder (150 mL), condenser, and a three-necked 500 mL round bottom solvent flask. The heating source used was an adjustable heating mantle (MRC Scientific Instruments model MNS-500, Holon, Israel).

2.4. Extraction and Sampling Procedures

To perform the extraction, 20 g of raw material was loaded into a cellulose extraction thimble (Whatman 603, diameter of 33 mm and length of 100 mm), 200 mL of the solvent was loaded into the round bottom solvent flask, and the extraction was run under full reflux conditions at a constant heating rate. Extraction times were measured from the first syphoning of the solvent. Samples of 5 mL each were taken at 30, 60, and 120 min directly from the round bottom solvent flask, the solvent was removed through evaporation in a vacuum oven, and samples were stored in airtight containers at 4 °C until analysis. Solvent boiling temperature was monitored using a thermocouple inserted through one of the necks of the round bottom solvent flask and recorded every 10 min, and the number of syphoning cycles during the extraction run was recorded.

2.5. Analytical Methods

Before sample analysis, stored samples were reconstituted in 5 mL demineralised water. All extraction samples were assayed for total phenolics and total flavonoids, and the ethanol extracts were further assayed for antioxidant activityaccording to the N,N-Dimethyl-p-phenylenediamine dihydrochloride (DMPD) assay.

2.5.1. Total Phenolic Assay

Total phenolics were determined according to the spectrophotometric Folin-Ciocalteu method of Singleton and Rossi [28], with slight modifications. Gallic acid was used as standard, and all values were expressed as gallic acid equivalents (GAE). Sample or standard solutions of 200 μL were added to a 4 mL cuvette, followed by 1000 μL of Folin-Ciocalteu reagent. The mixture was incubated for 8 min at room temperature and in the dark, after which 800 μL of a 7.5% sodium carbonate solution was added. A final amount of 1000 μL of demineralised water was then added, and the absorbance of the sample was measured with a spectrophotometer (A&E Lab, United Kingdom, model AE-S60-4U) at 765 nm. Blanks were prepared using demineralised water.

2.5.2. Total Flavonoid Assay

Total flavonoids were measured using the method described by Amado, et al. [29], with catechin as standard, and values were expressed as catechin equivalents (CE). A volume of 1000 μL of sample or standard was pipetted into a 4 mL cuvette, and 75 μL of 5% $NaNO_2$ solution was added and incubated at room temperature. After six minutes' incubation, 150 μL of 10% $AlCl_3$ was added to the solution and incubated for a further 5 min, after which 500 μL of 1 M NaOH was added. The solution was then made up to 2.5 mL by the addition of 775 μL of demineralised water, and incubated for 30 min before measuring the absorbance at a wavelength of 410 nm. Blanks were prepared using demineralised water.

2.5.3. DMPD Antioxidant Activity Assay

Only the 70% ethanol extracts were subjected to evaluation of antioxidant activity, due to difficulties in solubilisation of dried acetone and hexane extracts in the aqueous medium required to perform the antioxidant activity, and because the 70% ethanol extracts showed the highest polyphenolic and flavonoid content. The DMPD assay as described by Fogliano, et al. [30] was used for analysis. DMPD reagent was prepared by mixing 1000 μL of 100 mM DMPD solution, 200 μL of 0.05 M $FeCl_3$ solution, and 100 mL of pH 5.25 acetate buffer. This reagent was stored in the dark at 4 °C until use. To perform the assay, 100 μL of sample and 2 mL of the buffered 100 mM DMPD reagent were added to a cuvette, mixed, and incubated for 10 min at ambient temperature. Absorbance was then measured at 505 nm, with ascorbic acid used as standard and demineralised water as blank.

2.5.4. Identification of Phenolic Compounds

A Waters Synapt G2 quadrupole time-of-flight mass spectrometer connected to Waters Ultra pressure liquid chromatograph and photo diode array detection was used for LC-HRMS analysis. A previously published method [31] was used which employs a gradient specifically focusing on phenolic acids and flavonoids. The only difference was that a Waters BEH C18, 2.1 × 100 mm, 1.7 μm column was used. In short, a 0.1% formic acid (solvent A) to acetonitrile containing 0.1% formic acid (solvent B) gradient was applied up to 28% solvent B, followed by a wash step.

The instrument was operated using electrospray ionisation in negative MS^E mode, which consisted of a low collision energy scan (6 V) from m/z 150 to 1500, and a high collision energy scan from m/z 40 to 1500. Positive identification of compounds was based on retention time matching with authentic standards, accurate mass data, ultraviolet (UV) data, as well as mass spectrometry-mass spectrometry (MSMS) fragmentation data.

Ethanol extracts obtained via Soxhlet extraction were diluted five and ten fold in 50% methanol/water, centrifuged, and the supernatant injected directly into the system. A methanol extract was also prepared from the same raw material as used for Soxhlet extraction, and characterized for polyphenolic content. A cocktail of the standards were injected unto the system at (100, 50, 25, 10, 5 and 0.5 mg L^{-1}), and the application manager Targetlynx 4.1 (Waters, Milford, MA, USA) was used for the quantifications.

2.6. Statistical Analysis

Data on total phenolics, flavonoids, and antioxidant activity were analysed using the Statistica version 12 software package. Data were subjected to analysis of variance (ANOVA) and least significant difference (LSD) tests, using the Variance Estimation and Precision (VEPAC) module in Statistica. Main effects and interaction effects were estimated, and differences were deemed to be significant for $p < 0.05$.

3. Results

There were noticeable variations in the final colour of the extraction solvent collected in the round bottom flask between the solvents, with the 70% ethanol having an intense orange-red colour corresponding to that of the original raw material. Acetone extracts showed intermediate colour, while hexane extracts exhibited very little colour change.

Figure 1 shows the extraction of total phenolics over the course of 120 min, for all three solvents. Total phenolic content was significantly higher ($p < 0.05$) in the 70% ethanol extract than for the other solvents, at all sampling times during the extraction. Within the 70% ethanol extraction, total phenolics extracted increased significantly over time from 4312 ± 1819 mg L^{-1} GAE (mean $\pm$ SD) at 30 min to 6487 ± 1203 mg L^{-1} GAE at 120 min, but there was no significant difference between phenolics after 30 min and 60 min extraction time. No significant differences in total phenolics concentration were found between hexane and acetone extracts, and within each of these two solvents, the total phenolic concentration did not vary significantly between 30 min and 120 min extraction time. The interaction between solvent and time was found to be statistically insignificant for all solvents ($p > 0.05$).

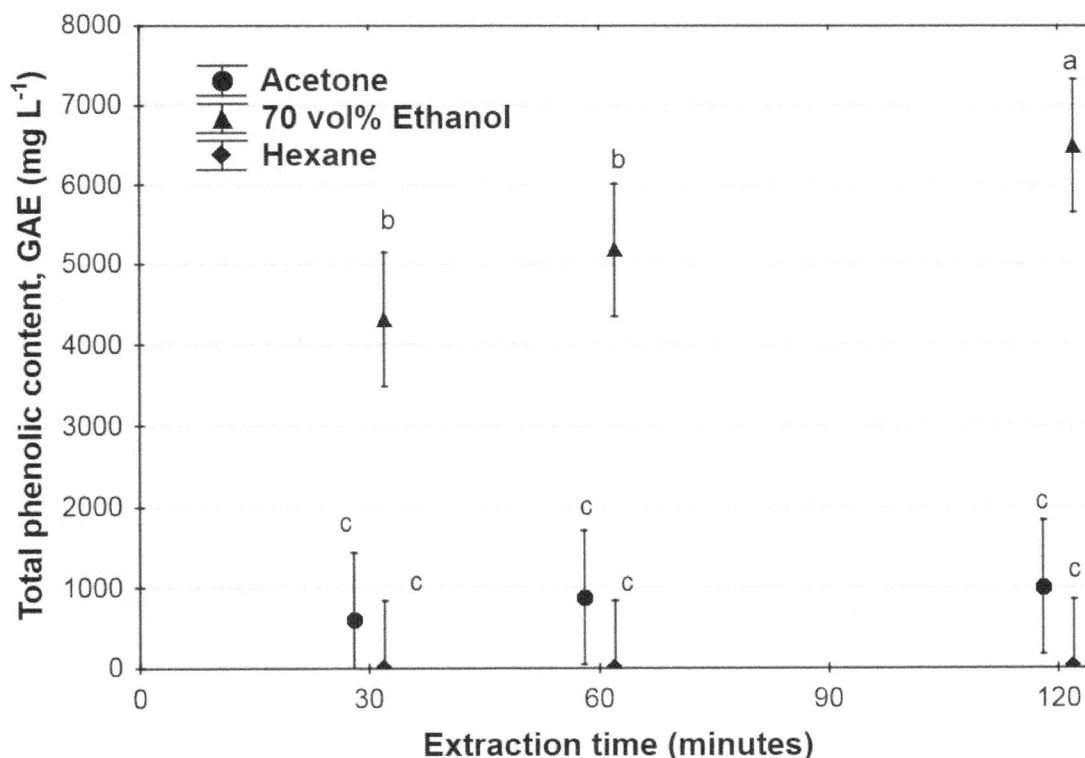

Figure 1. Total phenolic content of *Ximenia caffra* extracts over time, for different solvents, expressed as gallic acid equivalents (GAE). Data are represented as mean $\pm$ 95% confidence intervals. Values with common superscripts do not differ significantly.

Extraction of total flavonoids over time for all solvents is shown in Figure 2. Total flavonoid extraction was significantly higher for the 70% ethanol extraction than either acetone or hexane at all sampling times, and within the 70% ethanol, total flavonoid concentration increased significantly from 2571 ± 965 mg L^{-1} CE at 30 min, to 4000 ± 1480 mg L^{-1} CE at 120 min extraction time. There were no significant differences in flavonoid content between acetone and hexane extracts, and within each solvent type there were no significant increases in flavonoid concentration between 30 min and 120 min extraction time. No significant time-solvent interaction effect was found for flavonoid extraction.

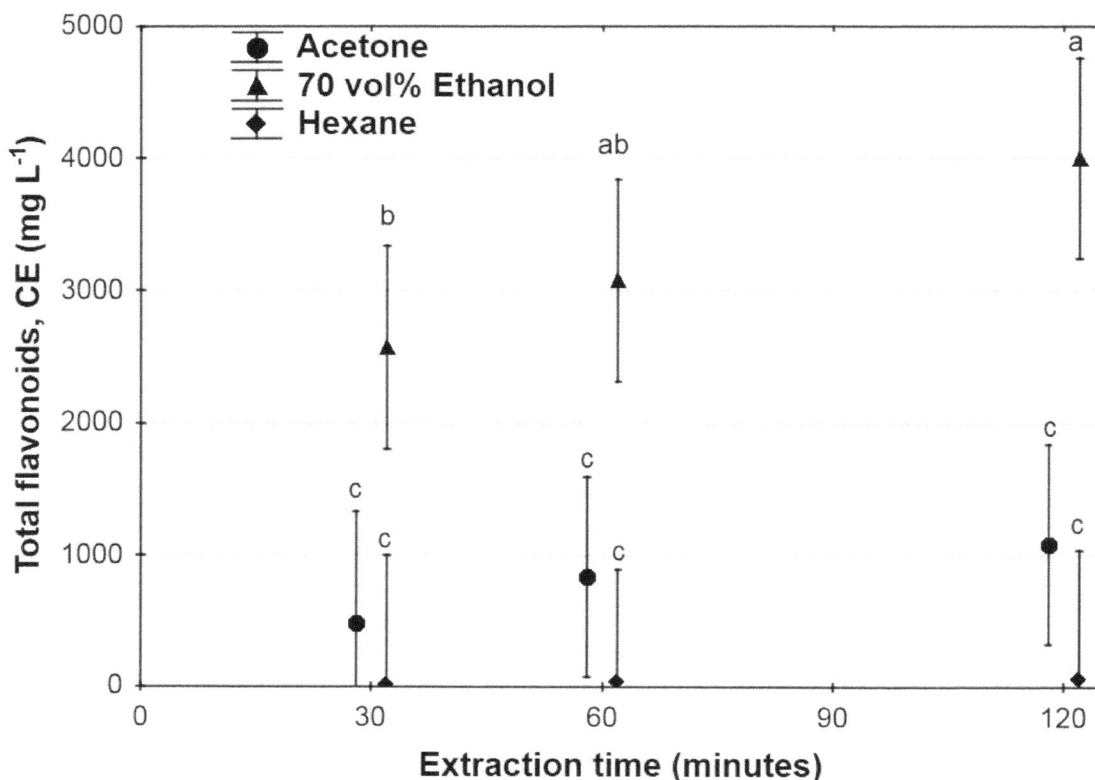

Figure 2. Total flavonoid content of *Ximenia caffra* extracts over time, expressed as catechin equivalents (CE). Data are represented as mean ± 95% confidence intervals. Values with common superscripts do not differ significantly.

Figure 3 shows the results of DMPD antioxidant activity, and the ratio of flavonoids to phenolics, for the 70% ethanol extracts between 30 min and 120 min extraction time. There was a numerical increase in antioxidant activity from 14.9 mg L^{-1} AAE at 30 min to 18.2 mg L^{-1} AAE at 120 min; however, the increase was not statistically significant. Within the 70% ethanol solvent, the mean values for the ratio of total flavonoids to total phenolics did not differ significantly over time, with a ratio 0.67 being obtained at 30 min, and a value of 0.66 at both 60 and 120 min.

Table 1 lists positively identified compounds obtained during extraction, along with concentrations of these compounds as extracted at different times using a 70% ethanol Soxhlet extraction run. Table 1 further indicates the retention times and other data used to identify individual compounds. The following compounds were positively identified: catechin, citric acid, epicatechin, gallic acid, hesperetin, hyperoside, isoquercitrin, kaemferol glucoside, luteolin-7-O-glucoside, procyanidin B1, procyanidin B2, quercetin-3-O-glucoside, quercetin-3-O-robinobioside, quercetin, rutin, and trilobatin. A number of compounds were tentatively identified, or could not be identified; concentrations of these compounds in the solvents were not determined. Please refer to Figure S1 for a chromatogram showing retention times and peaks of the positively identified compounds.

Table 1. LC-HRMS data obtained for the different extracts from *Ximenia caffra*, detailing compound identity and the time-dependent concentration for the ethanol extracts.

Compound Number	Compound Name	m/z [1]	Retention Time (min)	$[M-H]^-$	MS^E Fragments [2]	Individual Compound Concentrations (µg mL^{-1})			
						Ethanol: 30 min	Ethanol: 60 min	Ethanol: 120 min	Methanol Extraction
					Positively identified compounds				
1	Catechin	289.0713	11.48	$C_{15}H_{13}O_6$	289,125,203,245,151	36.8	51.9	54.9	68.0
2	Citric acid	191.0187	3.12	$C_6H_7O_7$	191,111,87,173	1042	1313	1288	2133
3	Epicatechin [3]	289.0698	13.57	$C_{15}H_{13}O_6$	weak	-	-	-	-
4	Gallic acid	169.0129	5.8	$C_7H_5O_5$	125,169,111	4.8	5.2	5.8	8.5
5	Hesperetin	301.1643	24.49	$C_{15}H_{25}O_6$	weak	0.1	0.1	0.1	0.1
6	Hyperoside	463.0878	17.51	$C_{21}H_{19}O_{12}$	300,463,271,255	34.6	42.9	40.8	102.8
7	Isoquercitrin	463.0876	17.51	$C_{21}H_{19}O_{12}$	300,463,271,301,255,	43.2	53.5	50.8	128.2
8	Kaempferol glucoside	447.0938	18.06	$C_{21}H_{19}O_{11}$	285,169,447	12.1	12.3	16.7	33.1
9	Luteolin-7-O-glucoside	447.0935	18.06	$C_{21}H_{19}O_{11}$	285,284,169,125,447	0.3	0.3	0.3	1.1
10	Procyanidin B1	577.1317	10.68	$C_{30}H_{25}O_{12}$	289,407,425,577	36.8	52.5	60.0	203.8
11	Procyanidin B2 [3]	577.1345	12.72	$C_{30}H_{25}O_{12}$	289,407,425,577	-	-	-	-
12	Quercetin-3-O-glucoside	463.0886	17.81	$C_{21}H_{19}O_{12}$	300,271,463,255,125	2.7	3.4	3.1	9.0
13	Quercetin-3-O-robinobioside	609.1432	17.06	$C_{27}H_{29}O_{16}$	300,609,271,125	3.9	3.7	5.8	15.4
14	Quercetin	301.0353	23.99	$C_{15}H_9O_7$	125,169	2.0	2.2	1.8	1.9
15	Rutin	609.1458	17.27	$C_{27}H_{29}O_{16}$	300,609,271,255	11.5	13.8	13.1	38.3
16	Trilobatin	435.1284	18.75	$C_{21}H_{23}O_{10}$	315,345	0.5	0.7	0.8	2.1
					Tentatively identified and unknown compounds [3]				
	Aconitic acid	173.0089	9.14	$C_6H_5O_6$	111				
	Dihydroxy hexadecanoic acid	287.2236	24.5	$C_{16}H_{31}O_4$	287				
	p-Coumaroylquinic acid	337.0916	11.18	$C_{16}H_{17}O_8$	163,119,191,337				
	Procyanidin	577.1344	10.68	$C_{30}H_{25}O_{12}$	289,407,425,577				
	Quercetin galloyl glucoside	615.0979	16.63	$C_{28}H_{23}O_{16}$	300,615,463,255,169				
	Quercetin galloyl glucoside	615.0977	16.94	$C_{28}H_{23}O_{16}$	300,463,615				
	Quercetin rhamnoside	447.0927	19.63	$C_{21}H_{19}O_{11}$	300,271,255,447,243				
	Quercetin rhamnoside	447.0927	18.89	$C_{21}H_{19}O_{11}$	300,271,255,447				
	Quercetin-3-O-pentoside	433.0764	18.83	$C_{20}H_{17}O_{11}$	300,271,255,433,315				
	unknown	340.1035	14.37	$C_{15}H_{18}NO_8$	161,101,85				
	unknown	443.1913	11.37	$C_{21}H_{31}O_{10}$	443,289,303				
	unknown	515.1246	5.49	$C_{18}H_{27}O_{17}$	515,111,173				
	unknown	515.1245	5.68	$C_{18}H_{27}O_{17}$	515,111,173				
	unknown	515.1255	5.83	$C_{18}H_{27}O_{17}$	515,111,173				
	unknown	515.1253	5.93	$C_{18}H_{27}O_{17}$	515,111,173				
	unknown	435.107	21.403	$C_{24}H_{19}O_8$	341,189,125,435				
	unknown	219.0506	9.37	$C_8H_{11}O_7$	111,219,87				

[1] The mass accuracy for all compounds was better than 5 ppm; [2] Most abundant fragment mentioned first; [3] Concentrations of epicatechin, procyanidin B$_2$ and all tentatively identified and unknown compounds were not determined.

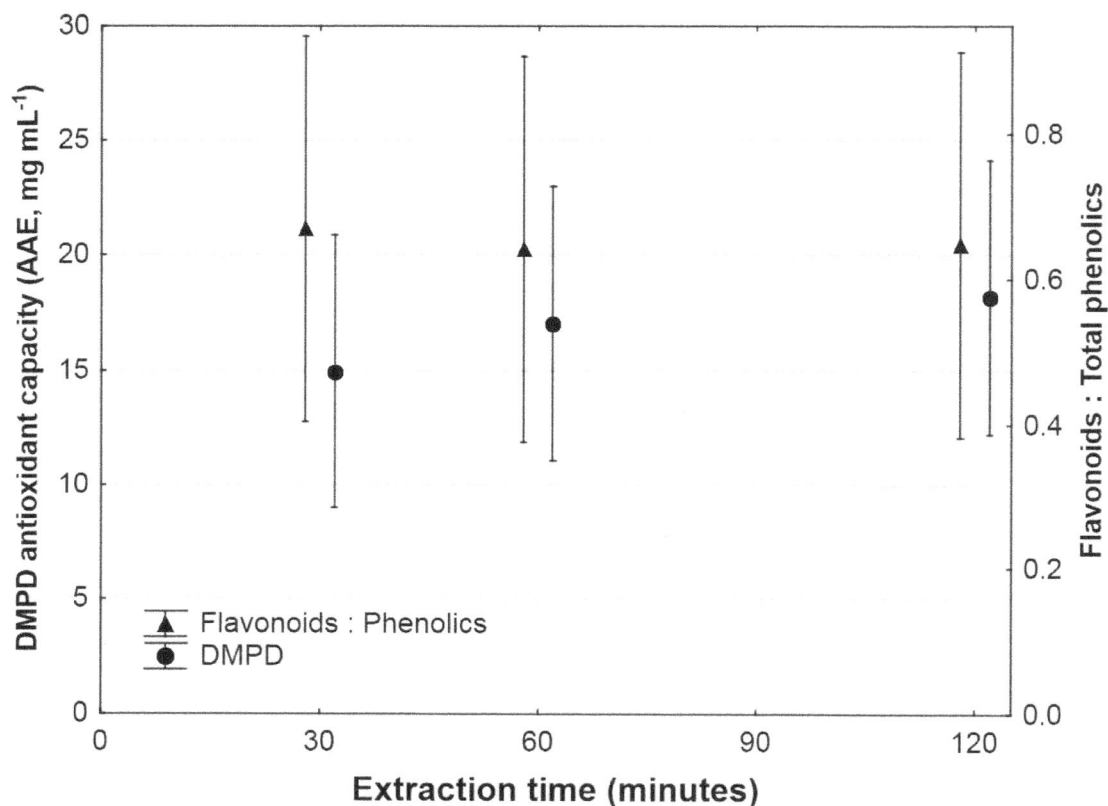

Figure 3. N,N-Dimethyl-p-phenylenediamine dihydrochloride (DMPD) antioxidant capacity and ratio of total flavonoids to total phenolics, for 70% ethanol extracts of *Ximenia caffra*. Data are represented as mean $\pm$ 95% confidence intervals.

Citric acid was the dominant compound extracted in all ethanol extractions, with a highest concentration of 1313 mg L^{-1} at 60 min extraction time, and a final concentration of 1288 mg L^{-1} at 120 min, followed by procyanidin B1 (60.0 mg L^{-1}), cathechin (54.9 mg L^{-1}), isoquercitrin (50.8 mg L^{-1}) and hyperoside (40.8 mg L^{-1}) after 120 min extraction time. For all compounds except quercetin-3-O-robinobioside, extracted concentrations increased from 30 min to 60 min extraction time. However, for hyperoside, rutin, quercitin, quercitin-3-O-glycoside, isoquercitrin and citric acid, the extracted concentrations decreased between 60 min and 120 min extraction time, while for all other compounds, the concentrations increased or remained constant.

4. Discussion

The current study reports findings on solvent extraction of polyphenols displaying high antioxidant activity from the fruits of *X. caffra*, and reports the identity of the individual compounds obtained in the ethanol extracts. There has recently been increased interest in the commercialisation of *X. caffra*, due to the range of different potential products which can be derived from this versatile plant species [6]; however, information on the individual compounds responsible for the high antioxidant capacity, and potential processing methods for specific product recovery from the different plant portions is lacking.

Optimal extraction of phenolic compounds and flavonoids, as measured with the spectrophotometric methods, was achieved using 70% aqueous ethanol as extraction solvent at 120 min extraction time. Phenolic acid and flavonoid recovery were both significantly affected by the choice of extraction solvent and length of extraction, while interaction effects between these two parameters were statistically insignificant. The results of the current study are in line with previous work on extraction of polyphenols from plant materials. It is known that the selection of an appropriate solvent is an important processing parameter during polyphenolic extraction, as extraction yield, total phenolic content, and antioxidant capacity of extracts, extraction kinetics and the bioactivity of the final extracts can all be affected by the choice of solvent [19,32,33]. The polarity of extraction solvents has been proposed to be one of the critical aspects resulting in differences in extraction efficiency [32,34]. The current study found large differences in extraction of polyphenol between the solvents, with the less-polar solvents hexane and acetone resulting in poor phenolics extraction. Previous work on *X. caffra* utilised methanol for extraction of phenolic compounds [1,35]; however, for the current study, ethanol was preferred, due to its decreased toxicity compared to methanol.

The significant effect of extraction time on the extraction of phenolics and flavonoids when using 70% ethanol as the solvent is apparent from Figures 1 and 2, where the optimal extraction time (based on spectrophotometric determination of total phenolics and total flavonoids) was found to be 120 min in both instances, with significant increases occurring throughout the entire extraction run. Time dependence of phenolic acids and flavonoid extraction was not found for either acetone or hexane as solvents; this is ascribed to the overall low extraction achieved using these solvents. However, despite longer extraction times indicating higher overall polyphenolic extraction, the data in Table 1 clearly indicates decreases in concentration of certain compounds between 60 and 120 min extraction time. These observed decreases in concentration may be due to the fact that some polyphenolics can degrade over time when kept at elevated temperatures [36–40], and it is clear from the data that compounds differed in this regard, e.g., the extracted concentrations of catechin and procyanidin B1 increased from 60 to 120 min extraction time, while extracted concentrations for hyperoside and isoquercitrin decreased over the same time period. Although further phenolic acid and/or flavonoid recovery may be achieved by extending extraction time beyond 120 min, this needs to be balanced against the potential time-dependent degradation of thermally labile components in the extracts [26].

The fruit of *X. caffra* are a good overall source of phenolic compounds. Relatively high amounts of total phenolics and flavonoids were extracted by the 70% ethanol solution from the raw material after 120 min of extraction time, corresponding to 6487 ± 1203 mg L^{-1} GAE and 4000 ± 1480 mg L^{-1} CE respectively in the extracts, which translates to 65 mg g^{-1} GAE dry sample weight for total phenolics, and 40 mg g^{-1} CE dry sample weight for total flavonoids. By way of comparison, total phenolics extracted from blueberries, a fruit generally acknowledged to be high in antioxidants and phenolics, amounted to a maximum of 9.44 ± 0.22 mg g^{-1} GAE per dry weight [41], and 6.94 ± 0.47 mg g^{-1} GAE per gram fresh fruit weight [42] in two different studies. *X. caffra* fruit pulp and peels have been reported to have high antioxidant capacity, and to contain high total phenolic and proanthocyanidin levels [1,35]; the findings in the current study are therefore in agreement with those of prior studies. The major individual polyphenolic compounds identified within the extracts were catechin, hyperoside, isoquercitrin, and procyanidin B1 (all at levels higher than 40 μg mL^{-1} after 120 min extraction time). Both hyperoside and procyanidin B1 are known as strong antioxidants [43,44], while catechin is associated with improved cardiovascular health [45]. Isoquercitrin is a glycoside of quercetin and has been demonstrated to exhibit a number of potentially beneficial biological effects linked to its ability to act as antioxidant [46].

The majority of the polyphenols recovered using Soxhlet extraction consisted of flavonoids. Among all the compounds which could be positively identified with LC-HRMS, only citric acid and gallic acid are neither flavonoids nor glycosides of flavonoids (see Table 1). Citric acid is not a polyphenol, but is retained in the data as it can act as antioxidant in food systems, and it contributes to the antioxidant activity measured using the DMPD method [47,48]. The ratio of total flavonoids to total phenolics seemed to remain fairly constant when calculated based on spectrophotometric analyses, and remained between 0.66 and 0.67 over the whole extraction time (Figure 3). This apparent constant ratio of total flavonoids to total phenolics indicates that there is no preferential extraction of flavonoids relative to other phenolic compounds, or that the proportion of non-flavonoid phenolics recovered are much lower relative to flavonoids, and therefore, any potential differences cannot be determined from spectrophotometric analyses. One potential practical implication of this is that optical process monitoring can be employed during extraction, as increased phenolic extraction corresponded with increased colour in the extraction solvent. As flavonoids particularly contribute to colour in fruit [49], the monitoring of extract colour can provide a rapid method for determination of approximate flavonoid concentration in extracts.

The DMPD antioxidant activity did not correspond to the increased extraction of total phenolics and flavonoids over time in this investigation. Even though Soxhlet extraction lead to a numerical increase in DMPD antioxidant activity from 30 to 120 min extraction, the increase was not statistically significant. Two contributing factors for this could be degradation of certain phenolic compounds in the extracts (and therefore decreased antioxidant activity), as seen in the data of Table 1, and the possibility that the majority of compounds that exhibit antioxidant activity were recovered within the first 30 min of the extraction. The data in Table 1 indeed confirm that, for all compounds which were positively identified, the majority of phenolics' extraction took place during the first 30 min. Additionally, it is also possible that the total phenolic content in the extract was not a good predictor of total antioxidant activity in this instance. Phenolics are known to be a very diverse group of plant compounds [2], and different phenolic compounds have different reactions with regards to total phenolic and antioxidant assays [16,50–52]. Further, phenolic compounds are not the only compounds in plant extracts that contribute toward total antioxidant activity; thus, even though there is generally a correlation between total phenolic content and antioxidant activity [53,54], there have been other reports where higher phenolic content in fruit extracts did not necessarily translate to higher antioxidant capacity [54]. All of these factors may have contributed toward the fact that the DMPD assay did not follow the same trends as those of total phenolics or total flavonoids in this investigation.

5. Conclusions

The present work has shown that the fruit skins of X. *caffra* contain high levels of total phenolics and flavonoids, and that relatively high levels of these compounds can be extracted using a 70% aqueous ethanol as solvent. Extraction was time-dependent, and prolonged extraction times, i.e., beyond 60 min, lead to decreases in extraction of certain phenolic compounds, presumably due to heat degradation. The majority of extracted phenolics consisted of flavonoids, and individual compounds were successfully identified and quantified using LC-HRMS. This work makes a contribution toward identifying compounds with high antioxidant activity—and with potentially high-value—that can be extracted from X. *caffra*, and in establishing appropriate extraction conditions for doing so. Future studies should focus on elucidating the antioxidant and bioactivity of the extracts.

Author Contributions: The various authors' individual contributions to the study were as follows: Conceptualization, N.J.G, A.D.I., M.-M.P., G.O.U. and T.A.; Methodology, M.A.S.; Validation, D.O., N.J.G., M.A.S.; Formal analysis, D.O., N.J.; Investigation, D.O.; Resources, N.J.G.; Writing–Original Draft Preparation, D.O.; Writing–Review and Editing, N.J.G., M.A.S.; Supervision, N.J.G.; Project Administration, N.J.G.; Funding Acquisition, N.J.G., A.D.I., M.-M.P., G.O.U. and T.A.

Funding: This research was funded by International Foundation for Science: J/5503-1.

Acknowledgments: This research was supported by the International Foundation for Science, Stockholm, Sweden, through Grant number J/5503-1. Dave Rushworth in his personal capacity, and Moloko Mojapelo from the South African Department of Agriculture, Forestry and Fisheries are gratefully acknowledged for assistance with sourcing and identification of the fruit used in this study.

Conflicts of Interest: The authors declare that there are no actual or potential conflicts of interest.

List of Compounds

Catechin	PubChem CID: 9064
Citric acid	PubChem CID: 311
Gallic acid	PubChem CID: 370
Hyperoside	PubChem CID: 5281643
Isoquercitrin	PubChem CID: 5280804
Procyanidin B1	PubChem CID: 11250133
Quercetin-3-*O*-glucoside	PubChem CID: 5748594
Quercetin-3-*O*-robinobioside	PubChem CID: 10371536
Rutin	PubChem CID: 5280805

References

1. Ndhlala, A.R.; Muchuweti, M.; Mupure, C.; Chitindingu, K.; Murenje, T.; Kasiyamhuru, A.; Benhura, M.A. Phenolic content and profiles of selected wild fruits of zimbabwe: *Ximenia caffra, Artobotrys brachypetalus* and *Syzygium cordatum. Int. J. Food Sci. Technol.* **2008**, *43*, 1333–1337. [CrossRef]

2. Haminiuk, C.W.I.; Maciel, G.M.; Plata-Oviedo, M.S.V.; Peralta, R.M. Phenolic compounds in fruits—An overview. *Int. J. Food Sci. Technol.* **2012**, *47*, 2023–2044. [CrossRef]

3. Scalbert, A.; Johnson, I.A.; Saltmarsh, M. Polyphenols: Antioxidants and beyond. *Am. J. Clin. Nutr.* **2005**, *81*, 215S–217S. [CrossRef] [PubMed]

4. Ganesan, K.; Xu, B. A critical review on polyphenols and health benefits of black soybeans. *Nutrients* **2017**, *9*, 455. [CrossRef] [PubMed]

5. Van Wyk, B.-E. The potential of South African plants in the development of new medicinal products. *S. Afr. J. Bot.* **2011**, *77*, 812–829. [CrossRef]

6. Maroyi, A. *Ximenia caffra* sond. (ximeniaceae) in sub-saharan africa: A synthesis and review of its medicinal potential. *J. Ethnopharmacol.* **2016**, *184*, 81–100. [CrossRef] [PubMed]

7. Chivandi, E.; Davidson, B.C.; Erlwanger, K.H. A comparison of the lipid and fatty acid profiles from the kernels of the fruits (nuts) of *Ximenia caffra* and *Ricinodendron rautenenii* from Zimbabwe. *Ind. Crops Prod.* **2008**, *27*, 29–32. [CrossRef]

8. Maroyi, A. Traditional use of medicinal plants in south-central Zimbabwe: Review and perspectives. *J. Ethnobiol. Ethnomed.* **2013**, *9*, 31. [CrossRef] [PubMed]

9. Nair, J.J.; Mulaudzi, R.B.; Chukwujekwu, J.C.; Van Heerden, F.R.; Van Staden, J. Antigonococcal activity of *Ximenia caffra* sond. (olacaceae) and identification of the active principle. *S. Afr. J. Bot.* **2013**, *86*, 111–115. [CrossRef]

10. Maroyi, A. An ethnobotanical survey of medicinal plants used by the people in Nhema communal area, Zimbabwe. *J. Ethnopharmacol.* **2011**, *136*, 347–354. [CrossRef] [PubMed]

11. Rangasamy, J. Antimicrobial Activity of *Zanthoxylum davyi* and *Ximenia caffra*. Ph.D. Thesis, University of Pretoria, Pretoria, South Africa, October 2016.

12. Motlhanka, D.M.T.; Motlhanka, P.; Selebatso, T. Edible indigenous wild fruit plants of eastern Botswana. *Int. J. Poult. Sci.* **2008**, *7*, 57–460. [CrossRef]

13. Mabogo, D.E.N. The Ethnobotany of the Vhavenda. Ph.D. Thesis, University of Pretoria, Pretoria, South Africa, July 1990.

14. Fu, L.; Xu, B.T.; Xu, X.R.; Gan, R.Y.; Zhang, Y.; Xia, E.Q.; Li, H.-B. Antioxidant capacities and total phenolic contents of 62 fruits. *Food Chem.* **2011**, *129*, 345–350. [CrossRef]

15. Liu, R.H. Health benefits of fruit and vegetables are from additive and synergistic combinations of phytochemicals. *Am. J. Clin. Nutr.* **2003**, *78*, 517S–520S. [CrossRef] [PubMed]

16. Ignat, I.; Volf, I.; Popa, V.I. A critical review of methods for characterisation of polyphenolic compounds in fruits and vegetables. *Food Chem.* **2011**, *126*, 1821–1835. [CrossRef] [PubMed]

17. Shahidi, F.; Ambigaipalan, P. Phenolics and polyphenolics in foods, beverages and spices: Antioxidant activity and health effects—A review. *J. Funct. Foods* **2015**, *18*, 820–897. [CrossRef]

18. Berdahl, D.; Nahas, R.I.; Barren, J.P. *Synthetic and Natural Additives in Food Stabilization: Current Applications and Future Research*; Woodhead Publishing: Oxford, UK, 2010; pp. 272–320.

19. Do, Q.D.; Angkawijaya, A.E.; Tran-Nguyen, P.L.; Huynh, L.H.; Soetaredjo, F.E.; Ismadji, S.; Ju, Y.-H. Effect of extraction solvent on total phenol content, total flavonoid content, and antioxidant activity of *Limnophila aromatica*. *J. Food Drug Anal.* **2014**, *22*, 296–302. [CrossRef] [PubMed]

20. Dai, J.; Mumber, R.J. Plant phenolics: Extraction, analysis and their antioxidant and anticancer properties. *Molecules* **2010**, *15*, 7313–7352. [CrossRef] [PubMed]

21. Zhao, J.; Lv, G.-P.; Chen, Y.W.; Li, S.P. Advanced development in analysis of phytochemicals from medicine and food dual purposes plants used in China. *J. Chromatogr.* **2011**, *1218*, 7453–7475. [CrossRef] [PubMed]

22. Pompeu, D.R.; Silva, E.M.; Rogez, H. Optimisation of the solvent extraction of phenolic antioxidants from fruits of *Euterpe oleracea* using response surface methodology. *Bioresour. Technol.* **2009**, *100*, 6076–6082. [CrossRef] [PubMed]

23. Carbonell-Capella, J.M.; Žlabur, J.Š.; Brnčić, S.R.; Francisco, J.B.; Grimi, N.; Koubaa, M.; Brnčić, M.; Vorobiev, E. Electrotechnologies, microwaves, and ultrasounds combined with binary mixtures of ethanol and water to extract steviol glycosides and antioxidant compounds from *Stevia rebaudiana* leaves. *J. Food Process. Preserv.* **2017**, *41*, e13179. [CrossRef]

24. Pellegrini, N.; Colombi, B.; Salvatore, S.; Brenna, O.V.; Galaverna, G.; Del Rio, D.; Bianchi, M.; Bennett, R.N.; Brighenti, F. Evaluation of antioxidant capacity of some fruit and vegetable foods: Efficiency of extraction of a sequence of solvents. *J. Sci. Food Agric.* **2007**, *87*, 103–111. [CrossRef]

25. Dhuique-Mayer, C.; Tbatou, M.; Carail, M.; Caris-Veyrat, C.; Dornier, M.; Amiot, M.J. Thermal degradation of antioxidant micronutrients in citrus juice: Kinetics and newly formed compounds. *J. Agric. Food Chem.* **2007**, *55*, 4209–4216. [CrossRef] [PubMed]

26. Aspé, E.; Fernández, K. The effect of different extraction techniques on extraction yield, total phenolic, and anti-radical capacity of extracts from *Pinus radiata* bark. *Ind. Crops Prod.* **2011**, *34*, 838–844. [CrossRef]

27. Kim, D.-O.; Lee, C.Y. Extraction and isolation of polyphenolics. *Curr. Protoc. Food Anal. Chem.* **2002**, *6*, I.1.2.1–I.1.2.12. [CrossRef]

28. Singleton, V.L.; Rossi, J.A. Colorimetry of total phenolics with phosphomolybdic-phosphotungstic acid reagents. *Am. J. Enol. Vitic.* **1965**, *16*, 144–158.

29. Amado, I.R.; Franco, D.; Sanches, M.; Zapata, C.; Vazquez, J.A. Optimisation of antioxidant extraction from *Solanum tuberosum* potato peel waste by surface response methodology. *Food Chem.* **2014**, *165*, 290–299. [CrossRef] [PubMed]

30. Fogliano, V.; Verde, V.; Randazzo, G.; Ritieni, A. Method for measuring antioxidant activity and its application to monitoring the antioxidant capacity of wines. *J. Agric. Food Chem.* **1999**, *47*, 1035–1040. [CrossRef] [PubMed]

31. Stander, M.A.; Van Wyk, B.-E.; Taylor, M.J.C.; Long, H.S. Analysis of phenolic compounds in rooibos tea (*Aspalathus linearis*) with a comparison of flavonoid-based compounds in natural populations of plants from different regions. *J. Agric. Food Chem.* **2017**, *65*, 10270–10281. [CrossRef] [PubMed]

32. Gironi, F.; Piemonte, V. Temperature and solvent effects on polyphenol extraction process from chestnut tree wood. *Chem. Eng. Res. Des.* **2011**, *89*, 857–862. [CrossRef]

33. Trabelsi, N.; Megdiche, W.; Ksouri, R.; Falleh, H.; Oueslati, S.; Soumaya, B.; Hajlaoui, H.; Abdelly, C. Solvent effects on phenolic contents and biological activities of the halophyte *Limoniastrum monopetalum* leaves. *LWT-Food Sci. Technol.* **2010**, *43*, 632–639. [CrossRef]

34. Hayouni, E.A.; Abedrabba, M.; Bouix, M.; Hamdi, M. The effects of solvents and extraction method on the phenolic contents and biological activities in vitro of tunisian *Quercus coccifera* L. and *Juniperus phoenicea* L. fruit extracts. *Food Chem.* **2007**, *105*, 1126–1134. [CrossRef]

35. Ndhlala, A.R.; Mupure, C.H.; Benhura, M.A.N.; Muchuweti, M. Antioxidant potentials and degrees of polymerization of six wild fruits. *Sci. Res. Essays* **2006**, *1*, 87–92.

36. Rohn, S.; Buchner, N.; Driemel, G.; Rauser, M.; Kroh, L.W. Thermal degradation of onion quercetin glucosides under roasting conditions. *J. Agric. Food Chem.* **2007**, *55*, 1568–1573. [CrossRef] [PubMed]

37. Crozier, A.; Lean, M.E.J.; McDonald, M.S.; Black, C. Quantitative analysis of the flavonoid content of commercial tomatoes, onions, lettuce, and celery. *J. Agric. Food Chem.* **1997**, *45*, 590–595. [CrossRef]

38. Buchner, N.; Krumbein, A.; Rohn, S.; Kroh, L.W. Effect of thermal processing on the flavonols rutin and quercetin. *Rapid Commun. Mass Spectrom.* **2006**, *20*, 3229–3235. [CrossRef] [PubMed]

39. De Castro, M.D.L.; García-Ayuso, L.E. Soxhlet extraction of solid materials: An outdated technique with a promising innovative future. *Anal. Chim. Acta* **1998**, *369*, 1–10. [CrossRef]

40. Spigno, G.; Tramelli, L.; De Faveri, D.M. Effects of extraction time, temperature and solvent on concentration and antioxidant activity of grape marc phenolics. *J. Food Eng.* **2007**, *81*, 200–208. [CrossRef]

41. Huang, W.-Y.; Zhang, H.-C.; Liu, W.-X.; Li, C.-H. Survey of antioxidant capacity and phenolic composition of blueberry, blackberry, and strawberry in Nanjing. *J. Zhejiang Univ. Sci. B* **2012**, *13*, 94–102. [CrossRef] [PubMed]

42. Rodrigues, E.; Poerner, N.; Rockenbach, I.I.; Gonzaga, L.V.; Mendes, C.R.; Fett, R. Phenolic compounds and antioxidant activity of blueberry cultivars grown in Brazil. *Food Sci. Technol.* **2011**, *34*, 911–917. [CrossRef]

43. Villaño, D.; Fernández-Pachón, M.S.; Moyá, M.L.; Troncoso, A.M.; García-Parrilla, M.C. Radical scavenging ability of polyphenolic compounds towards DPPH free radical. *Talanta* **2007**, *71*, 230–235. [CrossRef] [PubMed]

44. Park, J.Y.; Han, X.; Piao, M.J.; Oh, M.C.; Fernando, P.M.D.J.; Kang, K.A.; Ryu, Y.S.; Jung, U.; Kim, I.G.; Hyun, J.W. Hyperoside induces endogenous antioxidant system to alleviate oxidative stress. *J. Cancer Prev.* **2016**, *21*, 41–47. [CrossRef] [PubMed]

45. Williamson, G.; Manach, C. Bioavailability and bioefficacy of polyphenols in humans. II. Review of 93 intervention studies. *Am. J. Clin. Nutr.* **2005**, *81*, 243S–255S. [CrossRef] [PubMed]

46. Valentová, K.; Vrba, J.; Bancîřová, M.; Ulrichová, J.; Křen, K. Isoquercitrin: Pharmacology, toxicology, and metabolism. *Food Chem. Toxicol.* **2014**, *68*, 267–282. [CrossRef] [PubMed]

47. Gil, M.I.; Tomás-Barberán, F.A.; Hess-Pierce, B.; Holcroft, D.M.; Kader, A.A. Antioxidant activity of pomegranate juice and its relationship with phenolic composition and processing. *J. Agric. Food Chem.* **2000**, *48*, 4581–4589. [CrossRef] [PubMed]

48. Rostamzad, H.; Shabanpour, B.; Kashaninejad, M.; ShabaniI, A. Antioxidative activity of citric and ascorbic acids and their preventive effect on lipid oxidation in frozen Persian sturgeon fillets. *Lat. Am. Appl. Res.* **2011**, *41*, 135–140.

49. Lampila, P.; Van Lieshout, M.; Gremmen, B.; Lähteenmäki, L. Consumer attitudes towards enhanced flavonoid content in fruit. *Food Res. Int.* **2009**, *42*, 122–129. [CrossRef]

50. Prior, R.L.; Wu, X.; Schaich, K. Standardized methods for the determination of antioxidant capacity and phenolics in foods and dietary supplements. *J. Agric. Food Chem.* **2005**, *53*, 4290–4302. [CrossRef] [PubMed]

51. Chun, O.K.; Kim, D.-O. Consideration on equivalent chemicals in total phenolic assay of chlorogenic acid-rich plums. *Food Res. Int.* **2004**, *37*, 337–342. [CrossRef]

52. Galato, D.; Ckless, K.; Susin, M.F.; Giacomelli, C.; Ribeiro-do-Valle, R.M.; Spinelli, A. Antioxidant capacity of phenolic and related compounds: Correlation among electrochemical, visible spectroscopy methods and structure-antioxidant activity. *Redox Rep.* **2001**, *6*, 243–250. [CrossRef] [PubMed]

53. Kim, D.O.; Jeong, S.W.; Lee, C.Y. Antioxidant capacity of phenolic phytochemicals from various cultivars of plums. *Food Chem.* **2003**, *81*, 321–326. [CrossRef]

54. Tawaha, K.; Alali, F.Q.; Gharaibeh, M.; Mohammad, M.; El-Elimat, T. Antioxidant activity and total phenolic content of selected Jordanian plant species. *Food Chem.* **2007**, *104*, 1372–1378. [CrossRef]

10

The Energy Costs of Prematurity and the Neonatal Intensive Care Unit (NICU) Experience

John B. C. Tan [1], Danilo S. Boskovic [1] and Danilyn M. Angeles [2],* (ID)

[1] Division of Biochemistry, Department of Basic Sciences, Loma Linda University,
    Loma Linda, CA 92350, USA; jctan@llu.edu (J.B.C.T.); dboskovic@llu.edu (D.S.B.)
[2] Division of Physiology, Department of Basic Sciences, Loma Linda University, Loma Linda, CA 92350, USA
*   Correspondence: dangeles@llu.edu

Abstract: Premature neonates are in an energy deficient state due to (1) oxygen desaturation and hypoxia events, (2) painful and stressful stimuli, (3) illness, and (4) neurodevelopmental energy requirements. Failure to correct energy deficiency in premature infants may lead to adverse effects such as neurodevelopmental delay and negative long-term metabolic and cardiovascular outcomes. The effects of energy dysregulation and the challenges that clinicians in the Neonatal Intensive Care Unit (NICU) face in meeting the premature infant's metabolic demands are discussed. Specifically, the focus is on the effects of pain and stress on energy homeostasis. Energy deficiency is a complex problem and requires a multi-faceted solution to promote optimum development of premature infants.

Keywords: premature neonate; energy; nutrition; pain; sucrose

1. Introduction

Premature infants (less than 37 weeks gestational age) face numerous challenges during their stay in the neonatal intensive care unit (NICU). Not only do they face the challenge of being underdeveloped compared to term infants, they are also at risk to a variety of illnesses, as well as undernutrition and growth failure [1,2], These factors lead to a state of energy deficiency and catabolism, with potential long-term effects such as impaired neuronal development [3,4] and metabolic diseases [5,6]. Critically ill neonates and premature infants in particular, also undergo multiple (from 4 to 16) tissue damaging procedures (TDPs) for clinical care or diagnostic purposes [7–9]. These procedures include tape removal, heel-stick, venipuncture, intravenous or central catheter placement, injections and tracheal suctioning and intubation. Analgesic treatments for TDPs usually come in the form of 0.5 mL to 2 mL/kg per dose of a 24% oral sucrose solution given with a pacifier, lingually or at the buccal mucosa [10–13]. However, sucrose may play an indirect role in the modulation of the premature infant's stress physiology, metabolism and energy state [10,14–18]. With this in mind, the premature condition in the context of routine clinical procedures, energy metabolism and prospective long-term outcomes of energy deficit are of interest. The administration of oral sucrose and its potential effects on energy metabolism and stress physiology require particular attention. It is anticipated that, with improved understanding of the potential mechanisms of the development of energy deficit in premature neonates, rational preventive and treatment approaches will emerge. The objective of this narrative review is to summarize the complexity of the metabolic demands of the premature neonate, as well as the potential consequences of not meeting these demands, leading to energy deficit.

2. Premature Infants Are in an Energy-Deficit State

Preterm births steadily increased from 9.5% in 1981 to 12.7% in 2005 [19]. During the first few weeks of postnatal life, premature infants are most likely ill, physiologically unstable and lack adequate nutritional support [2]. Following birth, these infants simultaneously experience a loss of maternal nutritional support along with their own limited ability for energy storage [20,21]. Energy deficit occurs due to four possible reasons (see Figure 1 for a simplified diagram).

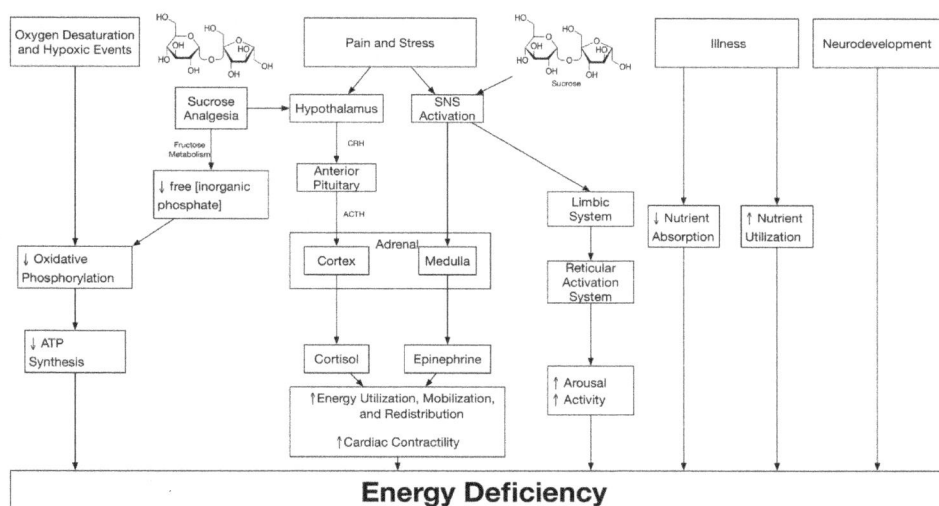

Figure 1. Causes of energy deficiency in the premature infant. (ATP, adenosine triphosphate; SNS, sympathetic nervous system).

First, there may be reduced energy stores due to oxygen desaturation events that occur frequently in the NICU setting, most often due to prematurity or respiratory disease [22]. Neonates experiencing multiple oxygen desaturation events are at risk for hypoxia, which refers to an inadequate oxygen supply to the tissues. This leads to a reduced rate of oxidative phosphorylation by aerobic respiration and to reduced adenosine triphosphate (ATP) synthesis [23]. Because of the lack of oxygen as a final electron acceptor, the mitochondria are unable to maintain the proton gradient necessary to form ATP from adenosine diphosphate (ADP) and inorganic phosphate [24]. Consequently, ATP production is reduced and possibly interrupted.

Second, energy stores may be reduced in response to stressful stimuli such as procedural pain. We explored the effects of tissue damaging procedures (TDPs) on ATP metabolism [25]. When the TDP was tape removal, performed along with the removal of a central or venous catheter, we found a significant increase in uric acid (UA) and malondialdehyde (MDA) thirty minutes after the painful stimulus. UA is a downstream product of ATP degradation. MDA is an oxidative stress marker formed by the oxidative degradation of polyunsaturated lipids by reactive oxygen species (ROS). The increase in ATP degradation in response to painful procedures may be due to energy expended through behavioral and physiological reactions to pain, such as crying, facial grimacing, flailing and tachycardia [26]. The increased oxidative stress could be due to increased purine degradation with concomitant production of ROS. Alternatively, oxidative stress could also be due to increased mitochondrial ATP synthesis activity, of which ROS is a byproduct, in order to meet the energy demands of increased ATP utilization [27]. Both the increased ATP utilization and oxidative stress can lead to energy deficit.

Third, energy stores can be reduced during illness [2]. Though current understanding for the neonatal population is modest, studies in adult and children show that critical illness changes metabolism significantly by decreasing the rate of absorption and utilization of nutrients [28–31]. Furthermore, elevated pro-inflammatory cytokines, such as TNF-α, IL-6 and IL-10 play a role in increasing metabolic demand [29,32]. Such pro-inflammatory cytokines were found to be elevated in critically ill neonates, implying that increased metabolic demand can also occur in the premature neonate population [32,33]. An increase in metabolic demand will further decrease energy stores.

Finally, an increase in metabolic demand due to the high energy demands of the brain [34–36] can further reduce a premature neonate's energy stores. The neonatal brain accounts for 60% of total metabolism [37]. Most brain energy is used in the maintenance and manipulation of ion gradients for synaptic transmissions and cortical development [34]. As the brain develops during the early neonatal period, certain connections are pruned and ATP must be spent for the creation of cell components [38].

To make up for increased metabolic requirements, clinicians need to respond appropriately by increasing nutritional availability to premature neonates. This can be a challenge because premature infants have immature digestive and absorptive capabilities [39]. Moreover, most immature infants must rely on total parenteral nutrition (TPN) for exogenous nutritional support [40]. TPN, however, can only safely provide a limited amount and concentration of nutrients. Furthermore, TPN use is associated with added potential complications which includes the following: (a) TPN may lead to a stunting of the neonatal intestinal development due to absence of trophic factors that are only released when nutrients are present in the intestinal lumen [41,42] and (b) Long-term use of TPN is associated with an increased risk of metabolic liver dysfunction [43]. Because of such concerns, premature neonates are given early trophic feedings, weaned off TPN gradually and are cautiously introduced to enteral nutrition through a nasogastric or an orogastric tube [42,44].

Despite these attempts to provide adequate nutrition, preterm infants tend to experience growth failure. Reali et al. found that in their cohort of premature infants born with a weight appropriate for gestational age (AGA, 2.5–4.0 kg), as many as 71.4% weighed less than the 10th percentile at discharge from the hospital [45]. It is currently unclear whether the cause of growth failure is due to inadequate nutrient supply to the infant or due to non-nutritional mechanisms that can also restrict growth and energy stores, such as inflammation or illness [2,3]. Nonetheless, it is clear that premature infants are frequently in an energy-deprived state due to increased metabolic demands combined with inadequate nutrition.

Under circumstances of frequent energy deprivation, premature infants compensate through tissue breakdown and protein loss [46]. Tissue and energy stores are converted into readily available fuel. Amino acids are recycled through the liver as carbon sources for gluconeogenesis or degraded into ketones, serving as the brain's alternative fuel source [2]. As energy supply becomes increasingly scarce, tissue breakdown and energy storage utilization becomes necessary to provide fuel even for baseline cellular processes [47]. Under hypoxic conditions anaerobic metabolism is engaged, converting pyruvate to lactate and allowing the regeneration of nicotinamide-adenine dinucleotide (NAD^+), so glycolysis can continue to generate ATP. Nonetheless, the resulting ATP is expended quickly, resulting in a steady decrease of ATP stores [23].

3. Energy Deficiency Affects Long-Term Outcomes

Energy deficits were shown to be detrimental to neurodevelopment and cognitive functions, especially in neonates [48]. The brain is a rapidly developing organ, which is responsible for 60% of total body's energy requirements [37]. During development, a critical growth phase occurs, which refers to the period of time when the neonatal brain experiences a significant degree of neuroplasticity [49]. During this phase, the neonatal brain is highly influenced by nutritional availability [50]. Critical periods of growth are accompanied by an increase in metabolic demand, requiring adequate nutrition to support it. Stephens et. al identified the first week of life as a period of critical growth in extremely low birth weight infants (ELBW, infants who are born weighing less than 1000 g) and observed that increasing protein or energy intake during that time period correlated with improved neurodevelopmental outcomes at 18 months corrected age [51].

Despite the significant relationship between nutrition and growth and development, few tools exist that measure energy utilization and adequacy of nutrient intake in premature neonates. Current markers of nutritional status include growth velocity (15 g/k/day), weight gain (10–30 g/day) and head circumference (1 cm/week) [50,52]. However, these measures, are shown to only be applicable to a limited range of postnatal age [53]. For example, Fenton et al. [53] has shown that the commonly used weight growth velocity goal of 15 g/kg/d was only consistent with the preterm infant growth reference curves at about 34 weeks. Tools that measure the energy states of premature neonates throughout the wide range of gestational ages are needed. These tools need to be individualized to gestational age, birth weight, gender, and illness severity. For example, our laboratory examined urinary biochemical markers as a measure of ATP utilization in premature neonates [10,54]. In the late pre-term neonates, we found urinary hypoxanthine to be highest in those with respiratory disease, showing the effect of illness on ATP degradation [54]. This data suggests that neonates with respiratory disease may require higher total energy intake [53]. In addition, we found an association between urinary allantoin levels and the incidence of severe intraventricular hemorrhage (IVH) [55]. Allantoin is an oxidation product of uric acid in the presence of reactive oxygen species, which may be produced during increased ATP utilization [10]. Few studies on IVH and nutrition exist but Sammallahti et al. [56] observed that those with IVH had lower total energy intake and lower energy intake from human milk. This data suggests the importance of careful monitoring and provision of adequate nutrition in this vulnerable population. An additional challenge for neonatal growth assessment is that optimal growth is currently not well defined. Additionally, the few reported studies in neonatal growth are impacted by confounding factors that reduce the value of their conclusions [57]. As previously described, current premature infant growth models only take into account simple measurements such as length, weight, head circumference and body mass index (BMI) [58]. Furthermore, it is unclear if these premature infant growth models are appropriate because they are based on a population of healthier term infants [2]. In view of the absence of correlation between rapid growth of premature neonates with long-term adult metabolic risks and clear association with a decreased infant morbidity and mortality, improved nutritional support may be warranted [59].

In contrast to the established long-term neurodevelopmental outcomes of energy deficit, evidence regarding long-term metabolic and cardiovascular outcomes is unclear. Once a premature infant is stabilized in the NICU, nutrition is given and accelerated catch-up growth may occur within the first 24 months of postnatal life [60,61]. It is currently believed that catch-up growth is beneficial for the first 2 years of life [62], especially for neurodevelopment [3,50] but may have negative long-term consequences in adult metabolism [63]. Unfortunately, studies on the non-neurodevelopmental effects of catch-up growth are few and of poor quality [57]. Despite the benefits of catch-up growth, there are reports that preterm infants with accelerated weight gain after the first two years of life have higher relative body adiposity and cardiovascular complications compared to term infants [64–66]. In adults, such increased body adiposity is a risk factor for cardiovascular morbidity and metabolic syndrome [67]. Because of this, it was suggested that quality assessment of neonatal growth should include more comprehensive measures of body composition, such as fat mass (FM) vs. fat-free mass (FFM), instead of simple body length, weight, head circumference and BMI [58,68,69]. However, it remains unclear whether the increased FM in early postnatal life independently alters cardiovascular and metabolic health in adulthood.

Long-term effects of fetal growth, postnatal growth and early nutrition were studied with respect to cardiovascular and metabolic outcomes in preterm infants [70]. Adults, who were born prematurely, were found to have a significantly greater risk of developing hypertension and insulin resistance compared to those born at term. This difference, however, was not associated with body size, body composition, or FM distribution. Furthermore, growth between birth or expected term age and 12 to 18 months post-term, had no significant influence on blood pressure or metabolic syndrome in adulthood. Instead, it was suggested that growth during late infancy and childhood may have a more significant influence on later cardiovascular and metabolic health. This is consistent with a recent longitudinal cohort study [71] of association between weight gain in infancy and childhood with biomarkers of metabolic syndrome in adolescents who were born preterm. No significant correlation between infant weight gain and long-term metabolic consequences was observed, regardless of catch-up growth rate. Instead, significant associations were reported between childhood weight gain (after 1 year of age) and later body composition changes ($p < 0.001$ for higher fat mass, high fat index, lean mass index and waist circumference), higher fasting insulin ($p = 0.002$), lower insulin sensitivity ($p < 0.001$), higher systolic and diastolic blood pressures (p = 0.006 and 0.005, respectively), lower high density lipoprotein (HDL) (p = 0.001) and a higher total cholesterol to HDL ratio (p < 0.001). These studies support the novel idea that the growth velocity after the first two years of life is a more accurate predictor of adult risk of metabolic disorders than the catch-up growth rate of premature infants during the first two years of life [3,4].

4. Prematurity and Chronic Stress, Energy Deficiency and Neuroplasticity

Preterm infants are in a state of chronic physiological and biochemical stress due to prematurity, illness, medications and many unavoidable environmental stressors in the NICU. When the relationship between clinical handling procedures, stress, pain and energy expenditure was examined, it was observed that as the level of intervention increased, infant energy expenditure increased as well [72]. Additionally, a negative correlation was found between energy expenditure and oxygen saturation, supporting the hypothesis that oxygen desaturation events are likely to result in hypoxia, resulting in decreased ATP synthesis coupled with an increased ATP utilization. Our lab found a similar association of increased ATP utilization in response to TDPs [25].

Because preterm infants lack the agency to limit external stressful stimuli, they must rely on their caregivers to limit their exposure to stressors. These environmental stressors include loud sounds and alarms from clinical equipment, noise from other infants, handling by the caregivers themselves and constant interruption of sleep for medical procedures. Furthermore, premature infants are also exposed to multiple tissue damaging procedures (TDPs) for clinical care or diagnostic purposes [8,73]. These can have long-term consequences, including neuroplastic modulation of the neonates' stress response.

The stress response can be represented by two concepts: allostasis and allostatic load [74]. Allostasis refers to the active process of metabolic or physiological adaptations in response to stressful stimuli. Allostatic load refers to the "wear and tear" of the body that increases over time in response to chronic stress [75]. Allostatic load can manifest itself as a dysregulation of the stress response due to a lack of adaptation, prolonged response, or inadequate response [75].

A key regulator of allostasis is the hypothalamic-pituitary-adrenal (HPA) axis. While the development and function of this axis still remains to be fully characterized in the newborn, stress regulation involves three main steps. First, the paraventricular nucleus of the hypothalamus synthesizes and secretes corticotrophin-releasing hormone (CRH). Second, the anterior lobe of the pituitary gland releases adrenocorticotropic hormone (ACTH) in response to CRH. Finally, cortisol is released by the adrenal glands in response to ACTH. For a healthy allostatic response, baseline hormone levels are restored through cortisol's negative feedback loop to the hypothalamus and the pituitary gland. In the premature infant, the allostatic response via the HPA axis may be irreversibly altered due to chronic stress exposure. The allostatic load may be elevated due to insufficient cortisol production caused by illness or an underdeveloped HPA axis [76]. Heckmann et al. found that a mature adrenal response, defined in clinically stable premature infants as a tripled level of cortisol in response to stress, was present only in 27% (12 out of 44) of ill preterm infants [77]. However, these high responders were more prone to central nervous system (CNS) bleeds. Additionally, it was demonstrated that during the first 7 days of life, the pituitary gland is responsive to human CRH but cortisol production was suboptimal [78]. This may be due to an underdeveloped adrenal cortex or cortisol synthesis. This cortisol deficiency disappeared by day of life 14 [78]. Thus, allostasis may be inadequate in early life.

The HPA axis also plays a role in energy homeostasis. As part of the allostatic response, the metabolic demand for energy is augmented to increase chances of survival. One group [72] showed a significant correlation between stress and energy expenditure in premature neonates. Stress was defined as (1) a heart rate of less than 100 bpm or more than 160 bpm or an increased baseline of 5 bpm or more, (2) irregular respiratory rate of less than 40 or more than 60 breaths/min, or a baseline increase of 7 breaths/min or more and (3) oxygen saturation of less than 90% or a decrease of 2.5% or more. Energy expenditure was measured as follows:

$$E = \frac{M \times t}{H_T}$$

where E = energy expenditure per heartbeat $\left(\frac{calories}{kg}\right)$, M = mean metabolic rate $\left(\frac{calories}{kg \cdot min}\right)$, t = duration of study (min) and H_T = total accumulated heartbeats.

Stressful experiences may also have lasting developmental impact. Allostatic load can manifest itself through the dysregulation and neuroplastic modification of the HPA axis. Recently, an "ACTH-cortisol" dissociation was reported in critically ill adults, referring to low circulating ACTH coupled with elevated plasma cortisol [79,80]. Furthermore, high levels of chronic stress can alter HPA axis reactivity and shift the baseline set point of cortisol, blunting the allostatic response to acute stress [81]. A prolonged period is required to return to pre-stress hormone levels and higher concentrations of cortisol is required to respond to subsequent stressors [82]. Prolonged exposure to elevated cortisol levels may lead to increased proteolysis, which can negatively impact the overall growth of the neonate [83]. Chronic stress may also be associated with increased cognitive and behavioral problems and metabolic risks [84–87]. This can modify the structure and synaptic connections of the prefrontal cortex, the area of the brain associated with personality expression, decision-making and social behavior [88]. In rats, chronic stress was shown to increase synaptic inhibition of prefrontal glutamatergic output neurons, resulting in decreased control of stress reactivity and behavior [89]. Furthermore, chronic stress decreases synaptic density in the prefrontal cortex as well as in the hippocampus [90]. Thus, there are good reasons to expect, even in the absence of human newborn studies, that allostatic modifications in response to chronic stress may influence the neuronal development of the premature infant's brain.

5. Sucrose and Stress Relief

Oral sucrose with non-nutritive sucking was shown in many studies to reduce procedural pain scores [11–13]. The evidence for the analgesic effects of sucrose is strongest for single event painful procedures such as heel lance, venipuncture, or intramuscular injection [7]. Analgesic benefits of sucrose for other painful procedures such as arterial puncture, subcutaneous injection, insertion of nasogastric or orogastric tubes, bladder catheterization, eye examinations or echocardiography examinations are less certain [7]. Most studies on sucrose examine pain behavior as the study variable. There is a limited amount of research on other outcome variables, such as cortisol. Some of these studies are outlined in Table 1.

Table 1. Summary table of studies that examined other variables besides pain response after sucrose administration. (CNS, central nervous system; ACTH, adrenocorticotropic hormone; CRH, corticotropin-releasing hormone; mRNA, messenger ribonucleic acid)

Population	Parameter Measured	Effect	Sucrose Dose	Control	References
Premature Infant	ATP Utilization	Increased	2 mL for neonates >2 kg 1.5 mL for neonates 1.5–2 kg 0.5 mL for neonates that were <1.5 kg	Placebo (Sterile Water)	[10]
	Oxidative Stress	Increased			
Premature Infant	Salivary Cortisol	No Significant Difference	0.1–0.3 mL per Painful Procedure	Placebo (Sterile Water)	[91]
Premature Infant	Plasma Cortisol	No Significant Difference	Pacifier Dipped in Sucrose	Water	[92]
Adult Human Females	Salivary Cortisol	Decreased	3 Servings of Study Beverage per Day	Aspartame	[93]
	Regional Brain Responses	Increased in Left Hippocampus			
Premature Infant	Neurodevelopmental Assessment	No Significant Difference	0.5 mL per Painful Procedure	Placebo (Sterile Water)	[94]
Mouse Pups	CNS White Matter Regions	Decreased	0.1–0.2 g Sucrose per kg Body Weight	Vehicle (Sterile Water)	[95]
	CNS Gray Matter Regions	Decreased			
Adult Rat	Plasma ACTH Corticosterone CRH mRNA	Decreased Decreased Decreased	Up to 4 mL Twice a Day	Saccharin and/or Water	[96,97]

A few studies in premature neonates measured the effects of sucrose administration on cortisol. Boyer et al. [91] found no significant difference in salivary cortisol concentration 30 min after a painful procedure in premature infants receiving either 24% sucrose or a placebo of sterile water. Stang et al. [92] found no significant difference in plasma cortisol 30 min after circumcision in groups receiving a dorsal penile nerve block agent and sucrose or water. Although sucrose had no significant effect on plasma cortisol levels, the pain scores decreased in both studies, which suggest that sucrose may only mask pain behavior with little effect on the glucocorticoid response [98]. A different response has been observed in animals. Ulrich-Lai and her colleagues showed that in rats exposed to chronic stress, sucrose consumption decreased corticotropin-releasing hormone messenger ribonucleic acid (CRH mRNA) in the paraventricular nucleus of the hypothalamus [96]. They also showed that the palatable and rewarding properties of sucrose are responsible for a decrease in adrenocorticotropic hormone (ACTH) and corticosterone [97]. The basolateral amygdala is altered in response to sucrose consumption and this alteration is long-lasting due to neuroplasticity [97]. Furthermore, increased duration and/or frequency of sucrose administration played a larger role in the dampening of the HPA axis than the volume of sucrose given, suggesting that sucrose may alter neuroplasticity and stress relief [99].

It was calculated that *"a 1000-gram infant receiving an average of 10 doses of 24% oral sucrose per day, at 0.5–1 mL per dose, is equal to a one year old infant receiving ½ can of regular Coke Classic per day"* [11]. The effect of this much sucrose on human premature infants is unknown. In adults, a 19-day study compared salivary cortisol levels between two groups that consumed either sucrose or aspartame along with a standardized, low-sugar baseline diet [93]. It was found that sucrose but not aspartame, reduced salivary cortisol levels after a comprehensive imaging stress test. In the same study, sucrose consumption correlated with a significant increase in activity levels in the left hippocampus, implying that sucrose inhibits stress induced deactivation of the hippocampus, perhaps through HPA axis suppression. These data suggest that oral sucrose consumption may modify the brain's response to stress, specifically in the paraventricular nucleus of the hypothalamus and the basolateral amygdala. Interestingly, Stevens et al. showed that preterm infants <31 weeks' gestational age who received >10 doses of sucrose per 24 h in the first week of life had poorer neurologic development compared with infants who received fewer sucrose doses [12]. However, in older premature neonates that are over 32 weeks gestational age, Banga et al. showed that repeated dosages of sucrose administration for procedural pain in premature infants for the first seven days after enrollment had no significant impact on neurobehavioral outcomes at 40 weeks post conception [94]. Additional studies are required to clarify the effect of sucrose analgesia on the newborn's brain.

The mechanism for sucrose's analgesic effect is unknown but is thought to be due to (a) the release of endogenous opioids two minutes after sucrose administration [100], although evidence to substantiate this hypothesis in humans is lacking, or (b) the occurrence of ingestion analgesia [101]. Ingestion analgesia occurs when hedonic foods are eaten and functions to defend eating from ending and stops when eating is over. Hedonic food is specific to the animal's homeostatic state. For example, sodium becomes hedonic when effective circulating volume is low [102]. In a complementary manner, the sensation of thirst increases when plasma osmolality rises above normal levels [103]. Similarly, sucrose, an inherently hedonic food due to its sweet taste, has been shown to reduce stress via brain reward pathways [97]. Chronic stress modifies the brain's reward pathway to increase the hedonic value of palatable high-calorie foods through the actions of glucocorticoids [16]. Incidentally, there is strong evidence that an animal's energy stores may play a role in the regulation of the HPA axis [16]. The hedonic value of oral sucrose may be elevated in chronically stressed premature infants that are energy deficient, which may contribute to its effectiveness in decreasing the behavioral signs of pain.

Though sucrose may have a role in pain and stress relief, it may come at the cost of long-term neurologic and metabolic consequences and altered brain stress and reward pathways. Acutely, a single dose of oral sucrose administration for heel lance has been associated with increased ATP utilization and oxidative stress [10], perhaps due to the high metabolic cost of the fructose moiety of sucrose [104]. In a mouse pup model, the effects of early repeated sucrose treatment before an intervention on long-term brain structure was examined [95]. These mice pups received an oral dose of vehicle (sterile water) or 24% sucrose via a micropipette, two minutes before an intervention. The mice pups were separated into three different intervention groups: a needle-prick on the paw, light tactile paw pressure with a cotton swab, or only handling in a similar manner as the other groups. The mice pups received 10 interventions daily from post-natal day 1 (P1) to P6 to model the NICU experience. Adult brains were collected between P85 and P95 and were scanned using magnetic resonance imaging (MRI). Early repetitive sucrose exposure in mice resulted in smaller white matter volumes in the corpus callosum, stria terminalis and fimbria ($p < 0.0001$) and smaller cortical and subcortical gray matter in the hippocampus and cerebellum ($p < 0.0001$), regardless of intervention. This suggests that sucrose may affect brain development independent of procedural pain. The modulation of the HPA axis and the increased hedonic values placed on sweet solutions may also play a role in the increased risk of long-term negative metabolic outcomes. In the interim, however, there is not enough evidence to recommend the cessation of oral sucrose administration for procedural pain in the NICU. More studies are required to examine the analgesic effectiveness of metabolically "cheaper" sweet solutions, such as glucose, as well as other pharmacologic and non-pharmacologic methods to reduce pain.

6. Conclusions

In conclusion, premature infants are in a state of energy deficiency due to hypoxia, pain and stress, illness and neurodevelopment. Each of these factors increases ATP utilization, reducing energy stores. In addition, oral sucrose, a commonly used intervention for pain was recently shown to acutely increase ATP utilization as evidenced by increased biochemical markers of hypoxia and oxidative stress over time [10]. Nutritional support specific to a neonate's age, weight, gender and illness severity needs to be provided to prevent energy deficit and tools that monitor energy states and efficacy of nutritional intake need to be developed and tested. Management of a neonate's nutritional status is complex and requires prospective studies that will yield evidence-based methods and techniques.

Acknowledgments: The authors gratefully acknowledge the Department of Basic Sciences, Loma Linda Medical School, for their support of this work. This work is partially supported by NIH NR011209-08.

Author Contributions: John B. C. Tan, initial primary author also involved in revisions. Danilyn M. Angeles and Danilo S. Boskovic, mentors contributing to the direction of topic, subject matter contained, revisions and editing.

Conflicts of Interest: The authors declare no conflicts of interest.

References

1. Dinerstein, A.; Nieto, R.M.; Solana, C.L.; Perez, G.P.; Otheguy, L.E.; Larguia, A.M. Early and aggressive nutritional strategy (parenteral and enteral) decreases postnatal growth failure in very low birth weight infants. *J. Perinatol.* **2006**, *26*, 436–442. [CrossRef] [PubMed]

2. Ramel, S.E.; Brown, L.D.; Georgieff, M.K. The Impact of Neonatal Illness on Nutritional Requirements—One Size Does Not Fit All. *Curr. Pediatr. Rep.* **2014**, *2*, 248–254. [CrossRef] [PubMed]

3. Ramel, S.E.; Demerath, E.W.; Gray, H.L.; Younge, N.; Boys, C.; Georgieff, M.K. The relationship of poor linear growth velocity with neonatal illness and two-year neurodevelopment in preterm infants. *Neonatology* **2012**, *102*, 19–24. [CrossRef] [PubMed]

4. Ehrenkranz, R.A.; Dusick, A.M.; Vohr, B.R.; Wright, L.L.; Wrage, L.A.; Poole, W.K. Growth in the neonatal intensive care unit influences neurodevelopmental and growth outcomes of extremely low birth weight infants. *Pediatrics* **2006**, *117*, 1253–1261. [CrossRef] [PubMed]

5. Lapillonne, A. Feeding the preterm infant after discharge. *World Rev. Nutr. Diet.* **2014**, *110*, 264–277. [CrossRef] [PubMed]

6. Vargas, J.; Junco, M.; Gomez, C.; Lajud, N. Early Life Stress Increases Metabolic Risk, HPA Axis Reactivity and Depressive-Like Behavior When Combined with Postweaning Social Isolation in Rats. *PLoS ONE* **2016**, *11*. [CrossRef] [PubMed]

7. Stevens, B.; Yamada, J.; Ohlsson, A.; Haliburton, S.; Shorkey, A. Sucrose for analgesia (pain relief) in newborn infants undergoing painful procedures. *Cochrane Database Syst. Rev.* **2016**, *7*. [CrossRef]

8. Carbajal, R.; Rousset, A.; Danan, C.; Coquery, S.; Nolent, P.; Ducrocq, S.; Saizou, C.; Lapillonne, A.; Granier, M.; Durand, P.; et al. Epidemiology and treatment of painful procedures in neonates in intensive care units. *JAMA* **2008**, *300*, 60–70. [CrossRef] [PubMed]

9. Angeles, D.M.; Ashwal, S.; Wycliffe, N.D.; Ebner, C.; Fayard, E.; Sowers, L.; Holshouser, B.A. Relationship between opioid therapy, tissue-damaging procedures and brain metabolites as measured by proton MRS in asphyxiated term neonates. *Pediatr. Res.* **2007**, *61*, 614–621. [CrossRef] [PubMed]

10. Asmerom, Y.; Slater, L.; Boskovic, D.S.; Bahjri, K.; Holden, M.S.; Phillips, R.; Deming, D.; Ashwal, S.; Fayard, E.; Angeles, D.M. Oral sucrose for heel lance increases adenosine triphosphate use and oxidative stress in preterm neonates. *J. Pediatr.* **2013**, *163*, 29–35. [CrossRef] [PubMed]

11. Holsti, L.; Grunau, R.E. Considerations for using sucrose to reduce procedural pain in preterm infants. *Pediatrics* **2010**, *125*, 1042–1047. [CrossRef] [PubMed]

12. Stevens, B.; Yamada, J.; Beyene, J.; Gibbins, S.; Petryshen, P.; Stinson, J.; Narciso, J. Consistent management of repeated procedural pain with sucrose in preterm neonates: Is it effective and safe for repeated use over time? *Clin. J. Pain* **2005**, *21*, 543–548. [CrossRef] [PubMed]

13. Taddio, A.; Shah, V.; Atenafu, E.; Katz, J. Influence of repeated painful procedures and sucrose analgesia on the development of hyperalgesia in newborn infants. *Pain* **2009**, *144*, 43–48. [CrossRef] [PubMed]

14. Muralidhara, D.V.; Shetty, P.S. Sucrose feeding stimulates basal metabolism & nonshivering thermogenesis in undernourished rats. *Indian J. Med. Res.* **1990**, *92*, 447–451. [PubMed]

15. Laugero, K.D. A new perspective on glucocorticoid feedback: Relation to stress, carbohydrate feeding and feeling better. *J. Neuroendocrinol.* **2001**, *13*, 827–835. [CrossRef] [PubMed]

16. Laugero, K.D. Reinterpretation of basal glucocorticoid feedback: Implications to behavioral and metabolic disease. *Vitam. Horm.* **2004**, *69*, 1–29. [CrossRef] [PubMed]

17. Goran, M.I.; Dumke, K.; Bouret, S.G.; Kayser, B.; Walker, R.W.; Blumberg, B. The obesogenic effect of high fructose exposure during early development. *Nat. Rev. Endocrinol.* **2013**, *9*, 494–500. [CrossRef] [PubMed]

18. Tappy, L.; Egli, L.; Lecoultre, V.; Schneider, P. Effects of fructose-containing caloric sweeteners on resting energy expenditure and energy efficiency: A review of human trials. *Nutr. Metab.* **2013**, *10*, 54. [CrossRef] [PubMed]

19. Goldenberg, R.L.; Culhane, J.F.; Iams, J.D.; Romero, R. Epidemiology and causes of preterm birth. *Lancet* **2008**, *371*, 75–84. [CrossRef]

20. Tchirikov, M.; Zhumadilov, Z.S.; Bapayeva, G.; Bergner, M.; Entezami, M. The effect of intraumbilical fetal nutrition via a subcutaneously implanted port system on amino acid concentration by severe IUGR human fetuses. *J. Perinat. Med.* **2017**, *45*, 227–236. [CrossRef] [PubMed]

21. Denne, S.C. Protein and energy requirements in preterm infants. *Semin. Neonatol. SN* **2001**, *6*, 377–382. [CrossRef] [PubMed]

22. Fairchild, K.; Mohr, M.; Paget-Brown, A.; Tabacaru, C.; Lake, D.; Delos, J.; Moorman, J.R.; Kattwinkel, J. Clinical associations of immature breathing in preterm infants: Part 1—Central apnea. *Pediatr. Res.* **2016**, *80*, 21–27. [CrossRef] [PubMed]

23. Plank, M.S.; Boskovic, D.S.; Sowers, L.C.; Angeles, D.M. Biochemical markers of neonatal hypoxia. *Pediatr. Health* **2008**, *2*, 485–501. [CrossRef]

24. Michiels, C. Physiological and pathological responses to hypoxia. *Am. J. Pathol.* **2004**, *164*, 1875–1882. [CrossRef]

25. Slater, L.; Asmerom, Y.; Boskovic, D.S.; Bahjri, K.; Plank, M.S.; Angeles, K.R.; Phillips, R.; Deming, D.; Ashwal, S.; Hougland, K.; et al. Procedural pain and oxidative stress in premature neonates. *J. Pain Off. J. Am. Pain Soc.* **2012**, *13*, 590–597. [CrossRef] [PubMed]

26. Holsti, L.; Grunau, R.E.; Oberlander, T.F.; Whitfield, M.F.; Weinberg, J. Body movements: An important additional factor in discriminating pain from stress in preterm infants. *Clin. J. Pain* **2005**, *21*, 491–498. [CrossRef] [PubMed]

27. Flatters, S.J. The Contribution of Mitochondria to Sensory Processing and Pain. *Prog. Mol. Biol. Transl. Sci.* **2015**, *131*, 119–146. [PubMed]

28. Steinhorn, D.M.; Green, T.P. Severity of illness correlates with alterations in energy metabolism in the pediatric intensive care unit. *Crit. Care Med.* **1991**, *19*, 1503–1509. [CrossRef] [PubMed]

29. Cerra, F.B.; Siegel, J.H.; Coleman, B.; Border, J.R.; McMenamy, R.R. Septic autocannibalism. A failure of exogenous nutritional support. *Ann. Surg.* **1980**, *192*, 570–580. [CrossRef] [PubMed]

30. Mehta, N.M.; Duggan, C.P. Nutritional Deficiencies during Critical Illness. *Pediatr. Clin. N. Am.* **2009**, *56*, 1143–1160. [CrossRef] [PubMed]

31. Dao, D.T.; Anez-Bustillos, L.; Cho, B.S.; Li, Z.; Puder, M.; Gura, K.M. Assessment of Micronutrient Status in Critically Ill Children: Challenges and Opportunities. *Nutrients* **2017**, *9*. [CrossRef] [PubMed]

32. De Albuquerque Wilasco, M.I.; Uribe-Cruz, C.; Santetti, D.; Fries, G.R.; Dornelles, C.T.L.; da Silveira, T.R. IL-6, TNF-α, IL-10 and nutritional status in pediatric patients with biliary atresia. *J. Pediatr. (Rio J.)* **2017**, *93*, 517–524. [CrossRef] [PubMed]

33. Harris, M.C.; Costarino, A.T.; Sullivan, J.S.; Dulkerian, S.; McCawley, L.; Corcoran, L.; Butler, S.; Kilpatrick, L. Cytokine elevations in critically ill infants with sepsis and necrotizing enterocolitis. *J. Pediatr.* **1994**, *124*, 105–111. [CrossRef]

34. Harris, J.J.; Jolivet, R.; Attwell, D. Synaptic energy use and supply. *Neuron* **2012**, *75*, 762–777. [CrossRef] [PubMed]

35. Brummelte, S.; Grunau, R.E.; Chau, V.; Poskitt, K.J.; Brant, R.; Vinall, J.; Gover, A.; Synnes, A.R.; Miller, S.P. Procedural pain and brain development in premature newborns. *Ann. Neurol.* **2012**, *71*, 385–396. [CrossRef] [PubMed]

36. Miller, S.P.; Ferriero, D.M. From selective vulnerability to connectivity: Insights from newborn brain imaging. *Trends Neurosci.* **2009**, *32*, 496–505. [CrossRef] [PubMed]

37. Kuzawa, C.W. Adipose tissue in human infancy and childhood: An evolutionary perspective. *Am. J. Phys. Anthropol.* **1998**, *27*, 177–209. [CrossRef]

38. Harris, J.J.; Reynell, C.; Attwell, D. The physiology of developmental changes in BOLD functional imaging signals. *Dev. Cogn. Neurosci.* **2011**, *1*, 199–216. [CrossRef] [PubMed]

39. Hay, W.W.; Brown, L.D.; Denne, S.C. Energy requirements, protein-energy metabolism and balance and carbohydrates in preterm infants. *World Rev. Nutr. Diet.* **2014**, *110*, 64–81. [CrossRef] [PubMed]

40. Neu, J. Gastrointestinal development and meeting the nutritional needs of premature infants. *Am. J. Clin. Nutr.* **2007**, *85*, 629S–634S. [CrossRef] [PubMed]

41. Burrin, D.G.; Stoll, B. Key nutrients and growth factors for the neonatal gastrointestinal tract. *Clin. Perinatol.* **2002**, *29*, 65–96. [CrossRef]

42. Jacobi, S.K.; Odle, J. Nutritional Factors Influencing Intestinal Health of the Neonate. *Adv. Nutr. Int. Rev. J.* **2012**, *3*, 687–696. [CrossRef] [PubMed]

43. Stoll, B.; Horst, D.A.; Cui, L.; Chang, X.; Ellis, K.J.; Hadsell, D.L.; Suryawan, A.; Kurundkar, A.; Maheshwari, A.; Davis, T.A.; et al. Chronic Parenteral Nutrition Induces Hepatic Inflammation, Steatosis and Insulin Resistance in Neonatal Pigs. *J. Nutr.* **2010**, *140*, 2193–2200. [CrossRef] [PubMed]

44. Tappenden, K.A. Mechanisms of enteral nutrient-enhanced intestinal adaptation. *Gastroenterology* **2006**, *130*, S93–S99. [CrossRef] [PubMed]

45. Reali, A.; Greco, F.; Marongiu, G.; Deidda, F.; Atzeni, S.; Campus, R.; Dessì, A.; Fanos, V. Individualized fortification of breast milk in 41 Extremely Low Birth Weight (ELBW) preterm infants. *Clin. Chim. Acta* **2015**, *451*, 107–110. [CrossRef] [PubMed]

46. Ibrahim, H.M.; Jeroudi, M.A.; Baier, R.J.; Dhanireddy, R.; Krouskop, R.W. Aggressive early total parental nutrition in low-birth-weight infants. *J. Perinatol. Off. J. Calif. Perinat. Assoc.* **2004**, *24*, 482–486. [CrossRef] [PubMed]

47. Shalak, L.; Perlman, J.M. Hypoxic-ischemic brain injury in the term infant-current concepts. *Early Hum. Dev.* **2004**, *80*, 125–141. [CrossRef] [PubMed]

48. Georgieff, M.K.; Brunette, K.E.; Tran, P.V. Early life nutrition and neural plasticity. *Dev. Psychopathol.* **2015**, *27*, 411–423. [CrossRef] [PubMed]

49. Hensch, T.K. Critical period regulation. *Annu. Rev. Neurosci.* **2004**, *27*, 549–579. [CrossRef] [PubMed]

50. Ramel, S.E.; Georgieff, M.K. Preterm nutrition and the brain. *World Rev. Nutr. Diet.* **2014**, *110*, 190–200. [CrossRef] [PubMed]

51. Stephens, B.E.; Walden, R.V.; Gargus, R.A.; Tucker, R.; McKinley, L.; Mance, M.; Nye, J.; Vohr, B.R. First-week protein and energy intakes are associated with 18-month developmental outcomes in extremely low birth weight infants. *Pediatrics* **2009**, *123*, 1337–1343. [CrossRef] [PubMed]

52. Isaacs, E.B.; Morley, R.; Lucas, A. Early diet and general cognitive outcome at adolescence in children born at or below 30 weeks gestation. *J. Pediatr.* **2009**, *155*, 229–234. [CrossRef] [PubMed]

53. Fenton, T.R.; Anderson, D.; Groh-Wargo, S.; Hoyos, A.; Ehrenkranz, R.A.; Senterre, T. An Attempt to Standardize the Calculation of Growth Velocity of Preterm Infants-Evaluation of Practical Bedside Methods. *J. Pediatr.* **2017**. [CrossRef] [PubMed]

54. Holden, M.S.; Hopper, A.; Slater, L.; Asmerom, Y.; Esiaba, I.; Boskovic, D.S.; Angeles, D.M. Urinary Hypoxanthine as a Measure of Increased ATP Utilization in Late Preterm Infants. *ICAN Infant Child Adolesc. Nutr.* **2014**. [CrossRef] [PubMed]

55. Esiaba, I.; Angeles, D.M.; Holden, M.S.; Tan, J.B.C.; Asmerom, Y.; Gollin, G.; Boskovic, D.S. Urinary Allantoin Is Elevated in Severe Intraventricular Hemorrhage in the Preterm Newborn. *Transl. Stroke Res.* **2016**, *7*, 97–102. [CrossRef] [PubMed]

56. Sammallahti, S.; Kajantie, E.; Matinolli, H.-M.; Pyhälä, R.; Lahti, J.; Heinonen, K.; Lahti, M.; Pesonen, A.-K.; Eriksson, J.G.; Hovi, P.; et al. Nutrition after preterm birth and adult neurocognitive outcomes. *PLoS ONE* **2017**, *12*. [CrossRef] [PubMed]

57. Martin, A.; Connelly, A.; Bland, R.M.; Reilly, J.J. Health impact of catch-up growth in low-birth weight infants: Systematic review, evidence appraisal and meta-analysis. *Matern. Child. Nutr.* **2016**. [CrossRef] [PubMed]

58. Rice, M.S.; Valentine, C.J. Neonatal Body Composition: Measuring Lean Mass as a Tool to Guide Nutrition Management in the Neonate. *Nutr. Clin. Pract. Off. Publ. Am. Soc. Parenter. Enter. Nutr.* **2015**, *30*, 625–632. [CrossRef] [PubMed]

59. Raaijmakers, A.; Allegaert, K. Catch-Up Growth in Former Preterm Neonates: No Time to Waste. *Nutrients* **2016**, *8*. [CrossRef] [PubMed]

60. Jaquet, D.; Deghmoun, S.; Chevenne, D.; Collin, D.; Czernichow, P.; Lévy-Marchal, C. Dynamic change in adiposity from fetal to postnatal life is involved in the metabolic syndrome associated with reduced fetal growth. *Diabetologia* **2005**, *48*, 849–855. [CrossRef] [PubMed]

61. Hay, W.W. Aggressive Nutrition of the Preterm Infant. *Curr. Pediatr. Rep.* **2013**, *1*. [CrossRef] [PubMed]

62. Victora, C.G.; Barros, F.C.; Horta, B.L.; Martorell, R. Short-term benefits of catch-up growth for small-for-gestational-age infants. *Int. J. Epidemiol.* **2001**, *30*, 1325–1330. [CrossRef] [PubMed]

63. Jain, V.; Singhal, A. Catch up growth in low birth weight infants: Striking a healthy balance. *Rev. Endocr. Metab. Disord.* **2012**, *13*, 141–147. [CrossRef] [PubMed]

64. Ramel, S.E.; Gray, H.L.; Ode, K.L.; Younge, N.; Georgieff, M.K.; Demerath, E.W. Body composition changes in preterm infants following hospital discharge: Comparison with term infants. *J. Pediatr. Gastroenterol. Nutr.* **2011**, *53*, 333–338. [CrossRef] [PubMed]

65. Olhager, E.; Törnqvist, C. Body composition in late preterm infants in the first 10 days of life and at full term. *Acta Paediatr.* **2014**, *103*, 737–743. [CrossRef] [PubMed]

66. Johnson, M.J.; Wootton, S.A.; Leaf, A.A.; Jackson, A.A. Preterm birth and body composition at term equivalent age: A systematic review and meta-analysis. *Pediatrics* **2012**, *130*, e640–e649. [CrossRef] [PubMed]

67. Franco, L.P.; Morais, C.C.; Cominetti, C. Normal-weight obesity syndrome: Diagnosis, prevalence and clinical implications. *Nutr. Rev.* **2016**, *74*, 558–570. [CrossRef] [PubMed]

68. Rigo, J.; de Curtis, M.; Pieltain, C. Nutritional assessment in preterm infants with special reference to body composition. *Semin. Neonatol.* **2001**, *6*, 383–391. [CrossRef] [PubMed]

69. Griffin, I.J. Nutritional assessment in preterm infants. *Nestlé Nutr. Workshop Ser. Paediatr. Programme* **2007**, *59*, 177–192. [CrossRef]

70. Lapillonne, A.; Griffin, I.J. Feeding preterm infants today for later metabolic and cardiovascular outcomes. *J. Pediatr.* **2013**, *162*, S7–S16. [CrossRef] [PubMed]

71. Embleton, N.D.; Korada, M.; Wood, C.L.; Pearce, M.S.; Swamy, R.; Cheetham, T.D. Catch-up growth and metabolic outcomes in adolescents born preterm. *Arch. Dis. Child.* **2016**. [CrossRef] [PubMed]

72. Peng, N.-H.; Bachman, J.; Chen, C.-H.; Huang, L.-C.; Lin, H.-C.; Li, T.-C. Energy expenditure in preterm infants during periods of environmental stress in the neonatal intensive care unit. *Jpn. J. Nurs. Sci. JJNS* **2014**, *11*, 241–247. [CrossRef] [PubMed]

73. Stevens, B.; Yamada, J.; Lee, G.Y.; Ohlsson, A. Sucrose for analgesia in newborn infants undergoing painful procedures. *Cochrane Database Syst. Rev.* **2013**, *1*. [CrossRef]

74. Atkinson, L.; Jamieson, B.; Khoury, J.; Ludmer, J.; Gonzalez, A. Stress Physiology in Infancy and Early Childhood: Cortisol Flexibility, Attunement and Coordination. *J. Neuroendocrinol.* **2016**, *28*. [CrossRef] [PubMed]

75. McEwen, B.S. Stress, adaptation and disease. Allostasis and allostatic load. *Ann. N. Y. Acad. Sci.* **1998**, *840*, 33–44. [CrossRef] [PubMed]

76. Fernandez, E.F.; Watterberg, K.L. Relative adrenal insufficiency in the preterm and term infant. *J. Perinatol. Off. J. Calif. Perinat. Assoc.* **2009**, *29*, S44–S49. [CrossRef] [PubMed]

77. Heckmann, M.; Hartmann, M.F.; Kampschulte, B.; Gack, H.; Bödeker, R.-H.; Gortner, L.; Wudy, S.A. Cortisol production rates in preterm infants in relation to growth and illness: A noninvasive prospective study using gas chromatography-mass spectrometry. *J. Clin. Endocrinol. Metab.* **2005**, *90*, 5737–5742. [CrossRef] [PubMed]

78. Ng, P.C. Effect of stress on the hypothalamic-pituitary-adrenal axis in the fetus and newborn. *J. Pediatr.* **2011**, *158*, e41–e43. [CrossRef] [PubMed]

79. Boonen, E.; Berghe, G.V. Novel insights in the HPA-axis during critical illness. *Acta Clin. Belg.* **2014**, *69*, 397–406. [CrossRef]

80. Peeters, B.; Boonen, E.; Langouche, L.; Van den Berghe, G. The HPA axis response to critical illness: New study results with diagnostic and therapeutic implications. *Mol. Cell. Endocrinol.* **2015**, *408*, 235–240. [CrossRef] [PubMed]

81. Stephens, M.A.C.; Wand, G. Stress and the HPA Axis. *Alcohol Res. Curr. Rev.* **2012**, *34*, 468–483.

82. McEwen, B.S.; Gianaros, P.J. Central role of the brain in stress and adaptation: Links to socioeconomic status, health and disease. *Ann. N. Y. Acad. Sci.* **2010**, *1186*, 190–222. [CrossRef] [PubMed]

83. Simmons, P.S.; Miles, J.M.; Gerich, J.E.; Haymond, M.W. Increased proteolysis. An effect of increases in plasma cortisol within the physiologic range. *J. Clin. Investig.* **1984**, *73*, 412–420. [CrossRef] [PubMed]

84. Haley, D.W.; Weinberg, J.; Grunau, R.E. Cortisol, contingency learning and memory in preterm and full-term infants. *Psychoneuroendocrinology* **2006**, *31*, 108–117. [CrossRef] [PubMed]

85. Quesada, A.A.; Tristão, R.M.; Pratesi, R.; Wolf, O.T. Hyper-responsiveness to acute stress, emotional problems and poorer memory in former preterm children. *Stress Amst. Neth.* **2014**, *17*, 389–399. [CrossRef] [PubMed]

86. Wadsby, M.; Nelson, N.; Ingemansson, F.; Samuelsson, S.; Leijon, I. Behaviour problems and cortisol levels in very-low-birth-weight children. *Nord. J. Psychiatry* **2014**, *68*, 626–632. [CrossRef] [PubMed]

87. Juruena, M.F. Early-life stress and HPA axis trigger recurrent adulthood depression. *Epilepsy Behav.* **2014**, *38*, 148–159. [CrossRef] [PubMed]

88. Yang, Y.; Raine, A. Prefrontal Structural and Functional Brain Imaging findings in Antisocial, Violent and Psychopathic Individuals: A Meta-Analysis. *Psychiatry Res.* **2009**, *174*, 81–88. [CrossRef] [PubMed]

89. McKlveen, J.M.; Morano, R.L.; Fitzgerald, M.; Zoubovsky, S.; Cassella, S.N.; Scheimann, J.R.; Ghosal, S.; Mahbod, P.; Packard, B.A.; Myers, B.; et al. Chronic Stress Increases Prefrontal Inhibition: A Mechanism for Stress-Induced Prefrontal Dysfunction. *Biol. Psychiatry* **2016**. [CrossRef] [PubMed]

90. Reser, J.E. Chronic stress, cortical plasticity and neuroecology. *Behav. Processes* **2016**, *129*, 105–115. [CrossRef] [PubMed]

91. Boyer, K.; Johnston, C.; Walker, C.-D.; Filion, F.; Sherrard, A. Does sucrose analgesia promote physiologic stability in preterm neonates? *Biol. Neonate* **2004**, *85*, 26–31. [CrossRef] [PubMed]

92. Stang, H.J.; Snellman, L.W.; Condon, L.M.; Conroy, M.M.; Liebo, R.; Brodersen, L.; Gunnar, M.R. Beyond dorsal penile nerve block: A more humane circumcision. *Pediatrics* **1997**, *100*, E3. [CrossRef] [PubMed]

93. Tryon, M.S.; Stanhope, K.L.; Epel, E.S.; Mason, A.E.; Brown, R.; Medici, V.; Havel, P.J.; Laugero, K.D. Excessive Sugar Consumption May Be a Difficult Habit to Break: A View From the Brain and Body. *J. Clin. Endocrinol. Metab.* **2015**. [CrossRef] [PubMed]

94. Banga, S.; Datta, V.; Rehan, H.S.; Bhakhri, B.K. Effect of Sucrose Analgesia, for Repeated Painful Procedures, on Short-term Neurobehavioral Outcome of Preterm Neonates: A Randomized Controlled Trial. *J. Trop. Pediatr.* **2016**, *62*, 101–106. [CrossRef] [PubMed]

95. Tremblay, S.; Ranger, M.; Chau, C.M.Y.; Ellegood, J.; Lerch, J.P.; Holsti, L.; Goldowitz, D.; Grunau, R.E. Repeated exposure to sucrose for procedural pain in mouse pups leads to long-term widespread brain alterations. *Pain* **2017**, *158*, 1586–1598. [CrossRef] [PubMed]

96. Ulrich-Lai, Y.M.; Ostrander, M.M.; Thomas, I.M.; Packard, B.A.; Furay, A.R.; Dolgas, C.M.; Van Hooren, D.C.; Figueiredo, H.F.; Mueller, N.K.; Choi, D.C.; et al. Daily limited access to sweetened drink attenuates hypothalamic-pituitary-adrenocortical axis stress responses. *Endocrinology* **2007**, *148*, 1823–1834. [CrossRef] [PubMed]

97. Ulrich-Lai, Y.M.; Christiansen, A.M.; Ostrander, M.M.; Jones, A.A.; Jones, K.R.; Choi, D.C.; Krause, E.G.; Evanson, N.K.; Furay, A.R.; Davis, J.F.; et al. Pleasurable behaviors reduce stress via brain reward pathways. *Proc. Natl. Acad. Sci. USA* **2010**, *107*, 20529–20534. [CrossRef] [PubMed]

98. Slater, R.; Cornelissen, L.; Fabrizi, L.; Patten, D.; Yoxen, J.; Worley, A.; Boyd, S.; Meek, J.; Fitzgerald, M. Oral sucrose as an analgesic drug for procedural pain in newborn infants: A randomised controlled trial. *Lancet* **2010**, *376*, 1225–1232. [CrossRef]

99. Ulrich-Lai, Y.M.; Ostrander, M.M.; Herman, J.P. HPA axis dampening by limited sucrose intake: Reward frequency vs. caloric consumption. *Physiol. Behav.* **2011**, *103*, 104–110. [CrossRef] [PubMed]

100. Blass, E.M.; Ciaramitaro, V. A new look at some old mechanisms in human newborns: Taste and tactile determinants of state, affect and action. *Monogr. Soc. Res. Child Dev.* **1994**, *59*, 1–81. [CrossRef]

101. Fitzgerald, M. What do we really know about newborn infant pain? *Exp. Physiol.* **2015**, *100*, 1451–1457. [CrossRef] [PubMed]

102. Foo, H.; Mason, P. Ingestion analgesia occurs when a bad taste turns good. *Behav. Neurosci.* **2011**, *125*, 956–961. [CrossRef] [PubMed]

103. Takamata, A.; Mack, G.W.; Gillen, C.M.; Nadel, E.R. Sodium appetite, thirst and body fluid regulation in humans during rehydration without sodium replacement. *Am. J. Physiol.* **1994**, *266*, R1493–R1502. [CrossRef] [PubMed]

104. Tappy, L.; Lê, K.-A. Metabolic effects of fructose and the worldwide increase in obesity. *Physiol. Rev.* **2010**, *90*, 23–46. [CrossRef] [PubMed]

11

Polyphenolic Compounds Analysis of Old and New Apple Cultivars and Contribution of Polyphenolic Profile to the In Vitro Antioxidant Capacity

Josephine Kschonsek, Theresa Wolfram, Annette Stöckl and Volker Böhm *

Institute of Nutrition, Friedrich Schiller University Jena, Dornburger Straße 25-29, 07743 Jena, Germany; Josephine.Kschonsek@uni-jena.de (J.K.); resi.leipzig@googlemail.com (T.W.); st_annette@gmx.de (A.S.)
* Correspondence: Volker.Boehm@uni-jena.de

Abstract: Polyphenols are antioxidant ingredients in apples and are related to human health because of their free radical scavenging activities. The polyphenolic profiles of old and new apple cultivars (n = 15) were analysed using high-performance liquid chromatography (HPLC) with diode array detection (DAD). The in vitro antioxidant capacity was determined by total phenolic content (TPC) assay, hydrophilic trolox equivalent antioxidant capacity (H-TEAC) assay and hydrophilic oxygen radical absorbance (H-ORAC) assay. Twenty polyphenolic compounds were identified in all investigated apples by HPLC analysis. Quercetin glycosides (203 $\pm$ 108 mg/100 g) were the main polyphenols in the peel and phenolic acids (10 $\pm$ 5 mg/100 g) in the flesh. The calculated relative contribution of single compounds indicated flavonols (peel) and vitamin C (flesh) as the major contributors to the antioxidant capacity, in all cultivars investigated. The polyphenolic content (HPLC data) of the flesh differed significantly between old (29 $\pm$ 7 mg/100 g) and new (13 $\pm$ 4 mg/100 g) cultivars, and the antioxidant capacity of old apple cultivars was up to 30% stronger compared to new ones.

Keywords: apple polyphenols; HPLC-DAD; Folin-Ciocalteu; TEAC; ORAC; vitamin C; relative antioxidant activity

1. Introduction

Apples (*Malus domestica*) have a growing scientific interest because many investigations have demonstrated their beneficial effects on human health. Through a variety of antioxidant ingredients, apples have been associated with reduced risks of degenerative and cardiovascular diseases, which are considered to be caused by oxidative stress, especially by free radicals and reactive oxygen species (ROS) [1]. Antioxidants have become even more a focus of research due to increased exposure to ROS.

Polyphenols are the most abundant antioxidants in the human diet and the major part of antioxidants in apples, rather than essential nutrients such as vitamin C [2,3]. Apples are one of the most important fruit sources of dietary polyphenolic compounds in the Western diet, due to the fact that they are consumed widely and are available throughout the year [4]. In Germany, they are the most popular type of fruit with an annual consumption of 25.9 kg per person [5]. Polyphenols represent a group of secondary metabolites with aromatic ring(s) bearing one or more hydroxyl moieties [6]. The large number of conjugated double bonds and hydroxyl groups is responsible for their antioxidant activity (AOA) [3,7]. There are five major groups of polyphenolic compounds found in apples: flavanols (catechin, epicatechin and procyanidins), phenolic acids (mainly chlorogenic acid), dihydrochalcones (phloretin glycosides), flavonols (quercetin glycosides) and anthocyanins (cyanidin) [8,9]. Various reports indicate that the polyphenolic profile and content as well as the antioxidant capacity (AOC) in apples are affected by different variables, such as cultivar, tissue zones, harvest time, geographic location and storage conditions [10–12].

In recent decades, new apple cultivars, such as Braeburn, Elstar, Golden Delicious, Granny Smith and Jonagold have become more popular among consumers in Germany and Western Europe, resulting in a gradual decrease of the cultivation of old cultivars. New cultivars are said to have a lower content of polyphenols. The contents of polyphenolic compounds of new cultivars were reduced by breeding due to the astringent taste and rapid enzymatic browning. Therefore, we hypothesize that the content of polyphenols and consequently the AOC of old apple cultivars are higher compared to new cultivars. The comparison of the polyphenol content as well as the occurrence and distribution of the main polyphenolic classes is barely reported for old and new apple cultivars. There is just one investigation that distinguished between old and new apple cultivars, but without separately analysing peel and flesh [13]. Apples provide a mixture of bioactive compounds, but the total phenolic or total flavonoid content often does not directly reflect the AOC [7]. There are some studies that have investigated the polyphenolic content of apple cultivars, using spectrophotometric assays or HPLC analysis. However, there is limited information about the relative contribution of each polyphenolic compound to the AOC because the number of standards used is restricted, especially with regard to the procyanidins and quercetin glycosides. In the present study, the contents of polyphenolic compounds in peel and flesh of different old and new apple cultivars were determined by using HPLC-DAD. Additionally, the in vitro AOC was measured using total phenolic content (TPC) assay, hydrophilic trolox equivalent antioxidant capacity (H-TEAC) assay and hydrophilic oxygen radical absorbance capacity (H-ORAC) assay. AOA data of 20 polyphenols and of vitamin C were determined and used to calculate the contribution of these antioxidants to the AOC.

2. Materials and Methods

2.1. Chemicals

Methanol and ethanol were from VWR (Darmstadt, Germany) and were like all other solvents used of HPLC grade. Trolox, 2,2′-azinobis-(3-ethylbenzothiazoline-6-sulphonic acid) diammonium salt (ABTS), Folin-Ciocalteu reagent, quercetin, (−)-epicatechin, procyanidin B1, procyanidin B2, procyanidin C1, p-coumaric acid, trans-cinnamic acid and phloridzin dihydrate were from Sigma–Aldrich (Taufkirchen, Germany). Gallic acid, (+)-catechin, chlorogenic acid, ferulic acid, coffeic acid, rutin trihydrate and acetic acid were purchased from Carl Roth (Karlsruhe, Germany). Avicularin was used from Phytolab (Vestenbergsgreuth, Germany). Protocatechuic acid, hyperoside, isoquercitrin, quercitrin and procyanidin A2 were from Extrasynthese (Genay, France). Reynoutrin was purchased from Carbosynth Limited (Berkshire, UK). 2,2′-Azobis(2-amidinopropane) dihydrochloride (AAPH) was from Fisher Scientific (Nidderau, Germany). HPLC grade water (18 MΩ) was prepared using a MicroPure purification system (Thermo Electron LED GmbH, Niederelbert, Germany). Sodium hydroxide, hydrochloric acid (Merck, Darmstadt, Germany), meta-phosphoric acid (Sigma–Aldrich) and all other chemicals were of analytical grade.

2.2. Sample Details and Preparation

Fifteen different apple cultivars were chosen for the investigation of polyphenolic compounds, vitamin C and AOC, including ten old apple cultivars (Berlepsch, Cox Orange, Dülmener Rosenapfel, Goldparmäne, Gravensteiner, James Grieve, Jonathan, Oldenburger, Ontario and Roter Boskoop) and five new apple cultivars (Braeburn, Elstar, Golden Delicious, Granny Smith and Jonagold). The new cultivars were picked at maturity, during harvest season in 2015, from a local market in Jena, Germany, and the old cultivars were from a private garden (Bad Blankenburg, Germany: 50° N–11° E). A pomologist authenticated the apple cultivars. One tree from each old cultivar was used for the gathering of fruits for the study. In total, three to five kg were harvested, depending on the size of the tree. The apples were picked from all sides of the tree. Fruit samples were peeled (2–3 mm thickness) and cored. The peel and flesh samples were homogenised separately, using a knife mill Grindomix GM 200 (Retsch, Haan, Germany), and stored at $-25\,°C$ until use. For all analyses (polyphenolic compounds, vitamin C and AOC), the peel and flesh samples were lyophilised.

2.3. Food Extraction

2.3.1. Polyphenolic Compounds Analysis

Each apple cultivar was weighed into a 50 mL Falcon tube. For the determination of content of polyphenols, freeze-dried samples of apple peel (0.5 ± 0.05 g) and apple flesh (2.0 ± 0.05 g) were used. Samples were hydrolysed, using a method slightly modified from [14], involving the stepwise addition of hydrochloric acid (1 M), followed by addition of sodium hydroxide solution in 75% methanol (2.0 M) and meta-phosphoric acid (0.75 M). A volume of 2 mL (apple peel) or 4 mL (apple flesh), respectively, was used of each solvent. All steps were accompanied by shaking (30 s) and heating in a water bath (30 min, $37\,°C$). After hydrolysis, the samples were centrifuged (5 min, $3000\times g$) (5702 R, Eppendorf, Hamburg, Germany). The supernatants were collected in 250 mL round-bottomed flasks. The remaining residues were extracted with 20 mL methanol/water (70/30, v/v), using an ultrasonic bath (20 min, $\leq 40\,°C$). After centrifugation (5 min, $3000\times g$), the supernatants were collected. The extraction was repeated twice, while the time of ultrasonic treatment was changed to 10 min (in both extractions) and the volume of methanol/water to 10 mL (only in the last extraction). The extraction procedure was performed according to a modified method from [15]. The supernatants of hydrolysis and the combined extracts were mixed and rotary-evaporated, under reduced pressure, at $35\,°C$, to a small volume. The dried residues were dissolved in methanol/water (70/30, v/v, 5 mL). After centrifugation (5 min, $19,000\times g$), the samples were used for HPLC analysis.

2.3.2. Antioxidant Capacity (AOC) Assays

Each apple cultivar was weighed into a 15 mL Falcon tube. For the AOC assays freeze-dried samples of apple peel (0.1 ± 0.01 g) and apple flesh (0.4 ± 0.05 g) were used. Samples were hydrolysed, as described in the previous Section 2.3.1, except that the volume of each solvent was decreased five-fold. After hydrolysis, the samples were centrifuged (5 min, $3000\times g$) (5702 R, Eppendorf, Hamburg, Germany) and the supernatants were collected in 10 mL volumetric flasks. The residues were extracted with 2 mL methanol/water (70/30, v/v) by shaking for 30 min. After centrifugation (5 min, $3000\times g$), the supernatants were collected and the extraction was repeated twice. The supernatants from hydrolysis and the combined extracts were mixed and used for AOC assays.

2.4. HPLC Analysis of Polyphenols

The polyphenolic composition was analysed using a diode array detector (L-7450A, Merck Hitachi, Darmstadt, Germany) according to the method from [16]. The column was a reversed-phase Luna C18 column (250 mm $\times$ 4.6 mm, particle size 5 μm, Phenomenex, Aschaffenburg, Germany) and was heated to $30\,°C$. An injection volume of 50 μL was used. The binary mobile phase consisted of 0.5% (v/v) acetic acid in water (solvent A) and methanol (solvent B), pumped at a flow rate of 0.8 mL/min, for a total run time of 160 min. Elution was performed using a gradient program: 0–2 min, 0% B isocratic; 2–6 min, linear gradient from 0% to 15% B; 6–12 min, 15% B isocratic; 12–17 min, linear gradient from 15% to 20% B; 17–35 min, 20% B isocratic; 35–90 min, linear gradient from 20% to 35% B; 90–132 min, 35% B isocratic, 132–150 min, linear gradient from 35% to 80% B, 150–160 min linear gradient from 80% to 0% B. The detector was set at 254, 280 and 320 nm for simultaneous monitoring of the different groups of polyphenols. The identification was performed by comparing retention times and DAD absorbance spectra with external standards (Table 1). Polyphenolic compound contents were quantified with a 7-point calibration curve of external standards. Linearity was given over the entire 7-point calibration curve. The limits of detection (LOD) and limits of quantification (LOQ) of the polyphenols were determined using the baseline noise signals in chromatograms of five solvent injections (Table S1).

Table 1. Characterization (retention time [t_R], absorption maximum [λ_{max}]) of 20 polyphenols of apples used as reference compounds in HPLC-DAD.

Group of Polyphenols	Phenolic Compound	Synonyms	t_R [min]	λ_{max} [nm]	λ [nm]
Flavanols	Procyanidin B1		21.09	281	280
	(+)-Catechin		25.71	281	280
	Procyanidin B2		29.04	281	280
	Procyanidin C1		39.87	275	280
	(−)-Epicatechin		43.11	280	280
	Procyanidin A2		68.85	280	280
Phenolic acids	Gallic acid		12.64	272	280
	Protocatechuic acid		18.80	261, 298	254
	5-O-Caffeoylquinic acid	Chlorogenic acid	31.12	326	320
	Caffeic acid		36.05	324	320
	p-Coumaric acid		57.10	310	320
	Ferulic acid		66.15	324	320
Dihydrochalcones	Phloretin-2-O-β-glucoside	Phloridzin *	106.84	287	280
Flavonols	Quercetin-3-O-galactoside	Hyperoside	94.19	259, 348	254
	Quercetin-3-O-glucoside	Isoquercitrin	96.96	259, 351	254
	Quercetin-3-O-rutinoside	Rutin *	97.68	259, 348	254
	Quercetin-3-O-xyloside	Reynoutrin	101.23	260, 348	254
	Quercetin-3-O-arabinoside	Avicularin	112.03	260, 347	254
	Quercetin-3-O-rhamnoside	Quercitrin	116.37	260, 347	254
	Quercetin		145.33	256, 372	254

* Phloridzin as Phloridzin dehydrate; Rutin as Rutin trihydrate; λ: wavelength used in HPLC-DAD.

2.5. Antioxidant Capacity (AOC)

The AOC assays were performed by using clear 96-well microplates (Kisker Biotech, Steinfurt, Germany) and a microplate reader FluoStar Optima (BMG Labtech, Offenburg, Germany), in accordance with [17].

2.5.1. Total Phenolic Content (TPC) Assay

The TPC was evaluated by using the Folin–Ciocalteu method [18]. Thirty microliters of methanol/water (70/30, v/v) extract were mixed with 150 µL 1:10 diluted Folin–Ciocalteu reagent and 120 µL sodium carbonate solution (75 g/L) in wells of a 96-well microplate. After 2 h in darkness, at room temperature, the absorbance was measured at 740 nm in the microplate reader, at 30 °C. Gallic acid monohydrate (8.51–170.12 mg/L) was used as the standard for calibration and construction of a linear regression line and water acted as the blank. The TPC is expressed as gallic acid equivalents (GAE) in mg/100 g.

2.5.2. Hydrophilic Trolox Equivalent Antioxidant Capacity (H-TEAC) Assay

The H-TEAC assay was performed using ABTS radical cation (ABTS$^{\bullet+}$) [19]. This stable radical cation was formed by mixing 10 mL ABTS solution (7 mM) with 10 mL potassium peroxodisulfate solution (2.45 mM). After 24 h at room temperature (darkness), the ABTS$^{\bullet+}$ stock solution was ready to use. The ABTS$^{\bullet+}$ working solution was prepared freshly each day by diluting the ABTS$^{\bullet+}$ stock solution with phosphate buffer (75 mM, pH 7.4) to an absorbance of 0.70 ± 0.05 at 730 nm. Twenty microliters of methanol/water (70/30, v/v) extract were mixed with 200 mL ABTS$^{\bullet+}$ working solution in a 96-well microplate. The decrease in absorbance at 730 nm, at 30 °C, was measured photometrically. Trolox solutions (12.5–250 µM) were used for constructing a regression line and water acted as blank. The AOC is expressed as trolox equivalents (TE) in mmol/100 g.

2.5.3. Hydrophilic Oxygen Radical Absorbance Capacity (H-ORAC) Assay

The H-ORAC assay was evaluated using fluorescein and AAPH [20]. The fluorescein working solution (1.2 µM) was prepared freshly each day by diluting the fluorescein stock solution (0.12 mM, stored in fridge) 1:100 with phosphate buffer (75 mM, pH 7.4). Ten microliters of methanol/water

(70/30, v/v) extract were mixed with 25 µL fluorescein working solution and 100 µL phosphate buffer, in microplate wells. Afterwards, the 96-well plate was pre-heated for 10 min at 37 °C. Following the addition of 150 µL of freshly prepared and ice-cooled AAPH solution (129 mM) in phosphate buffer, the reaction started, and the fluorescence intensity was measured each minute, for 4 h, at 37 °C. Fluorescence filters of 490 nm (excitation) and 520 nm (emission) were used in the microplate reader. Water acted as a blank and trolox standard solutions (0.1–2.0 mM) were used for calibration. Additionally, a negative control (water) was used for controlling the photostability of fluorescein. Therefore, 150 µL of phosphate buffer was utilised instead of AAPH solution. The calculation of the H-ORAC assay can be seen in the publication by [17]. The AOC is expressed as trolox equivalents (TE) in mmol/100 g.

2.6. Vitamin C Analysis

The vitamin C analysis was performed in accordance with [21]. Each apple cultivar was weighed into a screwed glass tube. Freeze-dried samples of apple peel (0.1 ± 0.01 g) and apple flesh (0.4 ± 0.05 g) were used. Samples were extracted three times with 5 mL meta-phosphoric acid (0.46 M) by shaking for 1 min. After each extraction, the samples were centrifuged (5 min, $3000 \times g$). The supernatants were collected in 20 mL volumetric flasks. Two hundred microliters of each sample, 200 µL of calibration solution (5.7–567.8 µM, respectively) and 200 µL of distilled water (blank) were mixed with 300 µL trichloroacetic acid (0.31 M) and centrifuged (5 min, $17,000 \times g$). Three hundred microliters of the supernatants were mixed with 100 µL DNP reagent (one volume of thiourea solution (0.83 M in distilled water), one volume of copper sulphate solution (24 mM in distilled water) and 20 volumes of 2,4-dinitrophenylhydrazine solution (0.11 M in 4.5 M sulfuric acid). The mixture was heated in a thermomixer (1 h, 60 °C). The samples were cooled in an ice bath for 5 min. Afterwards, 400 µL sulfuric acid (8.56 M) was added and mixed. The samples were placed into darkness for 20 min. Finally, the samples were decanted into semi-micro cuvettes and measured using a photometer at 520 nm.

2.7. Statistical Analysis

All analyses were done in triplicate. The data are expressed as mean ± standard deviation (SD) and were analysed using SPSS procedures (version 22.0, Statistical Package for the Social Sciences, Chicago, IL, USA). p-Values < 0.05 were considered significant. The homogeneity of variances for all data was assumed by Levene's test. The one factorial analysis of variance (ANOVA) was used followed by the Student-Newmann-Keuls (S-N-K) procedure for assessing differences between all 15 apple cultivars. The unpaired t-test was used to statistically compare the average out of all ten old cultivars and the average out of all five new cultivars. Correlations were tested by using the Pearson procedure, in which the p-value was considered to be significant at $p < 0.01$.

3. Results and Discussion

3.1. Quantification of Polyphenolic Compounds and Vitamin C

In the apples investigated, 20 polyphenolic compounds of four sub-classes (flavanols, phenolic acids, dihydrochalcones and flavonols) were identified by using retention times and absorption maxima of reference compounds (Table 1). The types of polyphenolic compounds detected in the apple cultivars were similar to previous studies, including the closely related quercetin glycosides that are often difficult to separate [13,15].

As shown in Tables 2 and 3, the content of polyphenolic compounds varied greatly between apple peel and flesh. The total polyphenols determined by HPLC ranged from 99.6 ± 5.4 to 495.3 ± 44.0 mg/100 g in the peel, whereas the flesh had a 3.0 to 28.4 times lower content (9.6 ± 0.6 to 41.6 ± 2.3 mg/100 g). These results are comparable with other investigations [9,11,22,23].

Table 2. Average content of vitamin C, polyphenolic compounds and antioxidant capacity values in the peel of different apple cultivars.

Apple Cultivars	1	2	3	4	5	6	7	8	9	10	11	12	13	14	15
vitamin C	207.5	215.7	196.9	155.5	186.4	124.3	225.8	99.2	117.4	184.0	189.1	210.2	256.0	300.9	204.4
procyanidin B1	n.d.	n.d.	1.3	4.8	n.d.	n.d.	0.9	n.d.	1.8	1.0	n.d.	0.9	n.d.	1.3	n.d.
(+)-catechin	2.3	4.9	2.7	6.8	9.0	1.5	3.5	3.4	3.2	3.0	8.3	7.4	11.7	7.4	3.6
procyanidin B2	7.5	7.2	7.8	5.2	9.0	8.2	9.6	5.1	4.4	6.8	7.6	8.3	8.2	6.2	6.7
procyanidin C1	6.6	7.0	5.2	6.6	9.5	n.d	6.6	6.9	n.d.	5.3	7.7	7.6	8.3	8.4	5.9
(−)-epicatechin	13.2	11.4	3.0	8.9	18.5	1.1	7.9	3.1	2.2	4.2	16.4	13.2	17.8	11.3	6.4
procyanidin A2	4.1	10.5	7.7	7.3	10.4	5.1	10.2	2.6	12.4	12.1	9.8	5.1	8.7	5.7	5.0
total flavanols	33.7	41.0	27.7	39.5	56.4	15.8	38.7	21.0	23.9	32.3	49.8	42.4	54.7	40.4	27.5
SD	±4.2	±2.7	±2.7	±1.5	±4.1	±3.3	±3.6	±1.8	±4.4	±3.8	±3.7	±4.1	±3.6	±3.3	±1.3
gallic acid	4.3	3.9	3.8	4.9	3.8	4.0	7.2	3.5	4.8	4.7	4.2	4.8	4.3	3.9	3.7
protocatechuic acid	1.0	1.3	1.5	2.3	1.9	0.6	1.9	0.8	1.1	1.3	2.0	3.8	1.9	2.4	2.5
chlorogenic acid	18.1	4.9	4.8	7.0	5.3	5.9	5.1	5.2	3.9	4.0	6.7	6.1	7.1	5.5	5.2
caffeic acid	6.6	1.1	0.4	11.1	1.2	0.6	6.2	0.1	3.2	0.8	1.2	1.4	10.4	3.5	2.2
p-coumaric acid	2.6	1.8	1.7	5.9	2.3	1.4	3.5	1.4	2.4	1.9	2.0	2.3	4.1	1.9	2.2
ferulic acid	1.1	0.4	1.0	2.3	0.7	1.3	2.3	0.7	0.7	0.7	1.4	1.4	1.4	1.0	1.4
total phenolic acids	33.6	13.5	13.2	33.6	15.2	13.7	26.2	11.7	16.1	13.4	17.5	19.7	29.3	18.1	17.1
SD	±6.5	±1.8	±1.7	±3.3	±1.7	±2.2	±2.1	±2.0	±1.6	±1.7	±2.1	±1.9	±3.4	±1.6	±1.4
phloridzin	37.1	4.6	1.5	6.1	8.3	1.5	63.8	0.8	15.3	6.1	8.8	14.5	6.8	6.9	8.0
hyperoside	94.7	103.5	91.1	44.7	102.8	18.31	83.4	28.6	8.0	80.3	168.1	190.9	60.2	189.4	79.3
isoquercitrin	30.9	19.1	8.1	12.6	18.5	4.87	44.8	11.0	5.6	9.7	29.6	18.9	13.8	24.5	9.8
Rutin	24.3	6.6	1.4	14.5	7.2	1.16	1.9	2.4	1.9	0.9	9.8	1.9	1.9	15.5	6.8
reynoutrin	18.6	19.6	15.6	10.6	19.3	6.99	15.7	11.2	4.1	10.2	27.9	39.8	20.1	40.0	15.4
avicularin	35.0	19.6	30.3	18.1	28.4	12.79	23.7	13.3	9.7	22.7	33.1	62.4	29.5	51.4	23.8
quercitrin	36.2	19.7	18.4	25.5	17.9	15.94	15.4	23.4	15.4	24.0	50.2	40.6	17.1	84.1	20.9
quercetin	17.7	13.5	16.9	7.6	13.8	8.54	12.5	8.8	7.3	14.0	22.4	32.5	12.0	25.1	9.5
total flavonols	257.3	201.6	181.8	133.4	207.9	68.6	197.4	98.6	52.0	161.8	340.9	386.9	154.4	430.0	165.5
SD	±26.6	±33.3	±30.1	±12.7	±32.8	±6.2	±27.7	±8.9	±4.3	±26.4	±54.0	±62.7	±18.8	±60.9	±25.3
total polyphenols	361.7	260.8	224.2	212.5	287.8	99.6	326.1	132.1	107.3	213.5	416.9	463.5	245.2	495.3	218.1
SD	±22.2	±22.7	±20.4	±9.7	±22.5	±5.4	±22.2	±7.8	±4.6	±17.7	±37.8	±42.9	±13.5	±44.0	±17.5
TPC	889.6	926.0	687.6	889.5	1320.4	521.9	1238.2	581.0	638.8	772.5	1224.2	1212.8	1590.5	1078.7	960.6
TEAC	5.3	6.0	4.4	5.9	8.5	2.4	7.7	3.4	3.4	5.0	9.1	9.9	12.8	8.3	6.1
ORAC	21.1	20.6	16.3	19.2	29.0	8.6	22.0	13.6	15.3	18.3	24.6	24.4	31.4	26.2	19.3

1. Berlepsch; 2: Braeburn; 3: Cox Orange; 4: Dülmener Rosenapfel; 5: Elstar; 6: Golden Delicious; 7: Goldparmäne; 8: Granny Smith; 9: Gravensteiner; 10: James Grieve; 11: Jonagold; 12: Jonathan; 13: Oldenburger; 14: Ontario; 15: Roter Boskoop; SD: standard derivation; n.d.: not detected; TPC: total phenolic content; TEAC: trolox equivalent antioxidant capacity; ORAC: oxygen radical antioxidant capacity; single compounds and total concentrations in mg/100 g freeze dried material; TPC in mg GAE/100 g freeze dried material; TEAC and ORAC in mmol TE/100 g freeze dried material; GAE: gallic acid equivalents; TE: trolox equivalents.

Table 3. Average content of vitamin C, polyphenolic compounds and antioxidant capacity values in the flesh of different apple cultivars.

Apple Cultivars	1	2	3	4	5	6	7	8	9	10	11	12	13	14	15
vitamin C	108.0	112.3	99.5	83.2	67.7	50.4	94.7	54.7	77.0	85.5	57.4	118.2	124.8	134.4	106.8
procyanidin B1	0.5	0.5	n.d.	6.8	n.d.	0.2	0.3	n.d.	0.8	0.7	n.d.	4.0	0.4	n.d.	n.d.
(+)-catechin	0.8	0.5	1.4	1.6	2.5	0.3	0.8	1.8	0.3	1.1	0.5	4.9	1.0	1.5	1.3
procyanidin B2	0.9	1.3	1.9	2.5	1.8	1.4	1.7	1.4	1.4	1.6	2.0	2.7	1.9	2.3	2.0
procyanidin C1	1.3	n.d.	n.d.	n.d.	n.d.	n.d.	n.d.	n.d.	n.d.	1.3	n.d.	1.7	n.d.	n.d.	n.d.
(−)-epicatechin	0.3	0.5	1.2	2.2	2.0	0.3	1.4	1.5	0.8	1.4	0.7	4.7	1.5	2.2	1.5
procyanidin A2	2.0	1.4	6.6	3.5	4.5	2.1	2.4	1.6	5.3	11.0	3.1	5.9	5.0	2.6	4.0
total flavanols	5.9	4.2	11.1	16.6	10.8	4.4	6.6	6.3	8.6	17.1	6.3	23.8	9.6	8.6	8.8
SD	±0.6	±0.5	±2.6	±2.1	±1.2	±0.9	±0.8	±0.2	±2.0	±4.0	±1.2	±1.5	±1.8	±0.5	±1.2
gallic acid	1.7	1.6	1.7	1.6	1.6	1.9	2.0	1.4	1.7	2.2	1.7	1.9	1.7	1.6	1.7
protocatechuic acid	0.2	0.1	0.	0.1	0.1	0.1	0.1	0.1	0.1	0.1	0.1	0.1	0.2	0.1	0.3
chlorogenic acid	8.4	2.0	3.2	10.8	3.6	1.4	5.8	1.7	3.3	3.3	2.1	4.4	8.3	7.6	8.6
caffeic acid	5.6	0.6	1.5	6.8	1.7	0.5	1.0	0.5	0.6	0.7	0.4	2.2	5.0	3.8	6.0
p-coumaric acid	0.7	0.4	0.6	0.8	0.6	0.4	0.7	0.4	0.7	0.6	0.5	0.7	0.9	0.7	0.8
ferulic acid	0.2	0.1	0.1	0.2	0.1	0.1	0.3	0.1	0.1	0.2	0.2	0.1	0.4	0.1	0.2
total phenolic acids	16.7	4.8	7.1	20.3	7.6	4.4	9.9	4.2	6.5	7.1	5.0	9.4	16.4	13.9	17.5
SD	±3.4	±0.8	±1.2	±4.4	±1.3	±0.7	±2.1	±0.7	±1.2	±1.3	±0.8	±1.6	±3.3	±2.9	±3.5
phloridzin	7.3	0.7	2.3	4.7	3.6	0.9	5.2	0.7	2.3	2.3	0.7	3.6	2.9	7.4	12.3
total polyphenols	29.8	9.6	20.5	41.6	20.8	9.6	21.7	11.2	17.4	26.5	12.0	36.8	28.9	29.9	38.6
SD	±2.8	±0.6	±1.8	±3.4	±1.4	±0.7	±2.9	±0.7	±1.5	±2.9	±1.0	±1.9	±2.5	±2.6	±3.9
TPC	220.7	143.6	219.8	300.3	276.4	136.5	252.0	163.3	174.9	246.3	177.5	361.7	242.9	217.6	334.1
TEAC	1.1	0.8	1.3	1.8	1.5	0.8	1.2	0.9	0.9	1.5	1.0	2.3	1.5	1.2	2.0
ORAC	5.7	4.9	5.2	6.1	6.7	2.4	4.5	4.0	4.5	5.9	5.0	8.1	5.4	4.7	6.9

1. Berlepsch; 2: Braeburn; 3: Cox Orange; 4: Dülmener Rosenapfel; 5: Elstar; 6: Golden Delicious; 7: Goldparmäne; 8: Gravensteiner; 9: Granny Smith; 10: James Grieve; 11: Jonagold; 12: Jonathan; 13: Oldenburger; 14: Ontario; 15: Roter Boskoop; SD: standard derivation; n.d.: not detected; TPC: total phenolic content; TEAC: trolox equivalent antioxidant capacity; ORAC: oxygen radical antioxidant capacity; single compounds and total concentrations in mg/100 g freeze dried material; TPC in mg GAE/100 g freeze dried material; TEAC and ORAC in mmol TE/100 g freeze dried material; GAE: gallic acid equivalents; TE: trolox equivalents.

The apple cultivars Ontario and Jonathan had the highest total polyphenol content in the peel and the cultivars Roter Boskoop and Dülmener Rosenapfel in the flesh. The cultivar Golden Delicious contained the significantly lowest content of total polyphenols in both peel and flesh, being in line with studies previously reported [12,24]. Furthermore, the occurrence and distribution of the main polyphenol classes differed between peel and flesh. Flavonols were the predominant group (72.2%) in the peel, followed by flavanols (14.7%), phenolic acids (8.3%) and the dihydrochalcone phloridzin (4.7%). The flavonols, which included quercetin and its glycosides, ranged from 52.0 ± 4.3 (Gravensteiner) to 430.0 ± 60.9 mg/100 g (Ontario). A high content of quercetin was found in the peel, due to hydrolysis with 1 M HCl, which efficiently released quercetin from sugar components [25,26]. The concentrations of the quercetin glycosides generally followed the order: hyperoside > quercitrin > avicularin > reynoutrin > isoquercitrin > rutin, with interchanging of avicularin and quercitrin depending on the apple cultivar, and is almost coincident with results of other studies [27–29]. The quercetin glycoside hyperoside was the major polyphenolic compound (30.3% of total polyphenols content) in the peel of all apple cultivars investigated and can be regarded as a marker for apple peel. Looking at the polyphenol profile in the flesh, the phenolic acids (43.0%) and the flavanols (41.1%) were the predominant groups, followed by the dihydrochalcon phloridzin (14.0%). The flavonols were missing in the flesh. The apple peel and flesh differed distinctly in the phenolic glycoside composition (Tables 2 and 3). The flesh contained the phloretin glycoside phloridzin, whereas peel possessed both phloridzin and quercetin glycosides [25]. Within the phenolic acids, chlorogenic acid was the major compound in the peel (6.3 ± 3.3 10 mg/100 g) and in the flesh (5.0 ± 3.0 mg/100 g).

As described by Guyot et al., (1998), the phenolic acid content decreased from the peel to the flesh [10]. A total of six flavanols could be quantified in both peel (36.3 ± 11.7 mg/100 g) and flesh (9.6 ± 5.0 mg/100 g), but their concentrations in the flesh were much lower than in the peel. In addition to (+)-catechin and (−)-epicatechin, the procyanidin isomers B1, B2, C1 and A2 were identified, even if they were not detectable in all apple cultivars. In previous studies, the flavanols, especially the procyanidins, were the major class of apple polyphenols in both flesh and peel, representing more than 80% of the total polyphenol content (HPLC data) [8,11,13,23,28]. However, the content and percentage of flavanols obtained in this study were lower than the quantities reported in other research. One possible reason for this may be the crushing of the apples without adding an antioxidant, like ascorbic acid. Flavanol monomers and procyanidins are good substrates for polyphenol oxidase and are directly involved in enzymatic oxidation, occurring when apples are crushed [10].

In addition to the determination of polyphenolic compounds, the vitamin C content of the apples was analysed. The vitamin C content in the peel ranged from 99.2 ± 10.0 (Granny Smith) to 300.9 ± 10.8 (Ontario) mg/100 g, and in the flesh from 50.4 ± 2.4 (Golden Delicious) to 143.4 ± 1.8 (Ontario) mg/100 g. The vitamin C results are similar to other investigations [13,30,31], but tended to be higher, which may be due to our method. In the spectrophotometric method with DNP reagent, used in this research, the total content of vitamin C was analysed, i.e., the content of ascorbic acid and dehydroascorbic acid present in the apples. The vitamin C concentration significantly correlated with the polyphenol content, in both flesh and peel ($r = 0.515$; $p < 0.001$ and $r = 0.736$; $p < 0.001$, respectively). Therefore, as with the polyphenols, the content of vitamin C in the peel was higher (1.5- to 3.3-fold greater), compared to the flesh. A possible reason for the higher content of polyphenols and vitamin C in the peel, compared to the flesh, might be the barrier function of the peel against external biotic and abiotic stress, to which apples are often exposed [32]. Thus, a higher concentration of antioxidants appears to be useful in the peel.

3.2. Antioxidant Capacity (AOC)

As shown in Tables 2 and 3, peel extracts had a stronger AOC than the flesh extracts, being comparable to studies previously reported [3,4,27,33,34]. The apple cultivar Oldenburger possessed the significantly highest AOC in the peel, and Jonathan in the flesh. The cultivars Golden Delicious and Braeburn had the significantly lowest AOC measured by all methods, in both peel and flesh. The total polyphenol content (HPLC data) significantly correlated with the values of the AOC results (TPC: 0.891; H-TEAC: 0.886; H-ORAC: 0.908; $p < 0.001$). The significant correlation between the vitamin C content and the AOC results (TPC: 0.867; H-TEAC: 0.861; H-ORAC: 0.883; $p < 0.001$) was lower compared to the polyphenols and suggest that the polyphenols have a more significant contribution to the AOC. The best correlation was found between the total polyphenols (HPLC data) and the H-ORAC results ($r = 0.908$; $p < 0.001$). The reaction mechanism of the ORAC assay is based on free peroxyl radicals, which are commonly found in the human body, making the reaction biologically relevant [34]. The H-ORAC values of the peel extracts showed the best positive linear correlation with the total flavanols ($r = 0.767$; $p < 0.001$) in the decreasing order of $(-)$-epicatechin > procyanidin C1 > $(+)$-catechin > procyanidin A2. Next to the flavanols, the total flavonols significantly correlated with the H-ORAC results ($r = 0.651$; $p < 0.001$), but the flavanols had an even better linear correlation. Similar observations for the flavanols were found in the flesh extracts ($r = 0.784$; $p < 0.001$), with some differences in the order: $(+)$-catechin > $(-)$-epicatechin > procyanidin A2 > procyanidin B2. These results show that the flavanols are major contributors to the AOC (H-ORAC), in both peel and flesh.

3.3. Relative Contribution to AOC

To indicate the relative contribution of single antioxidants to the AOC of each apple sample, the relative antioxidant activities (RAA) of the 20 polyphenolic compounds and vitamin C were calculated. The RAA resulted from the quotient of the molar AOA value of the H-ORAC assay of the corresponding polyphenol standard, and the molar concentration at which the H-ORAC was obtained.

$$RAA = AOA/C \tag{1}$$

The RAA of the polyphenols showed the following order: procyanidin B1 (10.4) and procyanidin C1 (10,4) > procyanidin B2 (9.6) > rutin trihydrate (9.1) > phloridzin dihydrate (8.7) > reynoutrin (8.6) > hyperoside (7.9) > isoquercitrin (7.2) > quercetin (6.8) > avicularin (6.7) > quercitrin (6.6) > procyanidin A2 (6.0) > $(-)$-epicatechin (5.0) > p-coumaric acid (4.9) and $(+)$-catechin (4.9) > chlorogenic acid (4.7) > protocatechuic acid (4.3) > caffeic acid (4.0) > ferulic acid (2.9) > gallic acid (1.7) > vitamin C (0.9).

The relative contribution of a single compound to the AOC of apple extracts was obtained as follows:

$$\text{contribution [\%]} = C_{HPLC} \times (RAA/AOC) \times 100 \tag{2}$$

C_{HPLC} is the molar concentration of an individual compound, determined by HPLC analysis, RAA is the RAA value of the corresponding standard and AOC is the H-ORAC value of the apple sample. The total relative contribution is a sum of all calculated relative contribution values of the polyphenols determined in each apple sample.

Vitamin C has been considered to be one of the most prevalent antioxidant components in apples. However, as Lee et al. (2003) reported, dietary polyphenols have much stronger antioxidant activities than vitamin C [7], being confirmed by our investigations. A comparison of the measured AOC with the calculated H-ORAC value (sum of contributions of polyphenols) showed that only 26.1% (between 15.4% and 37.4%) of the AOC of the apple peel and 15.9% (between 9.3% and 25.3%) of the AOC of the apple flesh were due to the compounds analysed (Figure 1).

All results calculated were smaller than those of the values measured, suggesting unquantified polyphenolic compounds and possible synergisms and/or antagonisms among the polyphenols [3,7]. The values calculated were smaller than those reported by other authors, due to possibly different apple cultivars, AOC assays and methods for extraction and quantification of polyphenolic compounds [3,35,36].

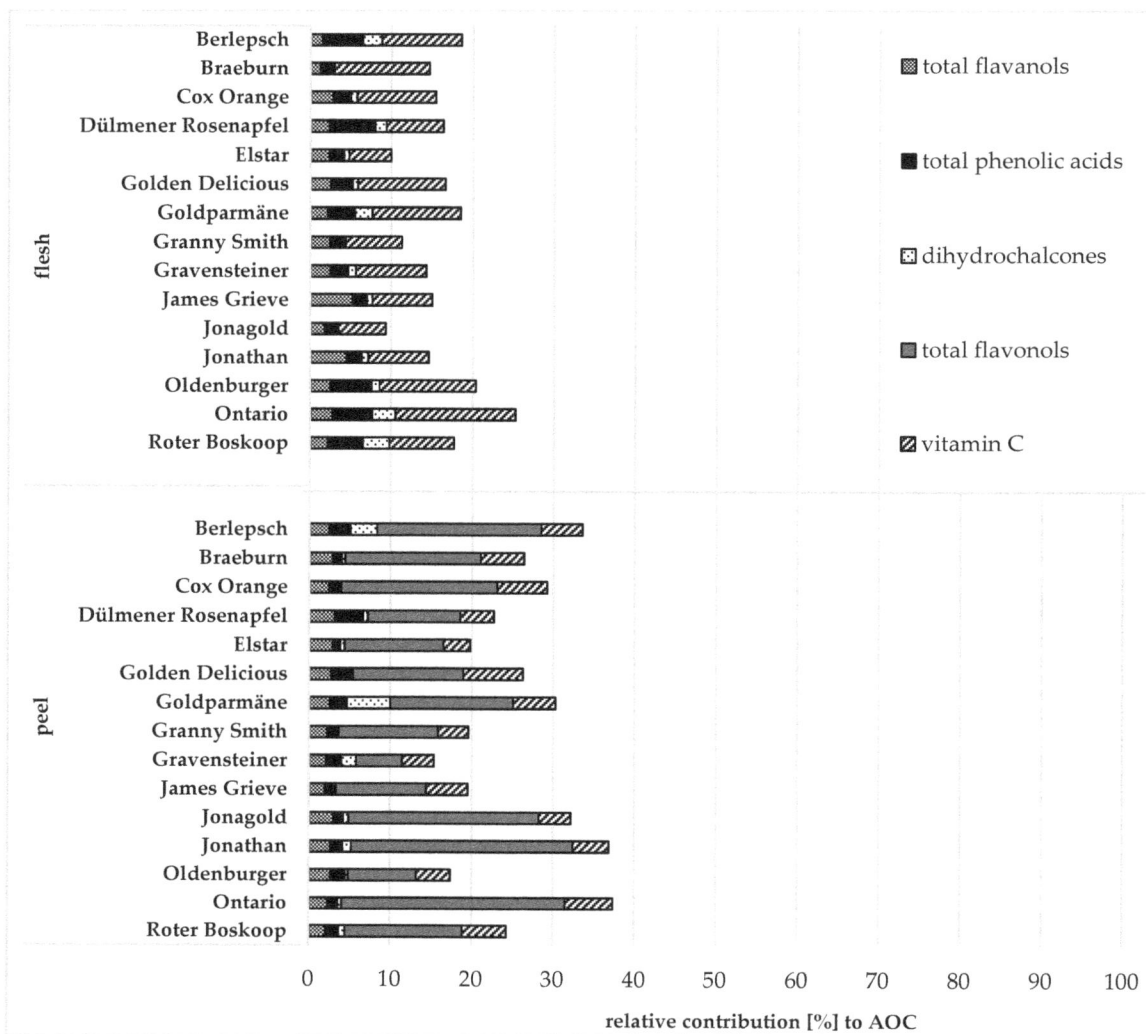

Figure 1. Relative contributions of the main polyphenol groups and vitamin C to the antioxidant capacity (AOC) of different apple cultivars in flesh and peel, calculated using H-ORAC results; H-ORAC: hydrophilic oxygen radical absorbance capacity.

Hyperoside had the highest contribution (6.8%) to the AOC in the peel, followed by quercitrin (2.1%) and avicularin (2.0%), whereas in the flesh, phloridzin and chlorogenic acid (1.2%) contributed the most, followed by caffeic acid (1.0%) and procyanidin A2 (0.8%). Considering the content of each polyphenolic compound, the total polyphenols had an average contribution of 21.2% (11.5–32.5%) to the AOC in the peel and of 6.8% (2.9–10.5%) to AOC in the flesh. In the apple peel, an average of 15.9% of the calculated AOC was due to the flavonols, 2.5% due to the flavanols, 1.7% due to the phenolic acids and 1.1% due to the dihydrochalcone phloridzin (Figure 1). Of the three polyphenolic groups identified in the flesh, the total phenolic acids provided 3.0%, followed by the total flavanols (2.6%) and the dihydrochalcone phloridzin (1.2%) (Figure 1). These results are in agreement with other publications, showing a strong AOA for flavanols and flavonols, being thus main contributors to the AOC of apples [3,7,8,36,37]. In addition to the polyphenols, vitamin C contributed to the AOC of peel (4.9%) and flesh (9.1%). These results clearly indicate that in the peel flavonols rather than vitamin C made the major contribution to AOC of apples, whereas in the flesh, vitamin C provided the highest contribution.

3.4. Comparison of Old and New Apple Cultivars

In the present study, the extracts of flesh and peel of old apple cultivars (n = 10) and new apple cultivars (n = 5) were analysed in terms of their polyphenolic profiles, vitamin C content and AOC. The flesh of old cultivars had significantly higher content of polyphenolic compounds (HPLC data) and vitamin C, compared to the flesh of new cultivars, which led also to a higher AOC in TPC, H-TEAC and H-ORAC assays for the old ones. In contrast to the flesh, the polyphenolic content and the AOC of the apple peel did not differ between old and new cultivars, whereas the vitamin C content was significantly higher in the peel of old cultivars. As shown in Table 4, the polyphenolic profile of the new apple cultivars was characterised by a lower content of total flavanols (flesh) and total phenolic acids (flesh and peel) and a lower content of phloridzin (flesh and peel), compared to the old ones. The lower content of flavanols and phloridzin resulted in a lower AOC in the new apple cultivars, because monomeric and oligomeric flavan-3-ols and phloridzin are strong antioxidants with high AOAs.

Table 4. Comparison of content of vitamin C, phenolic compounds and antioxidant capacity results between old apple cultivars (n = 10) and new apple cultivars (n = 5).

	Apple Flesh			Apple Peel		
	Old Cultivars	New Cultivars	p	Old Cultivars	New Cultivars	p
ascorbic acid	102.6 ± 19.3	68.5 ± 23.7	**<0.001**	203.5 ± 50.5	162.9 ± 45.9	**0.012**
procyanidin B1	1.0 ± 1.9	1.0 ± 0.1	0.081	1.9 ± 1.6	n.d.	-
(+)-catechin	1.5 ± 1.2	1.1 ± 0.9	0.351	5.1 ± 3.0	5.4 ± 3.0	0.745
procyanidin B2	1.9 ± 0.5	1.6 ± 0.3	0.061	7.1 ± 1.5	7.4 ± 1.4	0.427
procyanidin C1	1.5 ± 0.2	n.d.	-	6.7 ± 1.2	7.8 ± 1.1	**0.016**
(−)-epicatechin	1.7 ± 1.2	1.0 ± 0.7	**0.034**	8.8 ± 4.9	10.1 ± 7.2	0.543
procyanidin A2	4.8 ± 2.6	2.5 ± 1.2	**<0.001**	7.8 ± 2.9	7.7 ± 3.4	0.855
total flavanols	11.2 ± 5.2	6.4 ± 2.5	**<0.001**	36.1 ± 8.8	36.8 ± 16.5	0.883
gallic acid	1.8 ± 0.2	1.6 ± 0.2	0.054	4.6 ± 1.0	3.9 ± 0.3	**0.001**
protocatechuic acid	0.1 ± 0.1	0.1 ± 0.0	**0.005**	2.0 ± 0.8	1.3 ± 0.6	**0.012**
chlorogenic acid	6.4 ± 2.7	2.1 ± 0.8	**<0.001**	6.7 ± 4.0	5.6 ± 0.7	0.159
caffeic acid	3.3 ± 2.4	0.8 ± 0.5	**<0.001**	4.6 ± 3.7	0.8 ± 0.5	**<0.001**
p-coumaric acid	0.7 ± 0.1	0.5 ± 0.1	**<0.001**	2.8 ± 1.3	1.8 ± 0.4	**<0.001**
ferulic acid	0.2 ± 0.1	0.1 ± 0.1	**0.003**	1.3 ± 0.6	0.9 ± 0.4	**0.007**
total phenolic acids	12.5 ± 4.9	5.2 ± 1.3	**<0.001**	22.0 ± 7.7	14.3 ± 2.1	**<0.001**
phloridzin	5.0 ± 3.1	1.1 ± 0.7	**<0.001**	16.6 ± 18.7	4.8 ± 3.5	**0.002**
hyperoside	n.d.	n.d.	-	92.2 ± 55.8	84.2 ± 57.1	0.657
isoquercitrin	n.d.	n.d.	-	17.8 ± 11.9	16.6 ± 8.6	0.716
rutin	n.d.	n.d.	-	7.1 ± 7.9	5.4 ± 3.3	0.319
reynoutrin	n.d.	n.d.	-	19.0 ± 11.5	17.0 ± 7.6	0.550
avicularin	n.d.	n.d.	-	30.6 ± 15.2	21.4 ± 8.4	**0.035**
quercitrin	n.d.	n.d.	-	29.8 ± 20.3	25.4 ± 13.1	0.455
quercetin	n.d.	n.d.	-	15.5 ± 7.9	13.4 ± 5.2	0.366
total flavonols	n.d.	n.d.	-	212.1 ± 112.3	183.5 ± 99.6	0.410
total polyphenols	28.7 ± 7.4	12.6 ± 4.4	**<0.001**	286.8 ± 118.8	239.4 ± 118.6	0.214
TPC	257.0 ± 56.7	179.5 ± 52.3	**<0.001**	995.9 ± 281.6	914.7 ± 331.3	0.163
TEAC	1.5 ± 0.4	1.0 ± 0.3	**<0.001**	6.9 ± 2.8	5.9 ± 2.7	0.051
ORAC	5.7 ± 1.3	4.6 ± 1.6	**<0.001**	21.4 ± 5.4	19.2 ± 7.8	0.060

p-Values represent results from unpaired t-test ($p < 0.05$; significant values are shown in bold); n.d.: not detected; TPC: total phenolic content; TEAC: trolox equivalent antioxidant capacity; ORAC: oxygen radical antioxidant capacity; single compounds and total concentrations in mg/100 g freeze dried material; TPC in mg GAE/100 g freeze dried material; TEAC and ORAC in mmol TE/100 g freeze dried material; GAE: gallic acid equivalents; TE: trolox equivalents.

Phenolic acids and flavanols are responsible for an astringent taste and a rapid enzymatic browning of apples [38]. Since consumers prefer sweet-flavoured and low enzymatic browning apples, the content of phenolic acids and flavanols decreased by breeding new apple cultivars. New apple cultivars tend to be genetically impoverished because they are almost entirely due to six similar strain varieties, but old cultivars have a higher vitality [39]. Presumably, the flesh of old cultivars contains higher levels of polyphenolic compounds, vitamin C and AOC due to species diversity. Vrhovsek et al., (2004) also showed that old cultivars (whole fruit, without separation into peel and flesh) have a higher average content of total polyphenols and, in particular, of flavanols, compared to new cultivars [13]. A reason why there are no differences in the peel between old and new cultivars may be the protective function of antioxidants, like polyphenolic compounds, in the peel; thus, they are necessary ingredients to counter biotic and abiotic factors.

4. Conclusions

The results of this research clearly indicated that flavonols, rather than vitamin C, make the major contribution to AOC in apple peel, whereas in the flesh, vitamin C provides the highest contribution next to the flavanols. The flesh of old apple cultivars had a higher content of polyphenolic compounds and vitamin C, resulting in a higher AOC compared to new apple cultivars. For this reason, it is recommended to include preferably old apple cultivars, such as Jonathan, Ontario and Oldenburger, in the daily diet. Additionally, it is advisable to consume the apple with peel, due to its higher polyphenolic content and stronger AOC. Both aspects can help to increase the polyphenol intake and the AOC within the daily diet.

Author Contributions: Josephine Kschonsek and Volker Böhm conceived and designed the experiments; Josephine Kschonsek performed the experiments; Josephine Kschonsek, Theresa Wolfram and Annette Stöckel analysed the data; Josephine Kschonsek wrote the paper; Josephine Kschonsek and Volker Böhm critically read the manuscript and corrected it. All authors approved the final manuscript.

Conflicts of Interest: The authors declare no existing conflict of interest.

References

1. Hyson, D.A. A comprehensive review of apples and apple components and their relationship to human health. *Adv. Nutr.* **2011**, *2*, 408–420. [CrossRef] [PubMed]
2. Scalbert, A.; Morand, C.; Manach, C.; Rémésy, C. Absorption and metabolism of polyphenols in the gut and impact on health. *Biomed. Pharmacother.* **2002**, *56*, 276–282. [CrossRef]
3. Tsao, R.; Yang, R.; Xie, S.; Sockovie, E.; Khanizadeh, S. Which polyphenolic compounds contribute to the total antioxidant activities of apple? *J. Agric. Food. Chem.* **2005**, *53*, 4989–4995. [CrossRef] [PubMed]
4. Wolfe, K.; Wu, X.; Liu, R.H. Antioxidant activity of apple peels. *J. Agric. Food. Chem.* **2003**, *51*, 609–614. [CrossRef] [PubMed]
5. Bundesministerium für Ernährung und Landwirtschaft. Pressemitteilung Nr. 232, 2013. Available online: http://www.bmel.de/SharedDocs/Pressemitteilungen/2013/232-Zahl-der-Woche-Obstverbrauch. html?nn=312878 (accessed on 25 April 2017).
6. Han, X.; Shen, T.; Lou, H. Dietary polyphenols and their biological significance. *Int. J. Mol. Sci.* **2007**, *8*, 950–988. [CrossRef]
7. Lee, K.W.; Kim, Y.J.; Kim, D.; Lee, H.J.; Lee, C.Y. Major phenolics in apple and their contribution to the total antioxidant capacity. *J. Agric. Food. Chem.* **2003**, *51*, 6516–6520. [CrossRef] [PubMed]
8. Wojdyło, A.; Oszmiański, J.; Laskowski, P. Polyphenolic compounds and antioxidant activity of new and old apple varieties. *J. Agric. Food. Chem.* **2008**, *56*, 6520–6530. [CrossRef] [PubMed]
9. Łata, B.; Trampczynskab, A.; Paczesnaa, J. Cultivar variation in apple peel and whole fruit phenolic composition. *Sci. Hortic.* **2009**, *121*, 176–181. [CrossRef]
10. Guyot, S.; Marnet, N.; Djamel, L.; Sanoner, P.; Drilleau, J.F. Reversed-phase HPLC following thiolysis for quantitative estimation and characterization of the four main classes of phenolic compounds in different tissue zones of a French cider apple variety (*Malus domestica* Var. Kermerrien). *J. Agric. Food Chem.* **1998**, *46*, 1698–1705. [CrossRef]
11. Tsao, R.; Yang, R.; Young, J.C.; Zhu, H. Polyphenolic profiles in eight apple cultivars using High-Performance Liquid Chromatography (HPLC). *J. Agric. Food. Chem.* **2003**, *51*, 6347–6353. [CrossRef] [PubMed]

12. Van der Sluis, A.A.; Dekker, M.; de Jager, A.; Jongen, W. Activity and concentration of polyphenolic antioxidants in apple: Effect of cultivar, harvest year, and storage conditions. *J. Agric. Food. Chem.* **2001**, *49*, 3606–3613. [CrossRef] [PubMed]

13. Vrhovsek, U.; Rigo, A.; Tonon, D.; Mattivi, F. Quantitation of polyphenols in different apple varieties. *J. Agric. Food. Chem.* **2004**, *52*, 6532–6538. [CrossRef] [PubMed]

14. Bitsch, R.; Netzel, M.; Frank, T.; Strass, G.; Bitsch, I. Bioavailability and biokinetics of anthocyanins from red grape juice and red wine. *J. Biomed. Biotechnol.* **2004**, *5*, 293–298. [CrossRef] [PubMed]

15. Liaudanskas, M.; Viškelis, P.; Jakštas, V.; Raudonis, R.; Kviklys, D.; Milašius, A.; Janulis, V. Application of an optimized HPLC method for the detection of various phenolic compounds in apples from Lithuanian cultivars. *J. Chem.* **2014**, *2014*, 1–10. [CrossRef]

16. Abad-García, B.; Berrueta, L.A.; López-Márquez, D.M.; Crespo-Ferrer, I.; Gallo, B.; Vicente, F. Optimization and validation of a methodology based on solvent extraction and liquid chromatography for the simultaneous determination of several polyphenolic families in fruit juices. *J. Chromatogr. A* **2007**, *1154*, 87–96. [CrossRef] [PubMed]

17. Müller, L.; Gnoyke, S.; Popken, A.M.; Böhm, V. Antioxidant capacity and related parameters of different fruit formulations. *LWT-Food Sci. Technol.* **2010**, *43*, 992–999. [CrossRef]

18. Singleton, V.L.; Rossi, J.A. Colorimetry of total phenolics with phosphomolybdic-phosphotungstic acid reagents. *Am. J. Enol. Vitic.* **1965**, *16*, 144–158.

19. Re, R.; Pellegrini, N.; Proteggente, A.; Pannala, A.; Yang, M.; Rice-Evans, C. Antioxidant activity applying an improved ABTS radical cation decolorization assay. *Free Radic. Biol. Med.* **1999**, *26*, 1231–1237. [CrossRef]

20. Ou, B.; Hampsch-Woodill, M.; Prior, R.L. Development and validation of an improved oxygen radical absorbance capacity assay using fluorescein as the fluorescent probe. *J. Agric. Food. Chem.* **2001**, *49*, 4619–4626. [CrossRef] [PubMed]

21. Al-Duais, M.; Müller, L.; Böhm, V.; Jetschke, G. Antioxidant capacity and total phenolics of Cyphostemma digitatum before and after processing: Use of different assays. *Eur. Food. Res. Technol.* **2009**, *228*, 813–821. [CrossRef]

22. Petkovsek, M.M.; Stampar, F.; Veberic, R. Parameters of inner quality of the apple scab resistant and susceptible apple cultivars (*Malus domestica* Borkh). *Sci. Hortic.* **2007**, *114*, 37–44. [CrossRef]

23. Escarpa, A.; González, M.C. High-performance liquid chromatography with diode-array detection for the determination of phenolic compounds in peel and pulp from different apple varieties. *J. Chromatogr. A* **1998**, *823*, 331–337. [CrossRef]

24. Napolitano, A.; Cascone, A.; Graziani, G.; Ferracane, R.; Scalfi, L.; Di Vaio, C.; Ritieni, A.; Fogliano, V. Influence of variety and storage on the polyphenol composition of apple flesh. *J. Agric. Food Chem.* **2004**, *52*, 6526–6531. [CrossRef] [PubMed]

25. Oleszek, W.; Lee, C.Y.; Jaworski, A.W.; Price, K.R. Identification of some phenolic compounds in apples. *J. Agric. Food Chem.* **1988**, *36*, 430–432. [CrossRef]

26. Wach, A.; Pyrzynska, K.; Biesaga, M. Quercetin content in some food and herbal samples. *Food Chem.* **2007**, *100*, 699–704. [CrossRef]

27. Burda, S.; Oleszek, W.; Lee, C.Y. Phenolic compounds and their changes in apples during maturation and cold storage. *J. Agric. Food. Chem.* **1990**, *38*, 945–948. [CrossRef]

28. Khanizadeh, S.; Tsao, R.; Rekika, D.; Yang, R.; Charles, M.T.; Rupasinghe, V. Polyphenol composition and total antioxidant capacity of selected apple genotypes for processing. *J. Food Compos. Anal.* **2008**, *21*, 396–401. [CrossRef]

29. Raudone, L.; Raudonis, R.; Liaudanskas, M.; Viskelis, J.; Pukalskas, A.; Janulis, V. Phenolic profiles and contribution of individual compounds to antioxidant activity of apple powders. *J. Food Sci.* **2016**, *81*, C1055–C1061. [CrossRef] [PubMed]

30. Planchon, V.; Lateur, M.; Dupont, P.; Lognay, G. Ascorbic acid level of Belgian apple genetic resources. *Sci. Hortic.* **2004**, *100*, 51–61. [CrossRef]

31. Pissard, A.; Pierna, J.A.F.; Baeten, V.; Sinnaeve, G.; Lognay, G.; Mouteau, A.; Dupont, P.; Rondia, A.; Lateur, M. Non-destructive measurement of vitamin C, total polyphenol and sugar content in apples using near-infrared spectroscopy. *J. Sci. Food Agric.* **2013**, *93*, 238–244. [CrossRef] [PubMed]

32. Łata, B.; Tomala, K. Apple peel as a contributor to whole fruit quantity of potentially healthful bioactive compounds. Cultivar and year implication. *J. Agric. Food Chem.* **2007**, *55*, 10795–10802. [CrossRef] [PubMed]

33. Drogoudi, P.D.; Michailidis, Z.; Pantelidis, G. Peel and flesh antioxidant content and harvest quality characteristics of seven apple cultivars. *Sci. Hortic.* **2008**, *115*, 149–153. [CrossRef]

34. Giomaro, G.; Karioti, A.; Bilia, A.R.; Bucchini, A.; Giamperi, L.; Ricci, D.; Fraternale, D. Polyphenols profile and antioxidant activity of skin and pulp of a rare apple from Marche region (Italy). *Chem. Cent. J.* **2014**, *8*, 45. [CrossRef] [PubMed]

35. Van der Sluis, A.A.; Dekker, M.; Skrede, G.; Jongen, W.M.F. Activity and concentration of polyphenolic antioxidants in apple juice. 1. Effect of existing production methods. *J. Agric. Food. Chem.* **2002**, *50*, 7211–7219. [CrossRef] [PubMed]

36. Chinnici, F.; Bendini, A.; Gaiani, A.; Riponi, C. Radical scavening activities of pees and pulps from cv. Golden Delicious apples as related to their phenolic composition. *J. Agric. Food. Chem.* **2004**, *52*, 4684–4689. [CrossRef] [PubMed]

37. Stracke, A.B.; Rüfer, C.E.; Bub, A.; Weibel, F.P.; Kunz, C.; Watzl, B. Three-year comparison of the polyphenol contens and antioxidant capacities in organically and conventionally produced apples (*Malus domestica* Bork. Cultivar Golden Delicious). *J. Agric. Food Chem.* **2009**, *57*, 4598–4605. [CrossRef] [PubMed]

38. Renard, C.M.; Dupont, N.; Guillermin, P. Concentrations and characteristics of procyanidins and other phenolics in apples during fruit growth. *Phytochemistry* **2007**, *68*, 1128–1138. [CrossRef] [PubMed]

39. Bannier, H. Moderne Apfelzüchtung: Genetische Verarmung und Tendenzen zur Inzucht. Vitalitätsverluste erst bei Verzicht auf Fungizideinsatz sichtbar. *Erwerbs-Obstbau* **2011**, *52*, 85–110. [CrossRef]

12

Evening Primrose (*Oenothera biennis*) Biological Activity Dependent on Chemical Composition

Magdalena Timoszuk, Katarzyna Bielawska and Elżbieta Skrzydlewska *[iD]

Department of Inorganic and Analytical Chemistry, Medical University of Bialystok, 15-089 Bialystok, Poland; magdalena.timoszuk@umb.edu.pl (M.T.); katarzyna.bielawska@umb.edu.pl (K.B.)
* Correspondence: elzbieta.skrzydlewska@umb.edu.pl

Abstract: Evening primrose (*Oenothera* L.) is a plant belonging to the family Onagraceae, in which the most numerous species is *Oenothera biennis*. Some plants belonging to the genus *Oenothera* L. are characterized by biological activity. Therefore, studies were conducted to determine the dependence of biological activity on the chemical composition of various parts of the evening primrose, mainly leaves, stems, and seeds. Common components of all parts of the *Oenothera biennis* plants are fatty acids, phenolic acids, and flavonoids. In contrast, primrose seeds also contain proteins, carbohydrates, minerals, and vitamins. Therefore, it is believed that the most interesting sources of biologically active compounds are the seeds and, above all, evening primrose seed oil. This oil contains mainly aliphatic alcohols, fatty acids, sterols, and polyphenols. Evening primrose oil (EPO) is extremely high in linoleic acid (LA) (70–74%) and γ-linolenic acid (GLA) (8–10%), which may contribute to the proper functioning of human tissues because they are precursors of anti-inflammatory eicosanoids. EPO supplementation results in an increase in plasma levels of γ-linolenic acid and its metabolite dihomo-γ-linolenic acid (DGLA). This compound is oxidized by lipoxygenase (15-LOX) to 15-hydroxyeicosatrienoic acid (15-HETrE) or, under the influence of cyclooxygenase (COX), DGLA is metabolized to series 1 prostaglandins. These compounds have anti-inflammatory and anti-proliferative properties. Furthermore, 15-HETrE blocks the conversion of arachidonic acid (AA) to leukotriene A_4 (LTA_4) by direct inhibition of 5-LOX. In addition, γ-linolenic acid suppresses inflammation mediators such as interleukin 1β (IL-1β), interleukin 6 (IL-6), and cytokine - tumor necrosis factor α (TNF-α). The beneficial effects of EPO have been demonstrated in the case of atopic dermatitis, psoriasis, Sjögren's syndrome, asthma, and anti-cancer therapy.

Keywords: evening primrose oil; γ-linolenic acid; linoleic acid; omega-6 fatty acids; eicosanoids

1. Introduction

Evening primrose (*Oenothera* L.) is a plant belonging to the Onagraceae family. There are about 145 species in the genus *Oenothera* L., occurring in the temperate and tropical climate zones of North and South America. Some species have adapted to new areas, inhabiting the countries of the European continent, and about 70 species are now present in Europe. The most numerous species in the *Oenothera* L. family is *Oenothera biennis*, which also has the best-studied biological activity. It has been indicated that *Oenothera biennis* is beneficial in the treatment of many diseases. Therefore, research is ongoing to determine the chemical composition of these plants and how it relates to the biological activity of evening primrose. This research mainly concerns extracts from various parts of evening primrose (e.g., the leaves, stems, and seeds) [1].

2. Chemical Composition of Evening Primrose (*Oenothera biennis*)

Methanolic extracts prepared from the aerial parts of *Oenothera biennis* contain mainly phenolic acids and flavonoids. Phenolic acids present in the analyzed extracts include the following compounds: gallic acid and its ester derivatives (e.g., methyl gallate, galloylglucose, digalloylglucose, and tris-galloylglucose), 3-*p*-feruloylquinic acid, 3-*p*-coumaroylquinic acid, 4-*p*-feruloylquinic acid, caffeic acid pentoside, ellagic acid and its ester derivatives (e.g., ellagic acid hexoside and ellagic acid pentoside), and valoneic acid dilactone. Flavonoids present in the extracts include the following compounds: myricetin 3-*O*-glucuronide, quercetin 3-*O*-galactoside, quercetin 3-*O*-glucuronide, quercetin 3-*O*-glucoside, quercetin pentoside, quercetin dihexoside, quercetin glucuronylhexoside, quercetin 3-*O*-(2'-galloyl)-glucuronide, kaempferol 3-*O*-rhamnoglucoside, kaempferol 3-*O*-glucoside, kaempferol 3-*O*-glucuronide, kaempferol 3-*O*-(2'-galloyl)-glucuronide, and kaempferol pentoside [2].

The aqueous leaf extract of *Oenothera biennis* contains phenolic compounds (e.g., ellagitannins and caffeoyl tartaric acid) and flavonoids (quercetin glucuronide and kaempferol glucuronide) [3]. Among the tannins contained in the leaves of the evening primrose are oenothein A and oenothein B. The carbohydrates present in the extracts include arabinose, galactose, glucose, mannose, galacturonic acid, and glucuronic acid.

The roots of evening primrose contain the following sterols: sitosterol, oenotheralanosterol A, and oenotheralanosterol B. The triterpenes maslinic acid and oleanolic acid are also present in the root, along with the following carbohydrates: arabinose, galactose, glucose, mannose, galacturonic acid, and glucuronic acid. The following tannins are also found: gallic acid, tetramethylellagic acid, oenostacin, and 2,7,8-trimethylellagic acid [4]. The methanolic extract of the *Oenothera biennis* root also possesses significant amounts of xanthone (9H-xanthen-9-one) and its derivatives, such as dihydroxyprenyl xanthone and cetoleilyl diglucoside, which possess diverse biological and pharmacological properties [5].

Evening primrose seeds contain about 20% oil. The amount of oil depends on various factors, such as the age of the seed, the cultivar, and the growth conditions [6].

Generally, evening primrose oil is obtained from *Oenothera biennis* seeds using the cold-pressing method. The oil is a blend of about 13 triacylglycerol fractions, where the dominant combinations consist of the following fatty acids: linoleic–linoleic–linoleic (LLL, 40%), linoleic–linoleic–γ-linolenic (LLLnγ, approximately 15%), linoleic–linoleic–palmitic (LLP, approximately 8%), and linoleic–linoleic–oleic (LLO, approximately 8%) [7]. The oil consists of triacylglycerols—about 98%, with a small amount of other lipids and about 1–2% non-saponifiable fraction [6].

Evening primrose oil is very high in linoleic (70–74%) and γ-linolenic (8–10%) acids, and also contains other fatty acids: palmitic acid, oleic acid, stearic acid, and (in smaller amounts) myristic acid, oleopalmitic acid, vaccenic acid, eicosanoic acid, and eicosenoic acid (see Table 1) [8]. The phospholipid fraction comprises only 0.05% of the oil, and the following phospholipids have been identified in it: phosphatidylcholines (31.9%), phosphatidylinositols (27.1%), phosphatidylethanolamines (17.6%), phosphatidylglycerols (16.7%), and phosphatidic acids (6.7%) [6].

Table 1. Fatty acid composition of evening primrose oil (EPO) (*Oenothera biennis* L.) [8].

Compound Name	Contents (%)
linoleic acid	73.88 ± 0.09
γ-linolenic acid	9.24 ± 0.05
oleic acid	6.93 ± 0.02
palmitic acid	6.31 ± 0.14
stearic acid	1.88 ± 0.02
vaccenic acid	0.81 ± 0.03
eicosenoic acid	0.55 ± 0.01
eicosanoic acid	0.31 ± 0.03
behenic acid	0.10 ± 0.01

Evening primrose oil includes aliphatic alcohols, which make up about 798 mg/kg of the oil, 1-tetracosanol (about 237 mg/kg oil), and 1-hexacosanol (about 290 mg/kg oil) being present in the largest amount. The main triterpenes present are β-amyrin (about 996 mg/kg oil) and squalene (about 0.40 mg/kg oil) [8]. The oil contains a small amount of tocopherols: α-tocopherol (76 mg/kg oil), γ-tocopherol (187 mg/kg oil), and δ-tocopherol (15 mg/kg oil) [6].

Evening primrose seeds also contain phenolic acids, which are present in free acid form and as ester and glycoside derivatives (see Table 2) [9]. It has been shown that the seeds contain about 15% protein and 43% carbohydrates (in the form of cellulose, along with starch and dextrin). Lignin is also found in the seeds. In addition, the seeds contain amino acids: tryptophan (1.60%), lysine (0.31%), threonine (0.35%), cysteine (1.68%), valine (0.52%), isoleucine (0.41%), leucine (0.87%), and tyrosine (1.05%). Moreover, the seeds contain minerals, mainly calcium, potassium, and magnesium, and vitamins A, B, C, and E [10].

Table 2. Phenolic acid composition (mg/kg) in *Oenothera biennis* L. seed [9].

Acid Name	Included in			
	Free	Esters	Glycosides	Total
p-hydroxyphenyl acetic	n/a	1.03 ± 0.18	0.26 ± 0.05	1.29 ± 0.19
p-hydroxybenzoic	4.12 ± 0.25	0.38 ± 0.07	0.29 ± 0.10	4.79 ± 0.26
2-hydroxy-4-methoxybenzoic	6.52 ± 0.30	n/a	0.83 ± 0.28	7.35 ± 0.41
caffeic	6.48 ± 0.29	0.80 ± 0.14	n/a	7.51 ± 0.33
hydroxycaffeic	n/a	0.77 ± 0.18	n/a	0.77 ± 0.18
m-coumaric	4.90 ± 0.45	0.83 ± 0.21	n/a	5.73 ± 0.50
p-coumaric	1.32 ± 0.10	1.96 ± 0.23	0.06 ± 0.06	3.34 ± 0.25
ferulic	4.08 ± 0.30	0.72 ± 0.09	0.22 ± 0.06	5.02 ± 0.32
gallic	1.87 ± 0.22	7.03 ± 0.82	5.91 ± 1.56	14.81 ± 1.78
protocatechuic	50.28 ± 0.77	10.96 ± 0.34	2.16 ± 2.42	63.40 ± 2.56
vanillic	5.22 ± 0.28	0.06 ± 0.02	0.83 ± 0.28	7.35 ± 0.41
veratric	n/a	0.41 ± 0.03	0.47 ± 0.15	0.88 ± 0.15
homoveratric	n/a	0.43 ± 0.06	n/a	0.43 ± 0.06
salicylic	1.15 ± 0.04	1.40 ± 0.18	n/a	2.55 ± 0.18

n/a—not available.

Evening primrose oil also contains polyphenols, such as hydroxytyrosol (1.11 mg/kg oil), vanillic acid (3.27 mg/kg oil), vanillin (17.37 mg/kg oil), *p*-coumaric acid (1.75 mg/kg oil), and ferulic acid (25.23 mg/kg oil) [8].

The unsaponifiable matter of oil is composed partially of sterols, which comprise 53.16% of this fraction (see Table 3) [8].

Table 3. Sterol content of EPO (*Oenothera biennis* L.) [8].

Compound Name	Contents (mg/kg of Oil)
β-sitosterol	7952.00 ± 342.25
kampesterol	883.32 ± 0.45
Δ_5-avenasterol	429.65 ± 75.20
sitostanol	167.01 ± 39.77
clerosterol	120.44 ± 0.12
Δ_5-24-estigmastadienol	94.60 ± 5.68
Δ_7-estigmasterol	38.17 ± 14.33
Δ_7-avenasterol	27.80 ± 16.07

The seed ash contains a group of macroelements and microelements, including calcium, magnesium, potassium, phosphorus, manganese, iron, sodium, zinc, and copper (see Table 4) [10].

Table 4. Macroelements and microelements contributing to seed ash [10].

Macroelements	Contents (mg/100g of ash)
calcium	1800
magnesium	530
potassium	460
sodium	18
phosphorus	410

Microelements	Contents (mg/100g of ash)
iron	39
zinc	7
copper	1.1
manganese	0.5

3. Biological Activity of Evening Primrose Oil (*Oenothera biennis*)

The biological effect of evening primrose oil is a result of its composition and the biological properties of its components. Since the most important components in terms of quantity are polyunsaturated fatty acids (PUFAs), mainly linoleic acid (LA) and γ-linolenic acid (GLA) which belong to the group of omega-6 acids. The biological significance, especially of these acids, will be discussed in more detail.

Linoleic acid belongs to the group of essential fatty acids. These are also called exogenous fatty acids, because the human body does not synthesize them and it is necessary to obtain them from food [11]. Evening primrose oil contains over 70% linoleic acid (LA) and about 9% γ-linolenic acid (GLA) [10]. Linoleic acid and γ-linolenic acid contribute to the proper functioning of many tissues of the human body, because they are precursors of compounds that lead to the generation of anti-inflammatory eicosanoids, such as the series 1 prostaglandins and 15-hydroxyeicosatrienoic acid (15-HETrE). On the other hand, the enzymatic conversion of linoleic acid to arachidonic acid (AA) may form pro-inflammatory compounds, such as series 2 prostaglandins and series 4 leukotrienes [11]. With reference to the above, it is suggested that evening primrose oil may influence inflammatory diseases, including skin problems.

Linoleic acid [12], among others, plays an important role in the proper functioning of the skin, especially the stratum corneum, in which it is one of the main components of the ceramides building the lipid layer. It has been shown that the presence of this acid prevents the skin from peeling and the loss of water through the epidermis, while at the same time improving skin softness and elasticity and regulating the process of epidermal keratinization. A deficiency of linoleic acid, which is contained in large quantities in ceramide 1, leads to its replacement by oleic acid. This causes a deterioration in the protective properties of the epidermis [12,13].

Under the influence of Δ-6-desaturase (D6D), linoleic acid undergoes dehydrogenation to form γ-linolenic acid. The activity of Δ-6-desaturase in human cells depends on various factors and is reduced under the influence of nicotine, alcohol, magnesium deficiency, and a poor diet rich in saturated fatty acids, and under conditions of physiological aging of the body [12,14]. The basic component of evening primrose oil is linoleic acid, and the possibility of its metabolism to γ-linolenic acid due to the action of Δ-6-desaturase is an important point. Δ-6-Desaturase (D6D) activity is highest in the liver, the brain, the heart, and lung cells [15]. D6D activity is several times higher in the fetal human liver than in the adult human liver [11]. The fatty acid desaturase 2 (FADS2) gene encoding the Δ-6-desaturase enzyme is also expressed in skin cells: within the sebaceous gland, D6D desaturates palmitic acid to sapienic acid, which is the major fatty acid of human sebum [16,17]. On the other hand, the main epidermal cells—keratinocytes—are characterized by their lack of D6D and D5D activity [18] and the dermal fibroblasts express the D6D mRNA, which is capable of desaturation of the essential fatty acid (EFA) in the skin [19].

Δ-6-Desaturase is also present in evening primrose seeds. Huang et al. (2010) report that the cDNA sequence of the D6D gene was obtained from the developing seeds. The transformation of the plasmid DNA of a *Saccharomyces cerevisiae* strain then showed that after the addition of a medium containing linoleic acid to the yeast cells, a signal was obtained from γ-linolenic acid, indicating the presence of Δ-6-desaturase in seeds of the species *Oenothera biennis* [20,21].

A deficiency of γ-linolenic acid and other metabolites of linoleic acid was demonstrated in the plasma of patients with atopic dermatitis. This is linked to a decrease in Δ-6-desaturase activity, which makes the conversion of linoleic acid to γ-linolenic acid and the formation of its metabolites impossible [12,22]. It was found that oral treatment with evening primrose oil, which contains γ-linolenic acid, may lead to a reduction in the symptoms of atopic dermatitis [22]. However, subsequent studies have not confirmed that oral supplementation with evening primrose oil improves the skin condition in patients with atopic dermatitis [23].

The hydrocarbon chain of the emerging or supplied γ-linolenic acid under the influence of an elongase is elongated to dihomo-γ-linolenic acid (DGLA). The GLA elongation is faster than the desaturation of linoleic acid [24,25]. Dihomo-γ-linolenic acid is metabolized by cyclooxygenase (COX) to series 1 prostaglandins, which are eicosanoids with anti-inflammatory activity (see Table 5) [24]. Under the influence of 15-lipoxygenase (15-LOX), DGLA is oxidized to 15-hydroxyeicosatrienoic (15-HETrE) acid, which has anti-inflammatory and anti-proliferative properties [24,26]. Therefore, increased levels of GLA and DGLA, which are metabolized to anti-inflammatory compounds, suppress the inflammatory reaction. However, a decrease in these acids' levels may lead to the development of inflammatory diseases [24,27]. In addition, GLA suppresses inflammation mediators such as IL-1β, IL-6, and TNF-α cytokines [12,28]. In contrast, 15-HETrE acid, which is a product of the oxidation of dihomo-γ-linolenic acid by 15-LOX, has the ability to inhibit the synthesis of series 4 leukotrienes, whose elevated levels cause intensified pathological cell hyperproliferation [24]. This contributes to the inhibition of the pro-inflammatory action of leukotrienes, which are involved, among others, in the development of asthma [24,29] (see Figure 1).

Regardless of the metabolism of DGLA catalyzed by COXs and 15-LOX, dihomo-γ-linolenic acid under the influence of Δ-5-desaturase (D5D) is converted to arachidonic acid (AA), which is the precursor of many lipid mediators in the body, mainly pro-inflammatory [18,24]. Under physiological conditions, the sources of AA are membrane phospholipids, from which it is released by the hydrolysis of ester bonds, mainly via the action of phospholipase A_2 (PLA_2). There are two main ways that lead to the formation of free arachidonic acid. One pathway leads to the hydrolytic release of AA by the cytosolic isoform of PLA_2. The second way leads to the release of AA by the indirect action of phospholipase C (PLC) and diacylglycerol (DAG) lipase. DAG lipase and PLC result in the formation of inositol 1,4,5-triphosphate and DAG. The latter is then hydrolyzed by DAG lipase to form free arachidonic acid and monoacylglycerol (MAG) [18,30].

In pathological conditions and, for example, in the case of excessive exposure of the skin to UV radiation, the redox balance is disturbed and oxidative stress occurs, which results in the activation of cytosolic phospholipase A2 ($cPLA_2$) and PLC in the skin cells [18]. This leads to the excessive release of AA and the increased production of eicosanoids via cyclooxygenases and lipoxygenases. COX-1 and COX-2 catalyze the transformation of arachidonic acid into the series 2 prostanoids (PGE_2, PGD_2, PGI_2, TXA_2, and TXB_2). Moreover, 5-lipoxygenase (5-LOX) metabolizes arachidonic acid to series 4 leukotrienes (LTB_4, LTC_4, LTD_4, and LTE_4) [18,31]. Prostaglandins, series 2 thromboxanes, and series 4 leukotrienes belong to the pro-inflammatory eicosanoids [31]. However, 15-lipoxygenase (15-LOX) catalyzes the conversion of arachidonic acid to 15-hydroxyeicosatetraenoic acid (15-HETE), whose metabolites are lipoxins. These compounds have anti-inflammatory properties [18,31]. Moreover, 15-HETE can inhibit the formation of 12-HETE, which is a metabolite of 12-LOX's catalytic action on arachidonic acid [18].

Because DGLA can be metabolically converted via three different enzyme pathways, it is important to determine which enzyme has a higher affinity for arachidonic acid and which metabolites will dominate—pro-inflammatory or anti-inflammatory. Note that γ-linolenic acid, which is one of the main acids contained in evening primrose oil, is an important precursor of DGLA, which is a precursor of anti-inflammatory eicosanoids [32]. It has been shown that GLA or DGLA supplementation causes a modest increase in the prostaglandin E1 (PGE_1) level in tissues in relation to PGE_2, but the biological properties of PGE_1 are about 20 times stronger in comparison to PGE_2 [24]. However, GLA or DGLA supplementation may cause their conversion to AA and pro-inflammatory eicosanoids. Therefore, it is suggested that the metabolism should be directed to anti-inflammatory eicosanoids. An effective solution is an application of selective Δ-5-desaturase inhibitors, which may stop DGLA's conversion to AA and its further pro-inflammatory metabolites [24]. Moreover, as a polyunsaturated fatty acid, arachidonic acid undergoes peroxidation to form electrophilic aldehydes with low molecular weight and high reactivity, which may be a cause of the modification of both nucleophilic small molecules and high-molecular weight compounds, such as proteins, lipids, and DNA, which disturbs cellular metabolism [33].

Evening primrose oil has a high content of LA and GLA, and strengthens the epidermal barrier, normalizes the excessive loss of water through the epidermis, regenerates skin, and improves smoothness, after both topical and oral applications [12].

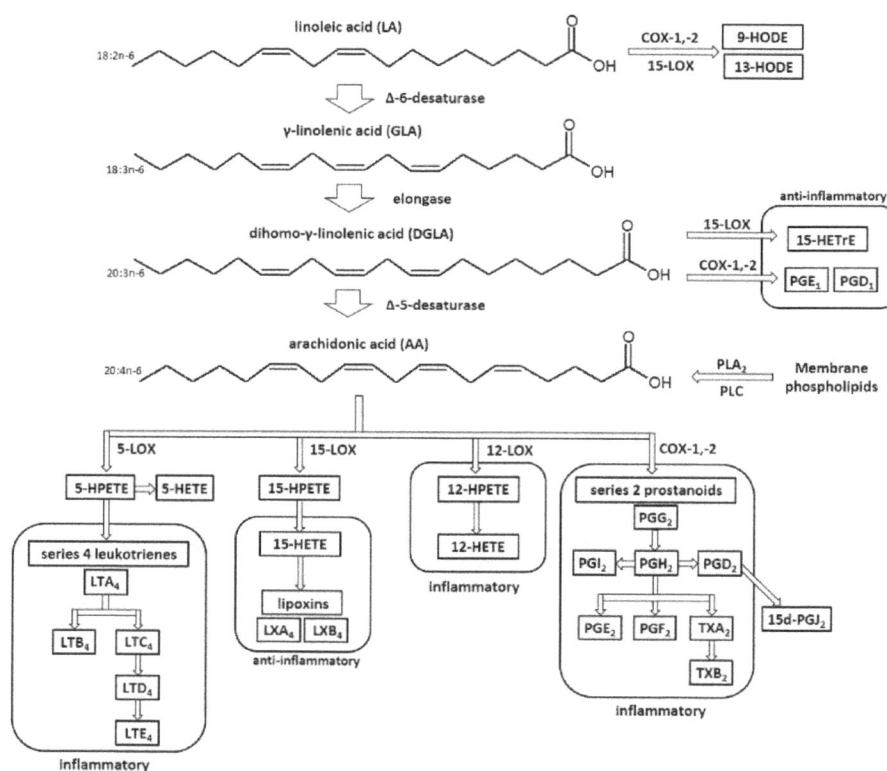

Figure 1. Linoleic acid (LA) metabolism. 9-HODE: 9-hydroxyoctadecadienoic acid; 13-HODE: 13-hydroxyoctadecadienoic acid; 15-HETrE: 15-hydroxyeicosatrienoic; PGE_1: prostaglandin E1; PGD_1: prostaglandin D1; PLA_2: phospholipase A2; PLC: phospholipase C; 5-HPETE: 5-hydroperoxyeicosatetraenoic acid; 5-HETE: 5-hydroxyeicosatetraenoic acid; LTA_4: leukotriene A4; LTB_4: leukotriene B4; LTC_4: leukotriene C4; LTD_4: leukotriene D4; LTE_4: leukotriene E4; 15-HPETE: 15-hydroperoxyeicosatetraenoic acid; 15-HETE: 15-hydroxyeicosatetraenoic acid; LXA4: lipoxin A_4; LXB_4: lipoxin B4; 12-HPETE: 12-hydroperoxyeicosatetraenoic acid; 12-HETE: 12-hydroxyeicosatetraenoic acid: PGG_2: prostaglandin G2; PGH_2: prostaglandin H2; PGI_2: prostaglandin I_2: PGD2: prostaglandin D2; 15-d-PGJ_2: 15-deoxy-delta-12,14-prostaglandin J2; PGE_2: prostaglandin E2: PGF_2: prostaglandin F2: TXA_2: thromboxane A2; TXB_2: thromboxane B2.

In addition, due to its linoleic acid content, evening primrose oil has a beneficial moisturizing effect on the mucous membrane in acne patients treated with isotretinoin [34]. This implies that skin supplementation with evening primrose oil improves the skin's water balance, which is weakened by treatment with isotretinoin. Moreover, γ-linolenic acid, contained in large amounts in the oil, is a source of the anti-inflammatory eicosanoids 15-HETrE and PGE_1, which have anti-proliferative properties that effectively prevent epidermal hyperproliferation [24,34]. In addition, these compounds inhibit the proliferation of smooth muscle cells and prevent the development of atherosclerotic plaque [24].

In recent years, it has been found that γ-linolenic acid is cytotoxic to glioma cells, and it can enhance gamma radiosensitivity [35,36]. It has been suggested that this effect is related to the accumulation of the toxic products of lipid peroxidation, which are cytotoxic to glioma cells. In cancer cells responsible for various types of cancer, the over-expression of the human epidermal growth factor receptor 2 (HER-2/neu) oncogene has been observed. This oncogene causes rapid and uncontrolled cell growth. However, γ-linolenic acid leads to an increase in the levels of polyomavirus enhancer activator 3 (PEA3), a transcriptional repressor of human epidermal growth factor receptor 2 (HER-2/neu) in cells, and a decrease in Her-2/neu promoter activity, thus reducing the likelihood of developing breast cancer [37]. Due to the inhibition of Her-2 expression, GLA administered together with transtuzumab, which as a monoclonal antibody binds to the Her-2 receptor, increases the process of the apoptosis of cancer cells and thus increases the effectiveness of pharmacotherapy with transtuzumab [37]. γ-Linolenic acid also causes an increase in the expression of the nm-23 metastasis-suppressor gene in cancer cells, which favors the inhibition of angiogenesis, cancer cell migration, and consequently, cancer metastasis [38,39]. The formation of these changes is also associated with a reduction in the expression of the vascular endothelial growth factor (VEGF), which plays a significant role in cancer (e.g., in the process of tumor angiogenesis) [40]. The above data suggest that evening primrose oil, as a rich source of gamma linolenic acid, supports anti-cancer therapy.

Moreover, it has been found that the oral supplementation of evening primrose oil (EPO) containing both linoleic acid and γ-linolenic acid reduces the inflammatory reaction and eases eye problems such as burning, dryness, and light sensitivity in people with Sjögren's syndrome [41]. Moreover, GLA reduces the levels of triacylglycerols and low-density lipoprotein (LDL) cholesterol in plasma [42]. It has been suggested that phytosterols, which are present in large quantities in EPO, also contribute to the above action [43].

Table 5. Biological effect and occurrence of selective eicosanoids [18,44,45].

	Metabolite	Biological Activity	Occurrence
anti-inflammatory	PGE_1	- anti-inflammatory - anti-proliferatory	keratinocytes fibroblasts sebocyte
	15-HETrE	- anti-inflammatory - anti-proliferatory	keratinocytes fibroblasts
	13-HODE	- anti-inflammatory - anti-proliferatory	keratinocytes fibroblasts
	15-HETE	- anti-inflammatory (lipoxin precursor) - anti-proliferatory - counteracts 12-HETE and LTB_4 effects - induces leukocyte chemotaxis	keratinocytes fibroblasts

Table 5. *Cont.*

	Metabolite	Biological Activity	Occurrence
inflammatory	LXA$_4$ LXB$_4$	- anti-inflammatory - LXA$_4$ inhibits expression of interleukin 6 (IL-6) and interleukin 8 (IL-8) - LXA$_4$ inhibits proliferation	neutrophils
	PGE$_2$	- proliferatory - chemotaxis - immunosuppression	keratinocytes fibroblasts
	5-HETE	- chemotaxis	keratinocytes
	LTB$_4$	- chemotaxis	leukocytes keratinocytes in chronic dermatitis (psoriasis, atopic dermatitis)
	Cys-LT (LTC$_4$ LTD$_4$ LTE$_4$)	- leukocyte activators - chemotaxis	leukocytes in chronic dermatitis (psoriasis, atopic dermatitis)
	12-HETE	- proliferatory - chemotaxis	keratinocytes fibroblasts Langerhans cells in chronic dermatitis (psoriasis)

Cys-LT: cysteinyl leukotrienes; LTC$_4$: leukotriene C4, LTD$_4$: leukotriene D4; LTE$_4$—leukotriene E4.

4. Conclusions

After analyzing the chemical composition of evening primrose (*Oenothera biennis*), especially the oil from its seeds and the biological activity of its components, it can be stated that it is a natural preparation supplementing the deficiency of essential fatty acids in the body. Therefore, it is beneficial in the treatment of chronic inflammation. It supports the metabolism of the body at various levels, especially in situations leading to the development of pathological conditions.

Author Contributions: M.T.: description of the biological activity of the evening primrose; K.B.: description of the chemical composition of the evening primrose; E.S.: major contribution in writing the manuscript. All authors read and approved the final manuscript.

Funding: This research received no external funding.

Conflicts of Interest: The authors declare no conflicts of interest.

References

1. Mihulka, S.; Pysek, P. Invasion history of Oenothera congeners in Europe: A comparative study of spreading rates in the last 200 years. *J. Biogeogr.* **2001**, *28*, 597–609. [CrossRef]
2. Granica, S.; Czerwińska, M.E.; Piwowarski, J.P.; Ziaja, M.; Kiss, A.K. Chemical composition, antioxidative and anti-inflammatory activity of extracts prepared from aerial parts of *Oenothera biennis* L. and Oenothera paradoxa Hudziok obtained after seeds cultivation. *J. Agric. Food Chem.* **2013**, *61*, 801–810. [CrossRef] [PubMed]

3. Johnson, M.T.J.; Agrawal, A.A.; Maron, J.L.; Salminen, J.P. Heritability, covariation and natural selection on 24 traits of common evening primrose (*Oenothera biennis*) from a field experiment. *J. Evol. Biol.* **2009**, *22*, 1295–1307. [CrossRef] [PubMed]

4. Singh, S.; Kaur, R.; Sharma, S.K. An updated review on the *Oenothera genus*. *J. Chin. Integr. Med.* **2012**, *10*, 717–725. [CrossRef]

5. Ahmad, A.; Singh, D.K.; Fatima, K.; Tandon, S.; Luqman, S. New constituents from the roots of *Oenothera biennis* and their free radical scavenging and ferric reducing activity. *Ind. Crops Prod.* **2014**, *58*, 125–132. [CrossRef]

6. Christie, W.W. The analysis of evening primrose oil. *Ind. Crops Prod.* **1999**, *10*, 73–83. [CrossRef]

7. Zadernowski, R.; Polakowska-Nowak, H.; Rashed, A.A.; Kowalska, M. Lipids from evening primrose and borage seeds. *Oilseed Crops* **1999**, *20*, 581–589.

8. Montserrat-de la Paz, S.; Fernandez-Arche, M.A.; Angel-Martin, M.; Garcia-Gimenez, M.D. Phytochemical characterization of potential nutraceutical ingredients from Evening Primrose oil (*Oenothera biennis* L.). *Phytochem. Lett.* **2014**, *8*, 158–162. [CrossRef]

9. Zadernowski, R.; Naczk, M.; Nowak-Polakowska, H. Phenolic Acids of Borage (*Borago officinalis* L.) and Evening Primrose (*Oenothera biennis* L.). *J. Am. Oil Chem. Soc.* **2002**, *79*, 335–338. [CrossRef]

10. Hudson, B.J.F. Evening primrose (*Oenothera* spp.) oil and seed. *J. Am. Oil Chem. Soc.* **1984**, *61*, 540–543. [CrossRef]

11. Białek, M.; Rutkowska, J. The importance of γ-linolenic acid in the prevention and treatment. *Adv. Hyg. Exp. Med.* **2015**, *69*, 892–904. [CrossRef]

12. Muggli, R. Systemic evening primrose oil improves the biophysical skin parameters of healthy adults. *Int. J. Cosmet. Sci.* **2005**, *27*, 243–249. [CrossRef] [PubMed]

13. Kendall, A.C.; Kiezel-Tsugunova, M.; Brownbridge, L.C.; Harwood, J.L.; Nicolaou, A. Lipid functions in skin: Differential effects of n-3 polyunsaturated fatty acids on cutaneous ceramides, in a human skin organ culture model. *Biochim. Biophys. Acta* **2017**, *1859*, 1679–1689. [CrossRef] [PubMed]

14. Mahfouz, M.M.; Kummerow, F.A. Effect of magnesium deficiency on delta 6 desaturase activity and fatty acid composition of rat liver microsomes. *Lipids* **1989**, *24*, 727–732. [CrossRef] [PubMed]

15. Zietemann, V.; Kröger, J.; Enzenbach, C.; Jansen, E.; Fritche, A.; Weiker, C.; Boeing, H.; Schylze, M.B. Genetic variation of the FADS1 FADS2 gene cluster and n-6 PUFA composition in erythrocyte membranes in the European Prospective Investigation into Cancer and Nutrition-Potsdam study. *Br. J. Nutr.* **2010**, *104*, 1748–1759. [CrossRef] [PubMed]

16. Ge, L.; Gordon, J.S.; Hsuan, C.; Stenn, K.; Prouty, S.M. Identification of the Δ-6 desaturase of human sebaceous glands: Expression and enzyme activity. *J. Investig. Dermatol.* **2003**, *120*, 707–714. [CrossRef] [PubMed]

17. Sampath, H.; Ntambi, J.M. The role of fatty acid desaturases in epidermal metabolism. *Dermatoendocrinol* **2011**, *3*, 62–64. [CrossRef] [PubMed]

18. Nicolaou, A. Eicosanoids in skin inflammation. *Prostaglandins Leukot. Essent. Fat. Acids* **2013**, *88*, 131–138. [CrossRef] [PubMed]

19. Williard, D.E.; Nwankwo, J.O.; Kaduce, T.L.; Harmon, S.D.; Irons, M.; Moser, H.W.; Raymond, G.V.; Spector, A.R. Identification of a fatty acid Δ⁶-desaturase deficiency in human skin fibroblasts. *J. Lipid Res.* **2001**, *42*, 501–508. [PubMed]

20. Huang, S.; Liu, R.; Niu, Y.; Hasi, A. Cloning and functional characterization of a fatty acid Δ6-desaturase from *Oenothera biennis*: Production of γ-linolenic acid by heterologous expression in *Saccharomyces cerevisiae*. *Russ. J. Plant Phys.* **2010**, *57*, 568–573. [CrossRef]

21. Cho, H.P.; Nakamura, M.T.; Clarke, S.D. Cloning, expression, and nutritional regulation of the mammalian Delta-6 desaturase. *J. Biol. Chem.* **1999**, *274*, 471–477. [CrossRef] [PubMed]

22. Senapati, S.; Sabyasachi, B.; Gangopadhyay, D.N. Evening primrose oil is effective in atopic dermatitis: A randomized placebo-controlled trial. *Indian J. Dermatol. Venereol. Leprol.* **2008**, *74*, 447–452. [CrossRef] [PubMed]

23. Schlichte, M.J.; Vandersall, A.; Katta, R. Diet and eczema: A review of dietary supplements for the treatment of atopic dermatitis. *Dermatol. Pract. Concept* **2016**, *6*, 23–29. [CrossRef] [PubMed]

24. Wang, W.; Lin, H.; Gu, Y. Multiple roles of dihomo-γ-linolenic acid against proliferation diseases. *Lipids Health Dis.* **2012**, *14*, 11–25. [CrossRef] [PubMed]

25. Fujiyama-Fujiwara, Y.; Ohmori, C.; Igarashi, O. Metabolism of γ-linolenic acid in primary cultures of rat hepatocytes and in Hep G2 cells. *J. Nutr. Sci. Vitaminol.* **1989**, *35*, 597–611. [CrossRef] [PubMed]

26. Ziboh, V.A.; Naguwa, S.; Vang, K.; Wineinger, J.; Morrissey, B.M.; Watnik, M.; Gershwin, M.E. Suppression of leukotriene B4 generation by ex-vivo neutrophils isolated from asthma patients on dietary supplementation with gammalinolenic acid-containing borage oil: Possible implication in asthma. *Clin. Dev. Immunol.* **2004**, *11*, 13–21. [CrossRef] [PubMed]

27. Belch, J.J.; Hill, A. Evening primrose oil and borage oil in rheumatologic conditions. *Am. J. Clin. Nutr.* **2000**, *71*, 352–356. [CrossRef] [PubMed]

28. Cao, D.; Luo, J.; Zang, W.; Chen, D.; Xu, H.; Shi, H.; Jing, H. Gamma-Linolenic Acid Suppresses NF-κB Signaling via CD36 in the Lipopolysaccharide-Induced Inflammatory Response in Primary Goat Mammary Gland Epithelial Cells. *Inflammation* **2016**, *39*, 1225–1237. [CrossRef] [PubMed]

29. Surette, M.E.; Koumenis, I.L.; Edens, M.B.; Tramposch, K.M.; Clayton, B.; Bowton, D.; Chilton, F.H. Inhibition of leukotriene biosynthesis by a novel dietary fatty acid formulation in patients with atopic asthma: A randomized, placebo-controlled, parallel-group, prospective trial. *Clin. Ther.* **2003**, *25*, 972–979. [CrossRef]

30. Khajeh, M.; Rahbarghazi, R.; Nouri, M.; Darabi, M. Potential role of polyunsaturated fatty acids, with particular regard to the signaling pathways of arachidonic acid and its derivatives in the process of maturation of the oocytes: Contemporary review. *Biomed. Pharmacother.* **2017**, *94*, 458–467. [CrossRef] [PubMed]

31. Larsson, S.C.; Kumlin, M.; Ingelman-Sunberg, M.; Wolk, A. Dietary long-chain n-3 fatty acids for the prevention of cancer: A review of potential mechanisms. *Am. J. Clin. Nutr.* **2004**, *79*, 935–945. [CrossRef] [PubMed]

32. Nilsen, D.W.T.; Aarsetoey, H.; Ponitz, V.; Brugger-Andersen, T.; Staines, H.; Harris, W.S.; Grundt, H. The prognostic utility of dihomo-gamma-linolenic acid (DGLA) in patients with acute coronary heart disease. *Int. J. Cardiol.* **2017**, *249*, 12–17. [CrossRef] [PubMed]

33. Łuczaj, W.; Gęgotek, A.; Skrzydlewska, E. Antioxidants and HNE in redox homeostasis. *Free Radic. Biol. Med.* **2017**, *111*, 87–101. [CrossRef]

34. Park, K.Y.; Ko, E.J.; Kim, I.S.; Li, K.; Kim, B.J.; Seo, S.J.; Kim, M.N.; Hong, C.K. The effect of evening primrose oil for the prevention of xerotic cheilitis in acne patients being treated with isotretinoin: A pilot study. *Ann. Dermatol.* **2014**, *26*, 706–712. [CrossRef] [PubMed]

35. Antal, O.; Peter, M.; Hackler, L., Jr.; Man, I.; Szebeni, G.; Ayaydin, F.; Hideghety, K.; Vigh, L.; Kitajka, K.; Balogh, G.; et al. Lipidomic analysis reveals a radiosensitizing role of gamma-linolenic acid in glioma cells. *Biochim. Biophys. Acta* **2015**, *1851*, 1271–1282. [CrossRef] [PubMed]

36. Das, U.N.; Rao, K.P. Effect of γ-linolenic acid and prostaglandins E1 on gamma-radiation and chemical-induced genetic damage to the bone marrow cells of mice. *Prostaglandins Leukot. Essent Fat. Acids* **2006**, *74*, 165–173. [CrossRef] [PubMed]

37. Menendez, J.A.; Vellon, L.; Colomer, R.; Lupu, R. Effect of γ-Linolenic Acid on the Transcriptional Activity of the Her-2/neu (erbB-2) Oncogene. *J. Natl. Cancer Inst.* **2005**, *2*, 1611–1615. [CrossRef] [PubMed]

38. Marshall, J.C.; Lee, J.H.; Steeg, P.S. Clinical-translational strategies for the elevation of Nm23-H1 metastasis suppressor gene expression. *Mol. Cell Biochem.* **2009**, *329*, 115–120. [CrossRef] [PubMed]

39. Jiang, W.G.; Hiscox, S.; Bryce, R.P.; Horrobin, D.F.; Mansel, R.E. The effects of n-6 polyunsaturated fatty acids on the expression of nm-23 in human cancer cells. *Br. J. Cancer* **1998**, *77*, 731–738. [CrossRef] [PubMed]

40. Miyake, J.A.; Benadiba, M.; Colquhoun, A. Gamma-linolenic acid inhibits both tumour cell cycle progression and angiogenesis in the orthotopic C6 glioma model through changes in VEGF, Flt1, ERK1/2, MMP2, cyclin D1, pRb, p53 and p27 protein expression. *Lipids Health Dis.* **2009**, *17*. [CrossRef] [PubMed]

41. Aragona, P.; Bucolo, S.; Spinella, R.; Giuffrida, S.; Ferreri, G. Systemic Omega-6 Essential Fatty Acid Treatment and PGE$_1$ Tear Content in Sjögren's Syndrome Patients, Investigative Ophthalmology & Visual Science. *Investig. Ophthalmol. Vis. Sci.* **2005**, *46*, 4474–4479. [CrossRef]

42. Dasgupta, S.; Bhattacharyya, D.K. Dietary effect of γ-linolenic acid on the lipid profile of rat fed erucic acid rich oil. *J. Oleo Sci.* **2007**, *56*, 569–577. [CrossRef] [PubMed]

43. Ras, R.T.; Geleijnse, J.M.; Trautwein, E.A. LDL-cholesterol-lowering effect of plant sterols and stanols across different dose ranges: A metaanalysis of randomized controlled studies. *Br. J. Nutr.* **2014**, *112*, 214–219. [CrossRef] [PubMed]

44. Sivamani, R.K. Eicosanoids and Keratinocytes in Wound Healing. *Adv. Wound Care* **2014**, *3*, 476–481. [CrossRef] [PubMed]

45. Guimaraes, R.F.; Sales-Campos, H.; Nardini, V.; da Costa, T.A.; Fonseca, M.T.C.; Júnior, V.R.; Sorgi, C.A.; da Silva, J.S.; Chica, J.E.L.; Faccioli, L.H.; et al. The inhibition of 5-Lipoxygenase (5-LO) products leukotriene B4 (LTB_4) and cysteinyl leukotrienes (cysLTs) modulates the inflammatory response and improves cutaneous wound healing. *Clin. Immunol.* **2018**, *190*, 74–83. [CrossRef] [PubMed]

13

Redistribution of Extracellular Superoxide Dismutase Causes Neonatal Pulmonary Vascular Remodeling and PH but Protects Against Experimental Bronchopulmonary Dysplasia

Laurie G. Sherlock [1], Ashley Trumpie [2], Laura Hernandez-Lagunas [2], Sarah McKenna [1], Susan Fisher [1], Russell Bowler [3], Clyde J. Wright [1], Cassidy Delaney [1,†] and Eva Nozik-Grayck [2,4,*,†] [iD]

[1]   Department of Pediatrics, Section of Neonatology, University of Colorado Anschutz Medical Campus, Aurora, CO 80045, USA; laura.sherlock@ucdenver.edu (L.G.S.); sarah.mckenna@ucdenver.edu (S.M.); susan.fisher@ucdenver.edu (S.F.); clyde.wright@ucdenver.edu (C.J.W.); cassidy.delaney@childrenscolorado.org (C.D.)
[2]   Cardiovascular Pulmonary Research Laboratories, University of Colorado Anschutz Medical Campus, Aurora, CO 80045, USA; Ashley.trumpie@ucdenver.edu (A.T.); ana-laura.hernandez@ucdenver.edu (L.H.-L.)
[3]   Department of Medicine, National Jewish Health, Denver, CO 80206, USA; bowlerr@njhealth.org
[4]   Pediatric Critical Care Medicine, University of Colorado Anschutz Medical Campus, Aurora, CO 80045, USA
*   Correspondence: eva.grayck@ucdenver.edu
†   Denotes equal senior author contribution.

Abstract: Background: A naturally occurring single nucleotide polymorphism (SNP), ($R_{213}G$), in extracellular superoxide dismutase (SOD3), decreases SOD3 matrix binding affinity. Humans and mature mice expressing the $R_{213}G$ SNP exhibit increased cardiovascular disease but decreased lung disease. The impact of this SNP on the neonatal lung at baseline or with injury is unknown. Methods: Wild type and homozygous $R_{213}G$ mice were injected with intraperitoneal bleomycin or phosphate buffered saline (PBS) three times weekly for three weeks and tissue harvested at 22 days of life. Vascular and alveolar development were evaluated by morphometric analysis and immunostaining of lung sections. Pulmonary hypertension (PH) was assessed by right ventricular hypertrophy (RVH). Lung protein expression for superoxide dismutase (SOD) isoforms, catalase, vascular endothelial growth factor receptor 2 (VEGFR2), endothelial nitric oxide synthase (eNOS) and guanosine triphosphate cyclohydrolase-1 (GTPCH-1) was evaluated by western blot. SOD activity and SOD3 expression were measured in serum. Results: In $R_{213}G$ mice, SOD3 lung protein expression decreased, serum SOD3 protein expression and SOD serum activity increased compared to wild type (WT) mice. Under control conditions, $R_{213}G$ mice developed pulmonary vascular remodeling (decreased vessel density and increased medial wall thickness) and PH; alveolar development was similar between strains. After bleomycin injury, in contrast to WT, $R_{213}G$ mice were protected from impaired alveolar development and their vascular abnormalities and PH did not worsen. Bleomycin decreased VEGFR2 and GTPCH-1 only in WT mice. Conclusion: $R_{213}G$ neonatal mice demonstrate impaired vascular development and PH at baseline without alveolar simplification, yet are protected from bleomycin induced lung injury and worsening of pulmonary vascular remodeling and PH. These results show that vessel bound SOD3 is essential in normal pulmonary vascular development, and increased serum SOD3 expression and SOD activity prevent lung injury in experimental bronchopulmonary dysplasia (BPD) and PH.

Keywords: extracellular superoxide dismutase; R213G single nucleotide polymorphism; neonate; bronchopulmonary dysplasia; pulmonary hypertension

1. Introduction

Bronchopulmonary dysplasia (BPD) is a disorder of lung development affecting preterm infants resulting in respiratory morbidities that can persist through adulthood [1]. Despite advances in neonatal care, the incidence of BPD is increasing [2]. A subset of infants with BPD also develop pulmonary hypertension (PH), characterized by impaired angiogenesis, pulmonary vascular remodeling and right ventricular failure, which significantly increases the morbidity and mortality [3,4]. Interventions to prevent and treat BPD complicated by PH are limited, thus there is an urgent need to improve understanding of the mechanisms contributing to the development of these frequent and burdensome diseases of prematurity.

Oxidative stress is central to the etiology of BPD and PH [5,6]. Antioxidant enzymes and essential nutrients that contribute to antioxidant status increase prior to birth and prepare infants for the increased partial pressure of oxygen with post-natal room air breathing [6]. Premature neonates have decreased antioxidant defenses, and increased oxidative stress due to oxygen therapy, infection, and mechanical ventilation [6]. However, despite compelling evidence that an imbalance of oxidative stress contributes to BPD and PH, generalized antioxidant therapies have not proven efficacious to preventing or treating these diseases [6]. An enhanced understanding of how antioxidants impact regional redox signaling may lead to more effective targeted antioxidant therapies that improve clinical outcomes.

A human single nucleotide polymorphism (SNP) of the antioxidant enzyme extracellular superoxide dismutase (EC-SOD or SOD3) provides insight into how the specific location of SOD3 influences human disease risk. The $R_{213}G$ SNP (rs1799895) is observed in 3–6% of studied populations; this SNP does not change enzyme activity, but lowers tissue binding [7]. SOD3 is typically tethered to the extracellular matrix (ECM) by a series of positively charged amino acids that bind to the negatively charged ligands in the ECM and glycocalyx of endothelial and epithelial cells [8,9]. The rs1799895 SNP leads to a single amino acid substitution from arginine to glycine at position 213 within the matrix binding region, lowering the matrix binding affinity of SOD3, and redistributing SOD3 from the lung parenchyma and vasculature into the plasma and epithelial lining fluid [7,10,11]. In humans, the $R_{213}G$ SNP is associated with decreased risk of chronic obstructive pulmonary disease (COPD) and asthma [12,13]. Adult mice harboring the same SNP are protected from intratracheal lipopolysaccharide (LPS) inflammation, bleomycin induced pulmonary fibrosis and PH, and ovalbumin (OVA) induced airway obstruction [7,12,14]. Conversely, this SNP is associated with worse outcomes in ischemic heart disease [15], and adult mice exhibit PH at baseline and exaggerated chronic hypoxia-induced PH [7,14]. The divergent risk profiles imparted by the $R_{213}G$ SNP in different diseases illustrates the importance of the site of oxidative stress and antioxidant defenses in disease pathogenesis.

SOD3 is developmentally regulated, and SOD3 deficient neonatal mice exhibit impaired alveolar and pulmonary vascular development at baseline [16]. The expression and activity of SOD3 is decreased in neonatal models of BPD and/or PH [17,18]. Overall SOD3 content influences response to disease, as overexpression of SOD3 ameliorates experimental BPD and/or PH [19–21], and SOD3 deficiency aggravates injury in experimental BPD and PH [16]. These findings provide evidence that SOD3 content is important in the normal developing lung and with neonatal lung injury, however the impact of the distribution of SOD3 on the developing lung and with injury is unknown. The $R_{213}G$ SNP provides a unique opportunity to interrogate the impact of SOD3 distribution as it only changes SOD3 location. We hypothesized that the redistribution of SOD3 from the lung and vasculature into the extracellular fluids due to the $R_{213}G$ SNP would impair baseline alveolar and/or vascular development and worsen neonatal BPD and PH.

2. Methods

2.1. Mouse Model

All animal studies were approved by the University of Colorado Denver Institutional Animal Care and Use Committee (IACUC) (B-7117(01)1E). C57BL/6 wild-type mice (Jackson Laboratory, Bar Harbor, ME, USA) and genetically engineered mice on the C57BL/6 background with knock-in of the human $R_{213}G$ SNP into the matrix binding region were raised in Denver altitude [7]. Bleomycin, a chemotherapeutic agent that induces significant lung fibrosis and inflammation in adults [22,23], has been adapted into a model of experimental BPD and PH in neonatal rodents, characterized by alveolar simplification, decreased vascular development, and vascular remodeling similar to infants with BPD complicated by PH [16,24–26]. Neonatal male and female mice were injected with 10 µL of intraperitoneal phosphate buffered saline (PBS) or bleomycin (3 units/kg/dose, dissolved in 10 µL PBS) (Hospira, Lake Forest, IL, USA), three times a week for three weeks for a total bleomycin exposure of 27 units/kg. Bleomycin was dosed per weight at each injection. Injections were started on day of life 2 and ended on day of life 22. Since the lungs of newborn mice are in the saccular stage of lung development, the 2-day old mouse at the onset of treatment models the stage of lung development of human infants born at 28–32 weeks [27]. Mice were anesthetized with 1.5% isoflurane, then euthanized with 100 µL of Fatal-Plus solution (Vortech Pharmaceuticals, Dearbon, MI, USA) and thoracotomy for tissue harvesting at 22 days of life, allowing for assessment during the late alveolar stage of development. Lungs were flushed with PBS and were either frozen in All-Protect (Qiagen, Valencia, CA, USA) for protein isolation, or inflation-fixed at 25 cm H_2O with 4% paraformaldehyde for paraffin embedding.

2.2. Immunohistochemistry

Immunohistochemistry for alpha smooth muscle actin (α-SMA)was performed as previously described with mouse monoclonal α-SMA antibody (1:1500, clone1A4; Sigma, St. Louis, MO, USA) and Mouse on Mouse (M.O.M.) immunodetection kit with ready-to-use anti-mouse secondary IgG antibody (Vector Laboratories, Burlingame, CA, USA) [16]. Additionally, lung sections were stained with rabbit anti-vWF (1:1500, Sigma-Aldrich, St. Louis, MO, USA), and ready-to- use horse radish peroxidase (HRP) conjugated anti-rabbit IgG (ImmPress Kit, Vector Laboratories, Burlingame, CA, USA). Slides were developed with Vector very intense purple (VIP) peroxidase (HRP) substrate kit (Vector Laboratories, Burlingame, CA, USA) and counterstained with methyl green.

2.3. Evaluation of Pulmonary Vascular Structure

Vessel density was assessed by counting the number of vessels <30 µm staining positive for von Willebrand Factor (vWF) per high-power field (20×). Lung fields containing large vessels or airways were excluded, and a minimum of 8 fields were included per mouse. Medial wall thickness was calculated for α-SMA stained vessels 30–100 µm located adjacent to airways [28]. The width of the medial wall was measured in four perpendicular locations and an average was calculated. The external diameter was measured in two locations, this was then averaged and divided by two to calculate the average radius. The medial wall thickness (MWT) was expressed as average width of the medial wall/average radius. The analysis was performed by an investigator blinded to the experiment group.

2.4. Evaluation of Alveolar Development

Radial alveolar counts (RACs) were calculated on hematoxylin and eosin stained lung sections by identifying the terminal bronchiole, drawing a perpendicular line to the lung periphery, and counting each intersection of lung alveoli [29]. At least five images were processed per mouse at 10× magnification. Mean linear intercept (MLI) was measured using Metamorph Basic (Molecular Devices Sunnyvale, San Jose, CA, USA). At least 7 non-overlapping sections per mouse were assessed at 20×

magnification. Fields with large airways or vessels were excluded. The analysis was performed by an investigator blinded to the experiment group.

2.5. Evaluation of Right Ventricular Hypertrophy

Fulton's index, defined as the ratio of right ventricle (RV) weight divided by left ventricle (LV) plus septum (S) (RV/(LV + S)), was determined as a measure of right ventricular hypertrophy. Hearts were stored in 4% paraformaldehyde until dissected, as previously described [16].

2.6. Protein Expression

Western blots were performed on 25 μg protein from total lung homogenates prepared in tissue protein extraction reagent (TPER) lysis buffer with protease and phosphatase inhibitors or 2 μL serum as previously described [30]. Blots were blocked for 1 h using 5% nonfat milk in $1\times$ TBST, then probed overnight at 4 °C using the following antibodies: catalase (1:500, Abcam, Cambridge, UK), superoxide dismutase 1 (SOD1) (1:1000, Abcam, Cambridge, UK), superoxide dismutase 2 (SOD2) (1:1000, Millipore, Billerica, MA, USA), SOD3 (1:1000, Santa Cruz Biotechnology, Santa Cruz, CA, USA), vascular endothelial growth factor receptor 2 (VEGFR2) (1:500, Cell Signaling, Danvers, MA, USA), endothelial nitric oxide synthase (eNOS) (1:1000, BD Biosciences, San Jose, CA, USA), guanosine triphosphate cyclohydrolase-1 (GTPCH-1) (1:1000, Abcam, Cambridge, UK). After washing, blots were incubated for 1 hour at room temperature with the species-appropriate secondary IgG antibody (1:10,000, Millipore, Billerica, MA, USA). They were then developed with SuperSignal Femto (ThermoScientific) or Western Lightning ECL. Blots were then stripped and reprobed with β-actin mouse monoclonal antibody (1:10,000, Sigma-Aldrich, St. Louis, MO, USA) as a loading control. Images were obtained on FluorChemM camera system. Densitometry was done using ImageJ (National Institute of Health, Bethesda, MD, USA) and subtracting for background.

2.7. SOD Activity Assay

SOD activity was measured on serum as previously described using a SOD activity assay kit (Dojindo Molecular Technologies, Santa Clara, CA, USA). Grossly hemolyzed samples were excluded to avoid elevated SOD activity resulting from the release of red blood cell SOD1. The standard curve was performed using bovine erythrocyte SOD1 (Sigma Aldrich, St Louis, MO, USA). SOD activity data were expressed as units of SOD activity per ml of serum [14].

2.8. Statistical Analysis

Data were analyzed using Prism (GraphPad Software, La Jolla, CA, USA) by unpaired t-test or two-way analysis of variance (ANOVA). Post-hoc analysis was performed using Tukey's test when significant differences were found between groups. Data are expressed as mean $\pm$ SD. Significance was defined as $p < 0.05$.

3. Results

3.1. The $R_{213}G$ SNP Redistributed SOD3 from The Lung to The Extracellular Fluid in Neonatal Mice

We first tested how the $R_{213}G$ SNP impacts SOD3 distribution in the immature lung. At 22 days, we observed significantly less SOD3 protein in the lungs of $R_{213}G$ mice (Figure 1a) and elevated serum SOD3 compared to wild type (WT) mice (Figure 1b), recapitulating what we reported previously in adult mice [7]. Serum SOD activity was also elevated in the $R_{213}G$ mice compared to WT (Figure 1c). We next evaluated if the $R_{213}G$ mice compensate for low lung SOD3 content by upregulating other key antioxidant enzymes in the neonatal lung. There was no change in lung SOD1 (Figure 1d,g), SOD2 (Figure 1e,g), or catalase (Figure 1f,g) at 22 days in mice expressing the SOD3 $R_{213}G$ SNP compared to WT mice.

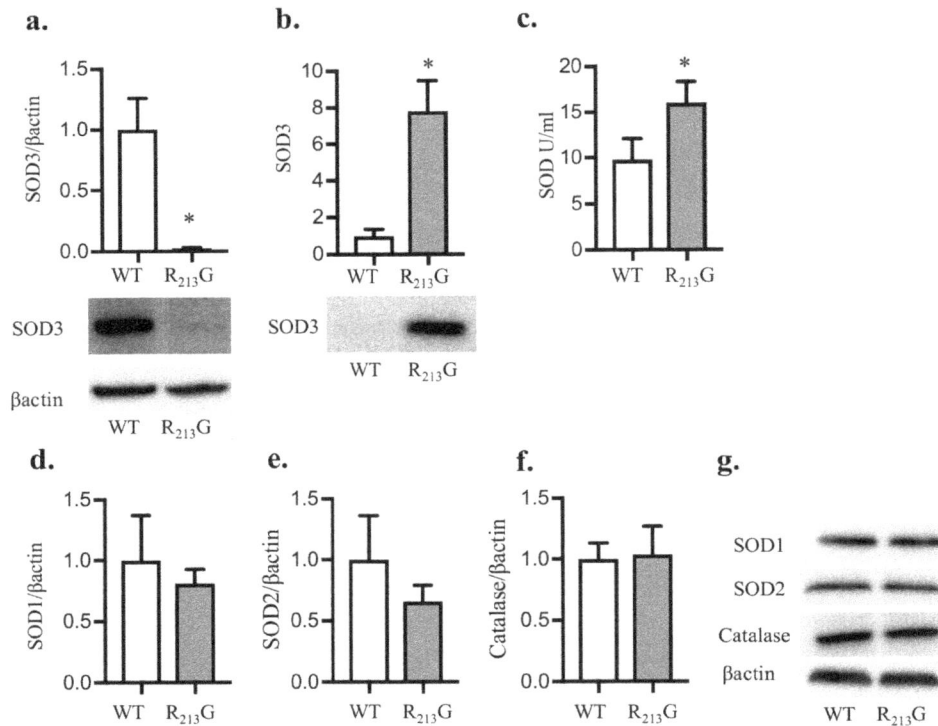

Figure 1. The $R_{213}G$ single nucleotide polymorphism (SNP) redistributed superoxide dismutase (SOD3) from the lung into the plasma at 22 days. SOD3 protein content in the lung and serum was evaluated by western blot analysis in control WT and $R_{213}G$ mice at 22 days of age. A quantity of 25 µg lung protein or 2 µL serum was loaded onto the gels. (**a**) Lung SOD3 (**b**) Serum SOD3. SOD activity in serum was measured using the SOD activity assay (Dojindo). Representative blots are shown below optical density normalized to β-actin and expressed relative to WT mice in Figure 1a,b. (**c**) Serum SOD Activity (units per mL). Several other key antioxidant enzymes were evaluated in the lung by western blot analysis. Representative blots are shown along with optical density normalized to β-actin and expressed relative to WT mice (**d**) Lung superoxide dismutase 1 (SOD1) (**e**) Lung superoxide dismutase 2 (SOD2) (**f**) Lung Catalase. (**g**) Representative blots for SOD1, SOD2, catalase and β-actin are shown).* $p < 0.05$ vs. WT PBS by unpaired t-test, $n = 5$–6 for all groups. WT: wild type.

3.2. Mice Expressing the $R_{213}G$ SNP Demonstrated Impaired Pulmonary Vascular Development and PH Under Control Conditions

In order to evaluate the redistribution of SOD3 on vascular development, we analyzed pulmonary vascular density and remodeling at 22 days. Vessel density (<30 µm) was decreased in the $R_{213}G$ mice (Figure 2c). Medial wall thickness (MWT) in vessels 30–150 µm, a marker of vascular remodeling, was increased in $R_{213}G$ mice (Figure 2f). As a surrogate for PH, we measured right ventricular hypertrophy (RVH) by Fulton's index and found RVH increased in mice expressing the $R_{213}G$ SNP compared to WT mice (Figure 2g). * $p < 0.05$ by unpaired t-test, $n = 5$–6.

3.3. Alveolar Development Was Not Altered in Mice Expressing the $R_{213}G$ SNP

To evaluate the impact of the $R_{213}G$ distribution on alveolar development, we performed morphometric assessment of alveolarization at 22 days with radial alveolar counts (RAC) and mean linear intercept (MLI). RAC and MLI were similar between $R_{213}G$ and WT control mice (Figure 3c,d).

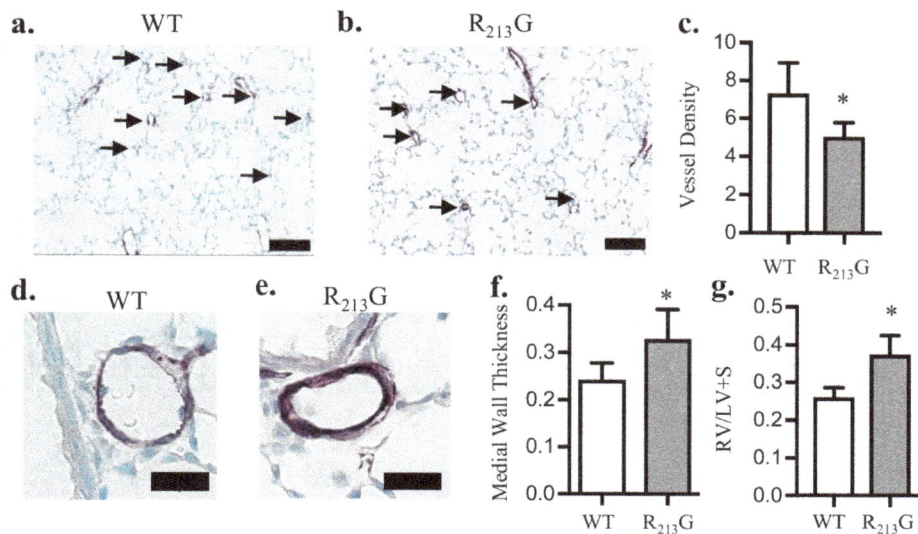

Figure 2. Mice expressing the $R_{213}G$ SNP had impaired pulmonary vascular development and pulmonary hypertension at 22 days. (**a,b**) Representative images of von willebrand factor (vWF) (purple) staining in (**a**) WT and (**b**) $R_{213}G$ control mice. Arrows indicate vessels < 30 μm, scale bar = 100 μm. (**c**) Vessel density in WT and $R_{213}G$ mice, * $p < 0.05$ by unpaired t-test, n= 5–6. (**d,e**) Representative images of alpha smooth muscle actin (αSMA) (purple) staining in (**d**) WT and (**e**) $R_{213}G$ mice, scale bar = 20 μm. (**f**) Medial wall thickness in WT and $R_{213}G$ mice; * $p < 0.05$ vs. WT phosphate buffered saline (PBS) by unpaired t-test, $n = 5$–6. (**g**) Right ventricular (RV)/left ventricular (LV) + septal (S) (RV/LV + S) weights in WT and $R_{213}G$ control mice, * $p < 0.05$ vs. WT PBS by unpaired t-test, $n = 5$–6.

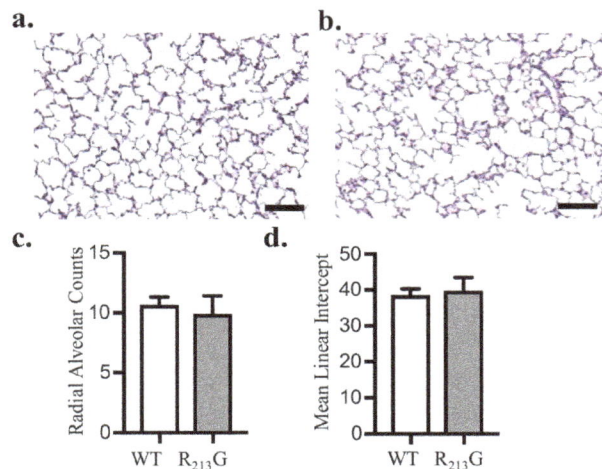

Figure 3. Mice expressing the $R_{213}G$ SNP exhibited normal alveolar development. Representative images of H & E stained lung in 22-day old (**a**) WT and (**b**) $R_{213}G$ control mice, scale bar = 100 μm. (**c**) Radial alveolar counts in control WT and $R_{213}G$ mice $p > 0.05$ by unpaired t-test, $n = 7$–8 (**d**) Mean linear intercepts in control WT and $R_{213}G$ mice. $p > 0.05$ vs. WT PBS by unpaired t-test, $n = 6$–8.

3.4. Bleomycin Did Not Alter Antioxidant Enzyme Expression in the Lung or Plasma in Either Strain

We next sought to determine how the $R_{213}G$ SNP impacts the response to bleomycin induced BPD and PH. First, we tested if bleomycin altered the content or distribution of SOD3 in the $R_{213}G$ mice by comparing bleomycin treated WT and $R_{213}G$ mice to the cohort of mice shown in Figures 1–3. By western blot analysis, bleomycin did not change lung or serum protein SOD3 levels in either mouse strain (Figure 4a,b). Bleomycin additionally did not impact the $R_{213}G$ redistribution of SOD3. Bleomycin did not change serum SOD activity in either strain compared to controls (Figure 4c). When evaluating the lung for changes in key antioxidant enzymes, we found no change in SOD1 (Figure 4d,g), SOD2 (Figure 4e,g), or catalase (Figure 4f,g) in the lungs of either strain after bleomycin exposure.

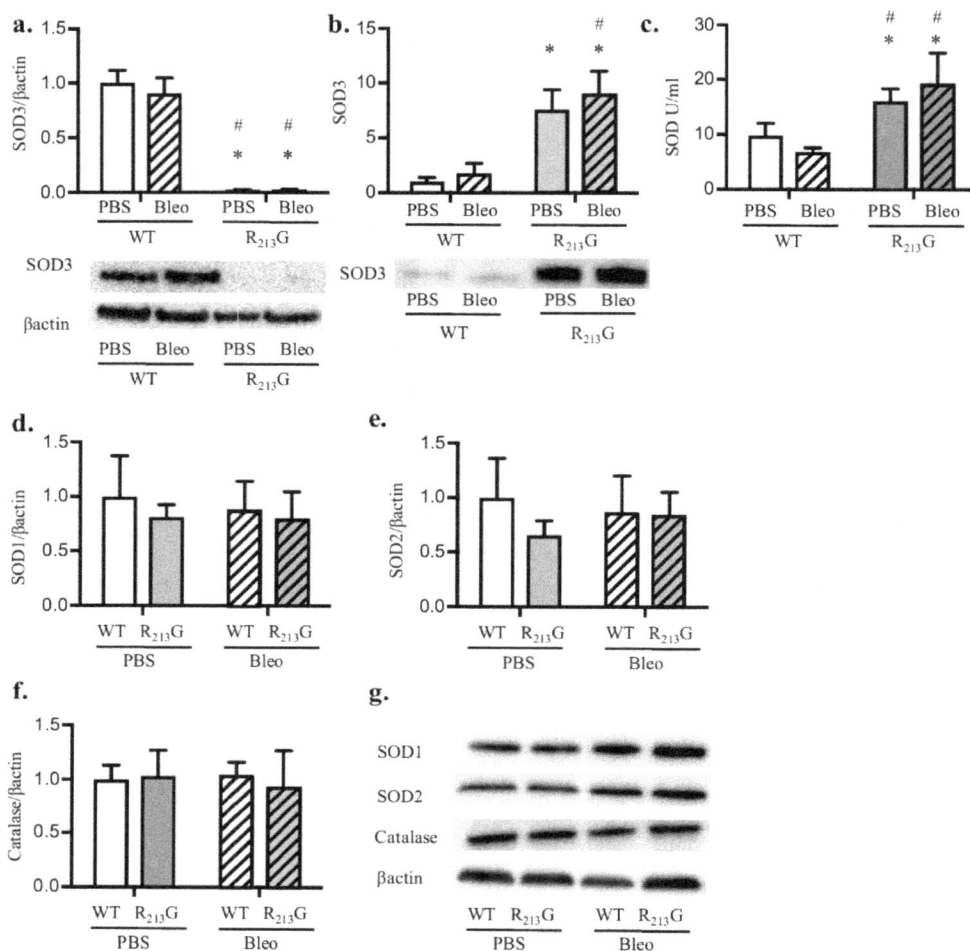

Figure 4. Bleomycin does not change $R_{213}G$ redistribution of SOD3. SOD3 protein content in the lung and serum was evaluated by western blot analysis in WT and $R_{213}G$ mice at 22 days of age after exposure to PBS (10 µL for 9 doses) or bleomycin (3 units/kg/dose dissolved in 10 µL of PBS for 9 doses). 25 µg lung protein or 2 µL serum was loaded onto the gels. (**a**) Lung SOD3 (**b**) Serum SOD3. Representative blots for Figure 4a,b are shown along with optical density normalized to β-actin and expressed relative to WT control mice. SOD activity was measured in serum. (**c**) Serum SOD Activity (units per ml). Several other key antioxidant enzymes were evaluated in the lung by western blot analysis. Representative blots are shown along with optical density normalized to β-actin and expressed relative to WT mice (**d**) Lung SOD1 (**e**) Lung SOD2 (**f**) Lung catalase. (**g**) Representative blots for SOD1, SOD2, catalase and β-actin. * $p < 0.05$ vs. WT PBS, # $p < 0.05$ vs. WT Bleo, all analysis by two-way ANOVA, $n = 5$–6 for all groups.

3.5. Mice Expressing the $R_{213}G$ SNP Do Not Have Further Worsening of Pulmonary Vascular Development or PH after Bleomycin Injury

Intraperitoneal bleomycin is used as a rodent model of BPD and PH. We tested if the redistribution of SOD3 due to the $R_{213}G$ polymorphism would worsen bleomycin induced pulmonary vascular remodeling and PH. Recapitulating our previous findings, in WT mice, bleomycin resulted in pulmonary vascular remodeling with decreased pulmonary vessel density (Figure 5e), and increased medial wall thickness (Figure 5j). Bleomycin also induced PH in WT mice, shown by RVH (Figure 5k). In contrast, bleomycin had no effect on vessel density, MWT, or RVH in the $R_{213}G$ mice compared to baseline (Figure 5e,j,k).

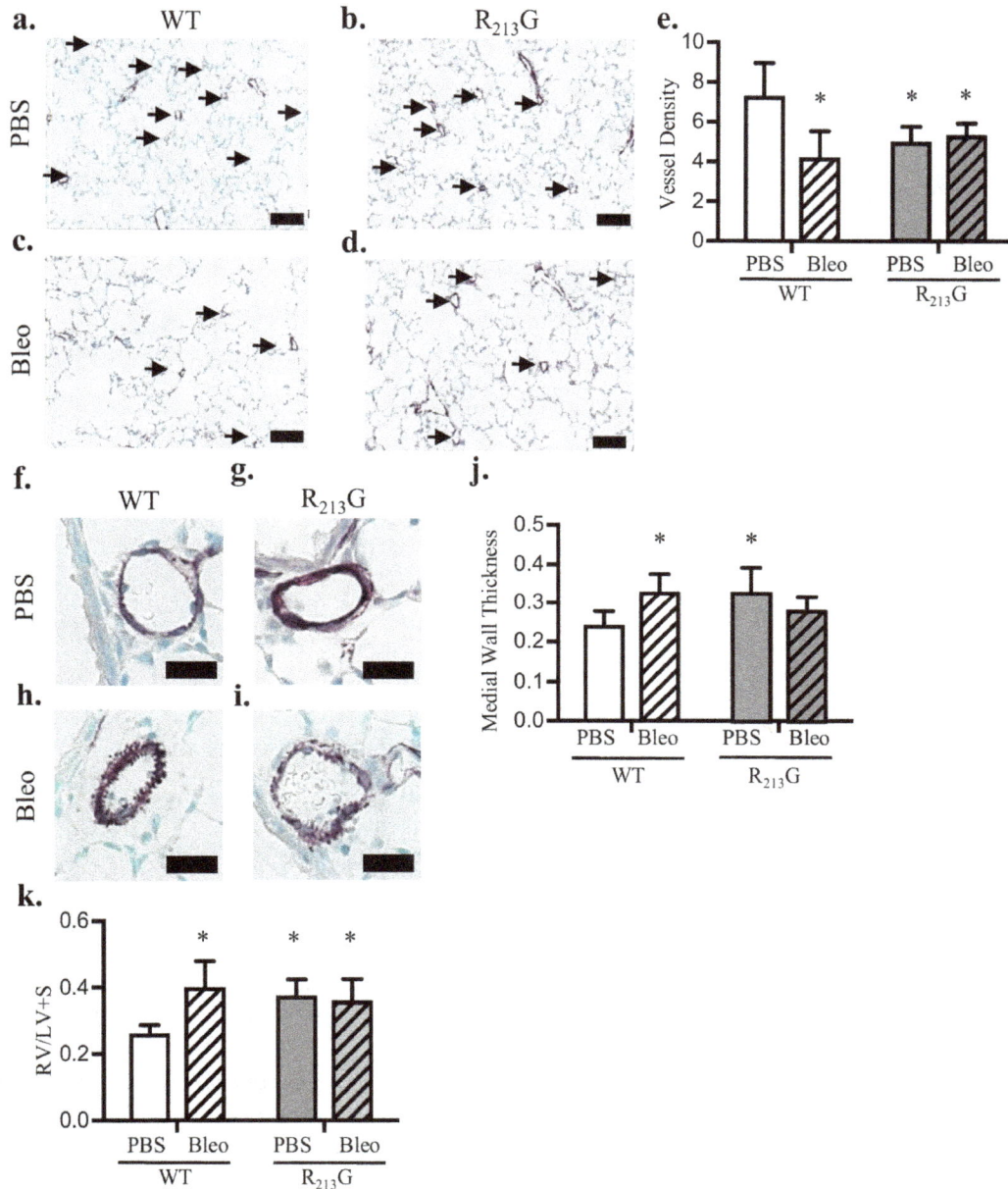

Figure 5. Bleomycin did not further impair the baseline pulmonary vascular impairment or worsen PH in the $R_{213}G$ mice. (**a–d**) Representative images of vWF (purple) staining in (**a**) WT PBS, (**b**) $R_{213}G$ PBS, (**c**) WT Bleo, (**d**) $R_{213}G$ Bleo. Arrows indicate vessels < 30 µm, scale bar = 100 µm. (**e**) Vessel density in WT and $R_{213}G$ mice following exposure to intraperitoneal (IP) PBS or bleomycin, * $p < 0.05$ vs. WT PBS by two-way ANOVA, $n = 6–9$. (**f–i**) Representative images of αSMA (purple) staining in (**f**) WT PBS, (**g**) $R_{213}G$ PBS, (**h**) WT Bleo, (**i**) $R_{213}G$ Bleo, scale bar = 20 µm. (**j**) Medial wall thickness in WT and $R_{213}G$ mice following IP PBS or bleomycin exposure, * $p < 0.05$ vs. WT PBS by two-way ANOVA, $n = 6–7$. (**k**) RV/LV + S weights in WT and $R_{213}G$ mice following IP PBS or bleomycin exposure, * $p < 0.05$ vs. WT PBS by two-way ANOVA, $n = 5–8$.

3.6. The $R_{213}G$ SNP Mitigated Bleomycin Induced Alveolar Simplification at 22 Days

Bleomycin causes impaired alveolar development in WT mice [16]. We performed morphometric assessment of WT mice and mice expressing the $R_{213}G$ SNP exposed to either bleomycin or PBS at 22 days with radial alveolar counts (RAC) and mean linear intercept (MLI). As we have previously shown, in WT mice, RAC decreased and MLI increased after bleomycin exposure (Figure 6e,f). Mice expressing the $R_{213}G$ SNP displayed no evidence of alveolar injury following bleomycin (Figure 6e,f).

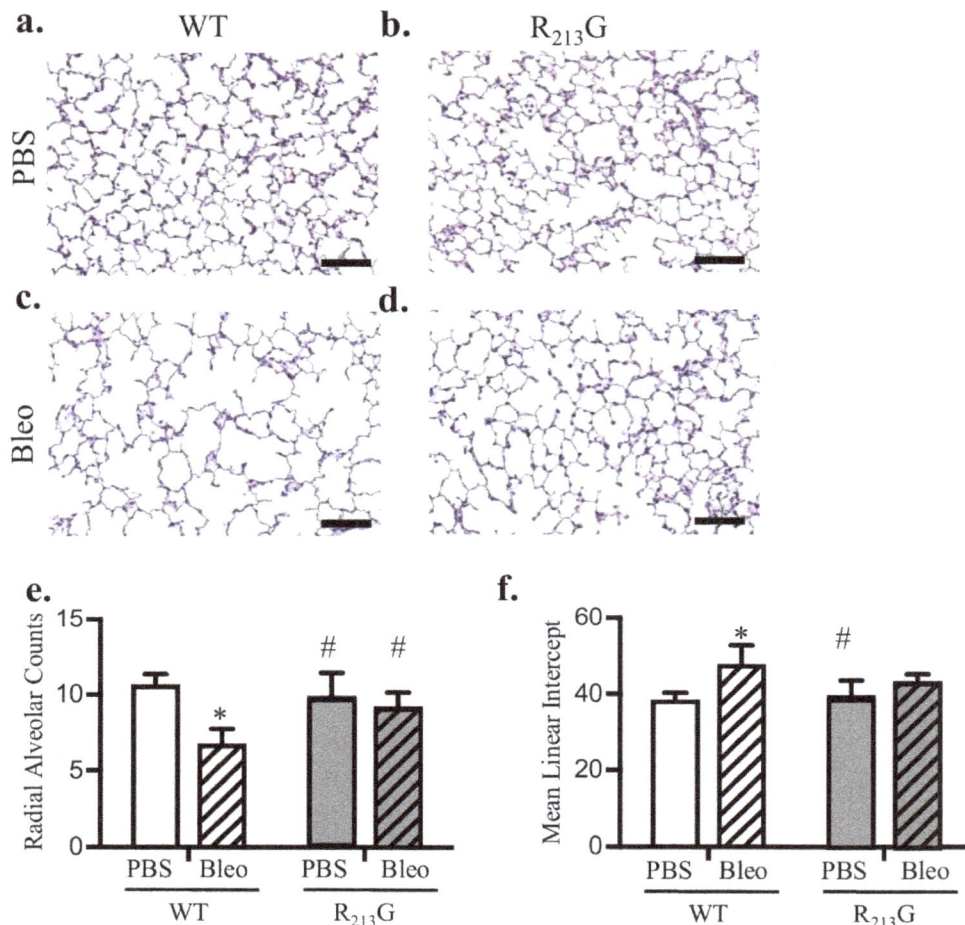

Figure 6. The SOD3 $R_{213}G$ SNP mitigated bleomycin induced alveolar simplification at 22 days. (**a–d**) Representative images of H&E staining in (**a**) WT PBS, (**b**) $R_{213}G$ PBS, (**c**) WT Bleo, (**d**) $R_{213}G$ Bleo, scale bar = 100 μm. (**e**) Radial alveolar counts in WT and $R_{213}G$ mice following IP PBS or bleomycin exposure, * $p < 0.05$ vs. WT PBS by two-way ANOVA, $n = 5$–8. (**f**) Mean linear intercept in WT and $R_{213}G$ mice following IP PBS or bleomycin exposure, scale bar = 200 μm * $p < 0.05$ vs. WT PBS by two-way ANOVA; # $p < 0.05$ vs. WT Bleo by two-way ANOVA $n = 7$–8.

3.7. Bleomycin Only Decreased VEGFR2 and GTPCH-1 Levels in WT Mice

We evaluated VEGFR2 and eNOS protein expression as evidence for impaired vascular endothelial growth factor/nitric oxide (VEGF/NO) signaling. We previously reported these two proteins were decreased in neonatal WT mice treated with bleomycin and mice lacking SOD3 at baseline [16]. We also tested GTPCH-1 expression as it is the rate-limiting enzyme responsible for tetrahydrobiopterin synthesis, a necessary cofactor for eNOS activity. GTPCH-1 is decreased in the setting of impaired SOD3 expression [30,31]. At baseline, VEGFR2 was not significantly different between $R_{213}G$ mice and WT mice (Figure 7a,c). We recapitulated our finding that bleomycin decreased lung VEGFR2 in WT mice (Figure 7a,c). In $R_{213}G$ mice, bleomycin did not decrease VEGFR2 compared to control (Figure 7a,c). There was a trend toward decreased eNOS in the bleomycin treated WT mice but no overall significant change between strain or exposure (Figure 7b,c). Bleomycin decreased GTPCH-1 in WT mice (Figure 7d,e). In the $R_{213}G$ mice GTPCH-1 expression did not change after bleomycin (Figure 7d,e).

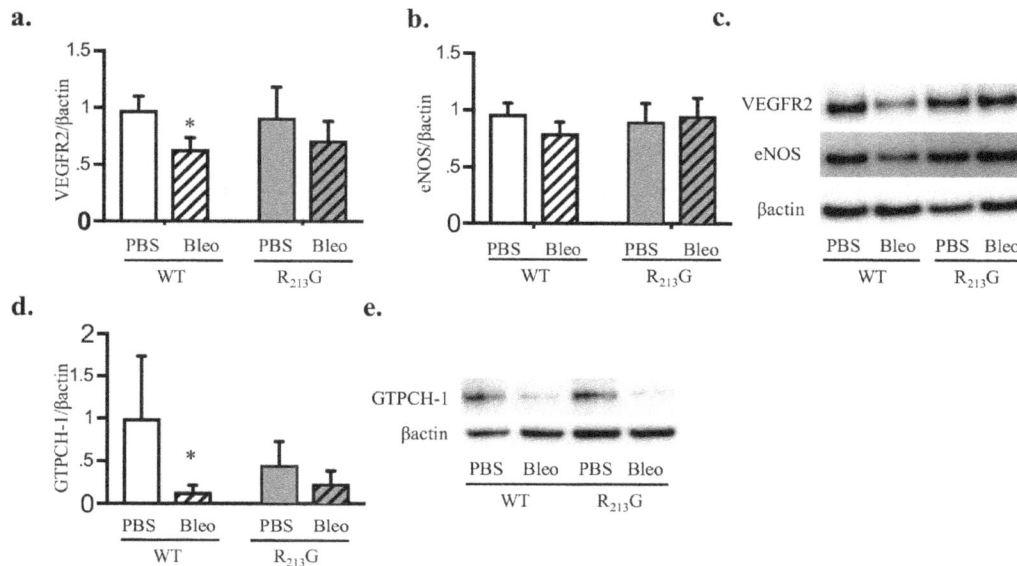

Figure 7. Bleomycin decreased vascular endothelial growth factor receptor 2 (VEGFR2) and guanosine triphosphate cyclohydrolase-1 (GTPCH-1) levels in WT mice. VEGFR2, endothelial nitric oxide synthase (eNOS) and GTPCH-1 protein content in the lung were evaluated by western blot analysis in WT and $R_{213}G$ mice at 22 days of age after exposure to PBS (10 μL for 9 doses) or Bleomycin (3 units/kg/dose dissolved in 10 μL of PBS for 9 doses). 25 μg lung protein was loaded onto the gels. Representative blots are shown along with optical density normalized to β-actin and expressed relative to WT control mice. (**a**) VEGFR2 (**b**) eNOS (**c**) Representative blots for VEGFR2 and eNOS (**d**) GTPCH-1, (**e**) Representative blot for GTPCH-1 * $p < 0.05$ vs. WT PBS, by two-way ANOVA, $n = 5$–6 for all groups.

4. Discussion

The human $R_{213}G$ SOD3 SNP decreases the ability for SOD3 to electrostatically tether to the extracellular matrix and vasculature, resulting in the release of SOD3 from the tissue (lung and vasculature) into the extracellular fluids. This SNP imparts a divergent disease susceptibility, with adult humans at higher risk for ischemic heart disease but lower risk for COPD and asthma [13,15]. Adult mice also exhibit parallel differences in disease susceptibility, demonstrating PH at baseline and aggravated hypoxia induced PH, but protection from LPS and bleomycin lung injury [7,12,14]. In this study, we test the impact of SOD3 redistribution on neonatal lung development and response to bleomycin induced BPD and PH. We report that immature $R_{213}G$ mice demonstrate a redistribution of active SOD3 from the lung into the circulation, similar to adult counterparts with consistent activity after bleomycin. The 22 day old $R_{213}G$ mice exhibit pulmonary vascular remodeling and PH under control conditions that persist but do not worsen in the setting of bleomycin induced lung injury. Despite the baseline vascular abnormalities, the $R_{213}G$ mice have normal alveolar development and are protected against alveolar injury in bleomycin induced BPD. Our study highlights the need to consider the compartmental redox-regulated signaling pathways that account for the discrepancy between vascular and alveolar development attributed to the altered distribution of SOD3. These findings have broad implications for a better understanding of the role for SOD3 in the neonatal lung and consideration of novel approaches to harness this information for more effective therapies.

SOD3 expression and activity are developmentally regulated, thus it was first necessary to evaluate SOD3 distribution in the immature $R_{213}G$ mouse. We observe that the distribution of SOD3 was similar in 22 day old and adult $R_{213}G$ mice, with decreased lung SOD3 and increased serum SOD3 expression and SOD activity [7,14]. Our next important finding is that the redistribution of SOD3 due to the $R_{213}G$ SNP impairs pulmonary vascular development and leads to PH in the developing lung but does not disrupt alveolar development. These findings are consistent with adult mice expressing the $R_{213}G$ SNP, who exhibit PH at baseline, however display normal pulmonary function, with normal airway reactivity and pulmonary mechanics [7,12,14]. In contrast, total body lack of SOD3 results in PH at Denver altitude, and impairs both pulmonary vascular development as well as alveolarization [16]. This suggests that the loss of bound SOD3 worsens vascular development but the presence of alveolar SOD3, despite low lung levels, is sufficient to allow normal alveolar development. Based on the known function of SOD3 to reduce superoxide, generate hydrogen peroxide and preserve nitric oxide (NO) bioactivity, we speculate that the loss of bound SOD3 due to the $R_{213}G$ SNP alters the local redox state in the vessel wall and contributes to abnormal vascular development and PH at baseline [32]. This could occur through a loss of NO bioactivity due to the inactivation of NO. Alternatively, insufficient vascular bound SOD3 may disrupt redox sensitive growth factors or cell adhesion molecules necessary for angiogenesis, either through increased local superoxide or insufficient vascular hydrogen peroxide [33–37]. As alveolar development is not impaired in the $R_{213}G$ mice, bound SOD3 must disrupt separate mechanisms than complete deficiency, where abnormal alveolar and vascular development occur in parallel. These findings add to the literature by demonstrating that in the neonatal lung, SOD3 localization as well as production is critical. This lays a foundation for further investigation to determine which redox regulated signaling pathways are mediated by the loss of vascular SOD3 during development.

We also show that the redistribution of SOD3 due to the $R_{213}G$ SNP prevents bleomycin induced lung injury and does not worsen the underlying pulmonary vascular abnormalities or PH. After bleomycin exposure, serum SOD3 and SOD activity in $R_{213}G$ mice remains elevated compared to WT mice. The mechanism for protection in $R_{213}G$ mice from bleomycin induced lung injury is currently unclear, however we speculate the elevated SOD3 in extracellular fluids attenuates bleomycin induced alveolar injury, pulmonary vascular development and PH by decreasing bleomycin induced oxidative stress. This is supported by work from our lab demonstrating the $R_{213}G$ adult mice exhibit decreased alveolar oxidative stress after intratracheal LPS, and preserved reduced glutathione in the lung after intratracheal bleomycin [7,14]. Alternatively, increased serum SOD3 may modulate lung inflammation, as adult $R_{213}G$ mice develop less alveolar inflammation following intratracheal LPS and show enhanced resolution of bleomycin induced inflammation [7,14]. These findings are in contrast to immature SOD3 knock out mice, who exhibit both aggravated BPD and worsened pulmonary vascular impairments and PH after bleomycin exposure [16]. These findings emphasize the need to understand the etiology of lung injury and PH in individuals, which may vary depending on the stimulus and individual genetic factors. Collectively, these results illustrate that while the total loss of SOD3 worsens both BPD and PH, the redistribution of SOD3 has a discordant effect on vascular vs. alveolar abnormalities in the setting of experimental BPD and PH.

Abnormalities in the VEGF/NO signaling pathway are widely implicated in the pathogenesis of BPD and PH [16,38–40]. VEGFR2 and eNOS expression are decreased in SOD3 knockout mice at baseline and in WT mice after bleomycin injury [16]. GTPCH-1 is the rate limiting enzyme for BH4, an essential cofactor for eNOS, and its deficiency leads to eNOS uncoupling. GTPCH-1 is decreased in ovine neonatal PH and is rescued by recombinant SOD [41–43]. Additionally, smooth muscle cell (SMC) selective knock down of SOD3 decreases GTPCH-1 in hypoxia induced PH [30]. We found bleomycin significantly decreases lung VEGFR2 and GTPCH-1 in WT mice, suggesting the impairment in VEGF/NO signaling is multifactorial, with both loss of VEGF signaling and eNOS uncoupling in the setting of vascular and alveolar injury. It is possible that altered NO signaling contributes to vascular abnormalities at baseline in the $R_{213}G$ mice as our data support an overall trend towards lower levels of lung GTPCH-1 compared to WT. Following bleomycin, there were no changes in lung VEGFR2, eNOS or GTPCH-1 in the $R_{213}G$ mice. This provides further support that the VEGF/NO signaling pathway is not solely responsible for the pathologic changes observed in bleomycin induced lung injury [24,26,44–48].

These data raise interesting observations regarding the relationship between alveolar and pulmonary vascular development. The findings in the $R_{213}G$ mice indicate that impaired vascular development does not always occur in parallel with impaired alveolar development. While numerous studies of neonatal BPD and PH demonstrate interdependent angiogenesis and alveolar development [38–40,49], other studies, such as a murine postnatal growth restriction and an ovine model of hypoxia induced neonatal PH, show normal alveolar growth despite neonatal vascular impairments and PH, consistent with this current study [50,51]. In addition, other models of neonatal lung injury are characterized by increased angiogenesis and highlight the importance of developmental stage as well as stimulus of injury [52,53]. To further illustrate that different mechanisms can drive alveolar and vascular impairments in the developing lung, multiple therapeutic strategies investigated in the bleomycin model of BPD and PH, including Rho-kinase inhibition, inhaled NO, and serotonin antagonism only ameliorate pulmonary vascular remodeling and PH, but fail to prevent bleomycin-induced alveolar damage [24,26,44–48]. These studies and ours highlight the complexity of normal pulmonary development and have important implications in understanding the risk factors and approach to treatment for at risk preterm infants.

A limitation of this study is that alveolar and vascular development are dynamic processes and only a single time point during the late alveolar stage was evaluated in this study. It is possible that we are missing subtle abnormalities in alveolarization at earlier time points in the $R_{213}G$ mice that have resolved with compensatory alveolar growth by 22 days of life, as is seen in some preterm infants with BPD who demonstrate improved airway abnormalities over time [54,55]. Sex differences are increasingly recognized as important in disease susceptibility, and have been demonstrated in neonatal hyperoxic lung injury as well as bleomycin induced lung injury in aged adult mice but not young adult mice [56,57]. While our preliminary analysis does not show a signal for any differences between sex at baseline or after exposure, we do not have a sufficient number of mice in each group to conclusively determine sex differences. In addition, while we did not find any effect of the $R_{213}G$ SNP on three key antioxidant enzymes, it is possible that a more comprehensive evaluation of the lung expression profile would identify a compensatory response to low lung SOD3 content in these mice. Additionally, due to technical challenges in neonatal mice, we did not measure bronchial alveolar lavage fluid (BALF) SOD3, though our prior studies in adult mice demonstrated elevated SOD3 in both serum and BALF in $R_{213}G$ mice at baseline and with bleomycin.

5. Conclusions

We conclude that a change in the distribution of SOD3 due to the $R_{213}G$ SNP leads to pulmonary vascular remodeling and PH at baseline, but protects against experimental neonatal lung injury. This has important therapeutic implications, as an improved understanding of where as well as how SOD3 is protective may lead to the development of more specifically targeted antioxidant therapies for the prevention and treatment of BPD and PH.

Acknowledgments: This study was supported by National Institute of Health/National Heart, Lung and Blood Institute (NIH/NHLBI) HL086680 and HL119533 to Eva Nozik-Grayck, NIH/NHLBI K08HL132014 to Cassidy Delaney, NIH/NHLBI HL132941 to Clyde J. Wright, by National Institute of Health/National Institute of Child Health and Human Development (NIH/NICHD) T32007186-32 to Laura G. Sherlock, the American Academy of Pediatrics (AAP) Marshall Klaus award and the Neonatal Cardiopulmonary Young Investigator award to Laura G. Sherlock. We gratefully thank Jeryl Sandoval and Joanna Maltzahn for technical support.

Author Contributions: Eva Nozik-Grayck, Cassidy Delaney, Russell Bowler and Laura G. Sherlock conceived and designed the experiments; Laura G. Sherlock, Clyde J. Wright, Laura Hernandez-Lagunas and Susan Fisher contributed to the experiments, Laura G. Sherlock, Eva Nozik-Grayck, Cassidy Delaney, Russell Bowler and Clyde J. Wright, analyzed the data, Laura G. Sherlock wrote the paper; Eva Nozik-Grayck, Cassidy Delaney, Russell Bowler and Clyde J. Wright revised the manuscript.

Conflicts of Interest: The authors declare no conflict of interest.

References

1.　Islam, J.Y.; Keller, R.L.; Aschner, J.L.; Hartert, T.V.; Moore, P.E. Understanding the short- and long-term respiratory outcomes of prematurity and bronchopulmonary dysplasia. *Am. J. Respir. Crit. Care Med.* **2015**, *192*, 134–156. [CrossRef] [PubMed]

2.　Stoll, B.J.; Hansen, N.I.; Bell, E.F.; Walsh, M.C.; Carlo, W.A.; Shankaran, S.; Laptook, A.R.; Sanchez, P.J.; Van Meurs, K.P.; Wyckoff, M.; et al. Trends in care practices, morbidity, and mortality of extremely preterm neonates, 1993–2012. *JAMA* **2015**, *314*, 1039–1051. [CrossRef] [PubMed]

3.　Jensen, E.A.; Schmidt, B. Epidemiology of bronchopulmonary dysplasia. *Birth Defects Res. Part A Clin. Mol. Teratol.* **2014**, *100*, 145–157. [CrossRef] [PubMed]

4.　Khemani, E.; McElhinney, D.B.; Rhein, L.; Andrade, O.; Lacro, R.V.; Thomas, K.C.; Mullen, M.P. Pulmonary artery hypertension in formerly premature infants with bronchopulmonary dysplasia: Clinical features and outcomes in the surfactant era. *Pediatrics* **2007**, *120*, 1260–1269. [CrossRef] [PubMed]

5.　Wedgwood, S.; Steinhorn, R.H. Role of reactive oxygen species in neonatal pulmonary vascular disease. *Antioxid. Redox Signal.* **2014**, *21*, 1926–1942. [CrossRef] [PubMed]

6.　Berkelhamer, S.K.; Farrow, K.N. Developmental regulation of antioxidant enzymes and their impact on neonatal lung disease. *Antioxid. Redox Signal.* **2014**, *21*, 1837–1848. [CrossRef] [PubMed]

7.　Hartney, J.M.; Stidham, T.; Goldstrohm, D.A.; Oberley-Deegan, R.E.; Weaver, M.R.; Valnickova-Hansen, Z.; Scavenius, C.; Benninger, R.K.; Leahy, K.F.; Johnson, R.; et al. A common polymorphism in extracellular superoxide dismutase affects cardiopulmonary disease risk by altering protein distribution. *Circ. Cardiovasc. Genet.* **2014**, *7*, 659–666. [CrossRef] [PubMed]

8.　Adachi, T.; Kodera, T.; Ohta, H.; Hayashi, K.; Hirano, K. The heparin binding site of human extracellular-superoxide dismutase. *Arch. Biochem. Biophys.* **1992**, *297*, 155–161. [CrossRef]

9.　Karlsson, K.; Lindahl, U.; Marklund, S.L. Binding of human extracellular superoxide dismutase C to sulphated glycosaminoglycans. *Biochem. J.* **1988**, *256*, 29–33. [CrossRef] [PubMed]

10.　Olsen, D.A.; Petersen, S.V.; Oury, T.D.; Valnickova, Z.; Thogersen, I.B.; Kristensen, T.; Bowler, R.P.; Crapo, J.D.; Enghild, J.J. The intracellular proteolytic processing of extracellular superoxide dismutase (EC-SOD) is a two-step event. *J. Biol. Chem.* **2004**, *279*, 22152–22157. [CrossRef] [PubMed]

11.　Petersen, S.V.; Olsen, D.A.; Kenney, J.M.; Oury, T.D.; Valnickova, Z.; Thogersen, I.B.; Crapo, J.D.; Enghild, J.J. The high concentration of Arg213→Gly extracellular superoxide dismutase (EC-SOD) in plasma is caused by a reduction of both heparin and collagen affinities. *Biochem. J.* **2005**, *385*, 427–432. [CrossRef] [PubMed]

12.　Gaurav, R.; Varasteh, J.T.; Weaver, M.R.; Jacobson, S.R.; Hernandez-Lagunas, L.; Liu, Q.; Nozik-Grayck, E.; Chu, H.W.; Alam, R.; Nordestgaard, B.G.; et al. The R213G polymorphism in SOD3 protects against allergic airway inflammation. *JCI Insight* **2017**, *2*. [CrossRef] [PubMed]

13.　Juul, K.; Tybjaerg-Hansen, A.; Marklund, S.; Lange, P.; Nordestgaard, B.G. Genetically increased antioxidative protection and decreased chronic obstructive pulmonary disease. *Am. J. Respir. Crit. Care Med.* **2006**, *173*, 858–864. [CrossRef] [PubMed]

14.　Mouradian, G.C.; Gaurav, R.; Pugliese, S.; El Kasmi, K.; Hartman, B.; Hernandez-Lagunas, L.; Stenmark, K.R.; Bowler, R.P.; Nozik-Grayck, E. Superoxide dismutase 3 R213G single-nucleotide polymorphism blocks murine bleomycin-induced fibrosis and promotes resolution of inflammation. *Am. J. Respir. Cell Mol. Biol.* **2017**, *56*, 362–371. [CrossRef] [PubMed]

15.　Juul, K.; Tybjaerg-Hansen, A.; Marklund, S.; Heegaard, N.H.; Steffensen, R.; Sillesen, H.; Jensen, G.; Nordestgaard, B.G. Genetically reduced antioxidative protection and increased ischemic heart disease risk: The copenhagen city heart study. *Circulation* **2004**, *109*, 59–65. [CrossRef] [PubMed]

16. Delaney, C.; Wright, R.H.; Tang, J.R.; Woods, C.; Villegas, L.; Sherlock, L.; Savani, R.C.; Abman, S.H.; Nozik-Grayck, E. Lack of EC-SOD worsens alveolar and vascular development in a neonatal mouse model of bleomycin-induced bronchopulmonary dysplasia and pulmonary hypertension. *Pediatric Res.* **2015**, *78*, 634–640. [CrossRef] [PubMed]

17. Giles, B.L.; Suliman, H.; Mamo, L.B.; Piantadosi, C.A.; Oury, T.D.; Nozik-Grayck, E. Prenatal hypoxia decreases lung extracellular superoxide dismutase expression and activity. *Am. J. Physiol. Lung Cell. Mol. Physiol.* **2002**, *283*, L549–L554. [CrossRef] [PubMed]

18. Poonyagariyagorn, H.K.; Metzger, S.; Dikeman, D.; Mercado, A.L.; Malinina, A.; Calvi, C.; McGrath-Morrow, S.; Neptune, E.R. Superoxide dismutase 3 dysregulation in a murine model of neonatal lung injury. *Am. J. Respir. Cell Mol. Biol.* **2014**, *51*, 380–390. [CrossRef] [PubMed]

19. Auten, R.L.; O'Reilly, M.A.; Oury, T.D.; Nozik-Grayck, E.; Whorton, M.H. Transgenic extracellular superoxide dismutase protects postnatal alveolar epithelial proliferation and development during hyperoxia. *Am. J. Physiol. Lung Cell. Mol. Physiol.* **2006**, *290*, L32–L40. [CrossRef] [PubMed]

20. Ahmed, M.N.; Suliman, H.B.; Folz, R.J.; Nozik-Grayck, E.; Golson, M.L.; Mason, S.N.; Auten, R.L. Extracellular superoxide dismutase protects lung development in hyperoxia-exposed newborn mice. *Am. J. Respir. Crit. Care Med.* **2003**, *167*, 400–405. [CrossRef] [PubMed]

21. Min, J.H.; Codipilly, C.N.; Nasim, S.; Miller, E.J.; Ahmed, M.N. Synergistic protection against hyperoxia-induced lung injury by neutrophils blockade and EC-SOD overexpression. *Respir. Res.* **2012**, *13*, 58. [CrossRef] [PubMed]

22. Della Latta, V.; Cecchettini, A.; Del Ry, S.; Morales, M.A. Bleomycin in the setting of lung fibrosis induction: From biological mechanisms to counteractions. *Pharmacol. Res.* **2015**, *97*, 122–130. [CrossRef] [PubMed]

23. Hecht, S.M. DNA strand scission by activated bleomycin group antibiotics. *Fed. Proc.* **1986**, *45*, 2784–2791. [PubMed]

24. Sewing, A.C.; Kantores, C.; Ivanovska, J.; Lee, A.H.; Masood, A.; Jain, A.; McNamara, P.J.; Tanswell, A.K.; Jankov, R.P. Therapeutic hypercapnia prevents bleomycin-induced pulmonary hypertension in neonatal rats by limiting macrophage-derived tumor necrosis factor-alpha. *Am. J. Physiol. Lung Cell. Mol. Physiol.* **2012**, *303*, L75–L87. [CrossRef] [PubMed]

25. Grasemann, H.; Dhaliwal, R.; Ivanovska, J.; Kantores, C.; McNamara, P.J.; Scott, J.A.; Belik, J.; Jankov, R.P. Arginase inhibition prevents bleomycin-induced pulmonary hypertension, vascular remodeling, and collagen deposition in neonatal rat lungs. *Am. J. Physiol. Lung Cell. Mol. Physiol.* **2015**, *308*, L503–L510. [CrossRef] [PubMed]

26. Lee, A.H.; Dhaliwal, R.; Kantores, C.; Ivanovska, J.; Gosal, K.; McNamara, P.J.; Letarte, M.; Jankov, R.P. Rho-kinase inhibitor prevents bleomycin-induced injury in neonatal rats independent of effects on lung inflammation. *Am. J. Respir. Cell Mol. Biol.* **2014**, *50*, 61–73. [PubMed]

27. Nardiello, C.; Mizikova, I.; Morty, R.E. Looking ahead: Where to next for animal models of bronchopulmonary dysplasia? *Cell Tissue Res.* **2017**, *367*, 457–468. [CrossRef] [PubMed]

28. Van Rheen, Z.; Fattman, C.; Domarski, S.; Majka, S.; Klemm, D.; Stenmark, K.R.; Nozik-Grayck, E. Lung extracellular superoxide dismutase overexpression lessens bleomycin-induced pulmonary hypertension and vascular remodeling. *Am. J. Respir. Cell Mol. Biol.* **2011**, *44*, 500–508. [CrossRef] [PubMed]

29. Cooney, T.P.; Thurlbeck, W.M. The radial alveolar count method of emery and mithal: A reappraisal 2–intrauterine and early postnatal lung growth. *Thorax* **1982**, *37*, 580–583. [CrossRef] [PubMed]

30. Nozik-Grayck, E.; Woods, C.; Taylor, J.M.; Benninger, R.K.; Johnson, R.D.; Villegas, L.R.; Stenmark, K.R.; Harrison, D.G.; Majka, S.M.; Irwin, D.; et al. Selective depletion of vascular EC-SOD augments chronic hypoxic pulmonary hypertension. *Am. J. Physiol. Lung Cell. Mol. Physiol.* **2014**, *307*, L868–L876. [CrossRef] [PubMed]

31. Farrow, K.N.; Lakshminrusimha, S.; Reda, W.J.; Wedgwood, S.; Czech, L.; Gugino, S.F.; Davis, J.M.; Russell, J.A.; Steinhorn, R.H. Superoxide dismutase restores eNOS expression and function in resistance pulmonary arteries from neonatal lambs with persistent pulmonary hypertension. *Am. J. Physiol. Lung Cell. Mol. Physiol.* **2008**, *295*, L979–L987. [CrossRef] [PubMed]

32. Oury, T.D.; Day, B.J.; Crapo, J.D. Extracellular superoxide dismutase: A regulator of nitric oxide bioavailability. *Lab. Investig.* **1996**, *75*, 617–636. [PubMed]

33. Langston, W.; Chidlow, J.H., Jr.; Booth, B.A.; Barlow, S.C.; Lefer, D.J.; Patel, R.P.; Kevil, C.G. Regulation of endothelial glutathione by ICAM-1 governs VEGF-A-mediated eNOS activity and angiogenesis. *Free Radic. Biol. Med.* **2007**, *42*, 720–729. [CrossRef] [PubMed]

34. Juarez, J.C.; Manuia, M.; Burnett, M.E.; Betancourt, O.; Boivin, B.; Shaw, D.E.; Tonks, N.K.; Mazar, A.P.; Donate, F. Superoxide dismutase 1 (SOD1) is essential for H_2O_2-mediated oxidation and inactivation of phosphatases in growth factor signaling. *Proc. Natl. Acad. Sci. USA* **2008**, *105*, 7147–7152. [CrossRef] [PubMed]

35. Murdoch, C.E.; Bachschmid, M.M.; Matsui, R. Regulation of neovascularization by S-glutathionylation via the Wnt5a/sFlt-1 pathway. *Biochem. Soc. Trans.* **2014**, *42*, 1665–1670. [CrossRef] [PubMed]

36. Kim, Y.M.; Kim, S.J.; Tatsunami, R.; Yamamura, H.; Fukai, T.; Ushio-Fukai, M. ROS-induced ROS release orchestrated by Nox4, Nox2, and mitochondria in VEGF signaling and angiogenesis. *Am. J. Physiol. Cell Physiol.* **2017**, *312*, C749–C764. [CrossRef] [PubMed]

37. Urao, N.; Sudhahar, V.; Kim, S.J.; Chen, G.F.; McKinney, R.D.; Kojda, G.; Fukai, T.; Ushio-Fukai, M. Critical role of endothelial hydrogen peroxide in post-ischemic neovascularization. *PLoS ONE* **2013**, *8*, e57618. [CrossRef] [PubMed]

38. Kunig, A.M.; Balasubramaniam, V.; Markham, N.E.; Morgan, D.; Montgomery, G.; Grover, T.R.; Abman, S.H. Recombinant human VEGF treatment enhances alveolarization after hyperoxic lung injury in neonatal rats. *Am. J. Physiol. Lung Cell. Mol. Physiol.* **2005**, *289*, L529–L535. [CrossRef] [PubMed]

39. Kunig, A.M.; Balasubramaniam, V.; Markham, N.E.; Seedorf, G.; Gien, J.; Abman, S.H. Recombinant human VEGF treatment transiently increases lung edema but enhances lung structure after neonatal hyperoxia. *Am. J. Physiol. Lung Cell. Mol. Physiol.* **2006**, *291*, L1068–L1078. [CrossRef] [PubMed]

40. Le Cras, T.D.; Markham, N.E.; Tuder, R.M.; Voelkel, N.F.; Abman, S.H. Treatment of newborn rats with a VEGF receptor inhibitor causes pulmonary hypertension and abnormal lung structure. *Am. J. Physiol. Lung Cell. Mol. Physiol.* **2002**, *283*, L555–L562. [CrossRef] [PubMed]

41. Wedgwood, S.; Lakshminrusimha, S.; Czech, L.; Schumacker, P.T.; Steinhorn, R.H. Increased p22(phox)/Nox4 expression is involved in remodeling through hydrogen peroxide signaling in experimental persistent pulmonary hypertension of the newborn. *Antioxid. Redox Signal.* **2013**, *18*, 1765–1776. [CrossRef] [PubMed]

42. Farrow, K.N.; Groh, B.S.; Schumacker, P.T.; Lakshminrusimha, S.; Czech, L.; Gugino, S.F.; Russell, J.A.; Steinhorn, R.H. Hyperoxia increases phosphodiesterase 5 expression and activity in ovine fetal pulmonary artery smooth muscle cells. *Circ. Res.* **2008**, *102*, 226–233. [CrossRef] [PubMed]

43. Farrow, K.N.; Lakshminrusimha, S.; Czech, L.; Groh, B.S.; Gugino, S.F.; Davis, J.M.; Russell, J.A.; Steinhorn, R.H. SOD and inhaled nitric oxide normalize phosphodiesterase 5 expression and activity in neonatal lambs with persistent pulmonary hypertension. *Am. J. Physiol. Lung Cell. Mol. Physiol.* **2010**, *299*, L109–L116. [CrossRef] [PubMed]

44. Gien, J.; Tseng, N.; Seedorf, G.; Kuhn, K.; Abman, S.H. Endothelin-1-Rho kinase interactions impair lung structure and cause pulmonary hypertension after bleomycin exposure in neonatal rat pups. *Am. J. Physiol. Lung Cell. Mol. Physiol.* **2016**, *311*, L1090–L1100. [CrossRef] [PubMed]

45. Baker, C.D.; Seedorf, G.J.; Wisniewski, B.L.; Black, C.P.; Ryan, S.L.; Balasubramaniam, V.; Abman, S.H. Endothelial colony-forming cell conditioned media promote angiogenesis in vitro and prevent pulmonary hypertension in experimental bronchopulmonary dysplasia. *Am. J. Physiol. Lung Cell. Mol. Physiol.* **2013**, *305*, L73–L81. [CrossRef] [PubMed]

46. Ee, M.T.; Kantores, C.; Ivanovska, J.; Wong, M.J.; Jain, A.; Jankov, R.P. Leukotriene B4 mediates macrophage influx and pulmonary hypertension in bleomycin-induced chronic neonatal lung injury. *Am. J. Physiol. Lung Cell. Mol. Physiol.* **2016**, *311*, L292–L302. [CrossRef] [PubMed]

47. Tourneux, P.; Markham, N.; Seedorf, G.; Balasubramaniam, V.; Abman, S.H. Inhaled nitric oxide improves lung structure and pulmonary hypertension in a model of bleomycin-induced bronchopulmonary dysplasia in neonatal rats. *Am. J. Physiol. Lung Cell. Mol. Physiol.* **2009**, *297*, L1103–L1111. [CrossRef] [PubMed]

48. Delaney, C.; Sherlock, L.; Fisher, S.; Maltzahn, J.K.; Wright, C.J.; Nozik-Grayck, E. Serotonin 2A receptor inhibition protects against the development of pulmonary hypertension and pulmonary vascular remodeling in neonatal mice. *Am. J. Physiol. Lung Cell. Mol. Physiol.* **2018**. [CrossRef] [PubMed]

49. Abman, S.H. Bronchopulmonary dysplasia: "A vascular hypothesis". *Am. J. Respir. Crit. Care Med.* **2001**, *164*, 1755–1756. [CrossRef] [PubMed]

50. De Wijs-Meijler, D.P.M.; van Duin, R.W.B.; Duncker, D.J.; Scherrer, U.; Sartori, C.; Reiss, I.K.M.; Merkus, D. Structural and functional changes of the pulmonary vasculature after hypoxia exposure in the neonatal period—A new swine model of pulmonary vascular disease. *Am. J. Physiol. Heart Circ. Physiol.* **2017**. [CrossRef] [PubMed]

51. Wedgwood, S.; Warford, C.; Agvateesiri, S.C.; Thai, P.; Berkelhamer, S.K.; Perez, M.; Underwood, M.A.; Steinhorn, R.H. Postnatal growth restriction augments oxygen-induced pulmonary hypertension in a neonatal rat model of bronchopulmonary dysplasia. *Pediatr. Res.* **2016**, *80*, 894–902. [CrossRef] [PubMed]

52. McCoy, A.M.; Herington, J.L.; Stouch, A.N.; Mukherjee, A.B.; Lakhdari, O.; Blackwell, T.S.; Prince, L.S. Ikkbeta activation in the fetal lung mesenchyme alters lung vascular development but not airway morphogenesis. *Am. J. Pathol.* **2017**, *187*, 2635–2644. [CrossRef] [PubMed]

53. Miller, J.D.; Benjamin, J.T.; Kelly, D.R.; Frank, D.B.; Prince, L.S. Chorioamnionitis stimulates angiogenesis in saccular stage fetal lungs via CC chemokines. *Am. J. Physiol. Lung Cell. Mol. Physiol.* **2010**, *298*, L637–L645. [CrossRef] [PubMed]

54. An, H.S.; Bae, E.J.; Kim, G.B.; Kwon, B.S.; Beak, J.S.; Kim, E.K.; Kim, H.S.; Choi, J.H.; Noh, C.I.; Yun, Y.S. Pulmonary hypertension in preterm infants with bronchopulmonary dysplasia. *Korean Circ. J.* **2010**, *40*, 131–136. [CrossRef] [PubMed]

55. Narayanan, M.; Beardsmore, C.S.; Owers-Bradley, J.; Dogaru, C.M.; Mada, M.; Ball, I.; Garipov, R.R.; Kuehni, C.E.; Spycher, B.D.; Silverman, M. Catch-up alveolarization in ex-preterm children: Evidence from (3)He magnetic resonance. *Am. J. Respir. Crit. Care Med.* **2013**, *187*, 1104–1109. [CrossRef] [PubMed]

56. Zhang, Y.; Jiang, W.; Wang, L.; Lingappan, K. Sex-specific differences in the modulation of growth differentiation factor 15 (GDF15) by hyperoxia in vivo and in vitro: Role of Hif-1alpha. *Toxicol. Appl. Pharmacol.* **2017**, *332*, 8–14. [CrossRef] [PubMed]

57. Redente, E.F.; Jacobsen, K.M.; Solomon, J.J.; Lara, A.R.; Faubel, S.; Keith, R.C.; Henson, P.M.; Downey, G.P.; Riches, D.W. Age and sex dimorphisms contribute to the severity of bleomycin-induced lung injury and fibrosis. *Am. J. Physiol. Lung Cell. Mol. Physiol.* **2011**, *301*, L510–L518. [CrossRef] [PubMed]

14

Phytochemicals in Human Milk and their Potential Antioxidative Protection

Apollinaire Tsopmo [1,2] (iD)

1 Food Science and Nutrition Program, Department of Chemistry, Carleton University, 1125 Colonel By Drive, Ottawa, ON K1S 5B6, Canada; apollinaire_tsopmo@carleton.ca
2 Institute of Biochemistry, Carleton University, 1125 Colonel By Drive, Ottawa, ON K1S 5B6, Canada

Abstract: Diets contain secondary plant metabolites commonly referred to as phytochemicals. Many of them are believed to impact human health through various mechanisms, including protection against oxidative stress and inflammation, and decreased risks of developing chronic diseases. For mothers and other people, phytochemical intake occurs through the consumption of foods such as fruits, vegetables, and grains. Research has shown that some these phytochemicals are present in the mother's milk and can contribute to its oxidative stability. For infants, human milk (HM) represents the primary and preferred source of nutrition because it is a complete food. Studies have reported that the benefit provided by HM goes beyond basic nutrition. It can, for example, reduce oxidative stress in infants, thereby reducing the risk of lung and intestinal diseases in infants. This paper summarizes the phytochemicals present in HM and their potential contribution to infant health.

Keywords: oxidative stress; human milk; infant; phytochemicals

1. Introduction

Plant secondary metabolites, often referred to as phytochemicals, are believed to play an important role in human health. Benefits include the protection against oxidative stress, inflammation; and reduction in risks factors of chronic conditions, such as heart diseases, cancer, diabetes, and neurodegenerative disorders [1,2]. Oxidative stress is present in all of these ailments and antioxidant phytochemicals have been widely investigated in the adult population for their roles in quenching or reducing excess oxidants, thereby restoring the redox balance. For newborns, human milk (HM) represents the primary and preferred source of nutrition and there are data in the literature showing that the benefits of HM go beyond basic nutrition [3].

Human milk from well-nourished mothers is believed to meet the nutrient requirements of infants for up to six months because its composition is dynamic and varies with the mother's diet and time postpartum. The dynamic changes in the composition of HM with time of lactation is to match the changing needs of growing infants. Proteins in HM are sources of nitrogen, amino acids and peptides for the newborn. Proteins, specifically those from the whey fraction are also involved in the development of the immune system, while lactoferrin from the casein group contributes to non-immunologic defence [4]. HM proteins can also serve as a source of antioxidant peptides [5,6]. As well, glutamate, present in HM, can act as a major oxidative fuel for enterocytes and promote gastrointestinal barrier function [7]. Oligosaccharides and polysaccharides in HM can inhibit the adhesion of bacteria to the surface of epithelial cells or promote the development of bifidus flora, thereby contributing to the prevention of infectious diseases in the newborn [8,9]. Oligosaccharides can also decrease the likelihood of injury to the retina and the lung in premature infants with respiratory distress syndrome [10,11]. HM lipids contain a considerable amount of long chain polyunsaturated fatty acids, which are precursors of prostaglandin-like prostacyclins that can improve ventricular function in infants [12]. These fatty acids are also essential components of membrane-rich tissues, such as the brain and the retina photoreceptor membrane [13]. HM provides bioactive agents that include antimicrobial (e.g., immuloglobulins), anti-inflammatory (e.g., lactoferrin) and bioactive peptides. In addition, there are data demonstrating that breastfeeding promotes the development of the infant immune system and this might confer long-term health outcomes [14]. However, the benefit of HM goes beyond that of proteins, oligosaccharides and lipids because phytochemicals from mothers' diets are transferred to their milk. Several of the phytochemicals in HM have antioxidant activities that may help the infant cope with oxidative stress. The aim of this review is to describe antioxidant phytochemicals present in the mother's milk and their potential contribution to redox balance in infants.

2. Phytochemicals in Human Milk

Polyphenols are one of the largest groups of phytochemicals present in crops. Thousands of phenolic structures have been identified, of which about half belong to the class of flavonoids. This class is further sub-divided into flavones, isoflavones, flavanones, catechins and anthocyanins. Polyphenols have been studies in various systems (in vitro and in vivo) and they possess biological activities, such as anti-inflammatory and antioxidant activities. In addition, they can regulate the activity of many enzymes [15,16]. These activities are associated with the promotion of vascular health, cognitive function, redox balance, hormonal balance, or neuronal function [15,17]. One of the most common biological functions of polyphenols is their ability to act as antioxidants, thereby potentially protecting adults against oxidative stress and inflammation, while, at the same time, decreasing the risk of developing chronic and degenerative diseases (e.g., macular degeneration, cancer, obesity, diabetes) [18,19]. Oxidative stress is also present in infants and is associated with respiratory and intestinal diseases [20,21].

2.1. Flavonoids in Human Milk

Secondary metabolites are classified into classes including polyphenols, of which flavonoids constitute the largest sub-group. Structures of some flavonoids identified in the mother's milk are presented in Figure 1 and their concentrations in Table 1. A study conducted by Song et al. [18] detected seven flavonoids—epicatechin, epicatechin gallate, epigallocatechin gallate, naringenin, kaempferol, hesperetin, and quercetin—in milk of mothers who gave birth to full term babies. Mean concentrations at one week postpartum varied from 15.7 nmol/L for kaempferol to 1118.8 nmol/L for epigallocatechin gallate. An ingestion of roasted soybeans (20 g, equivalent to 37 mg isoflavones) resulted in mean total isoflavone concentrations of about 0.2 µmol/L in breast milk, with the main constituents being daidzein and genistein [22]. In the work of Khymenets et al. [23], the consumption of dark chocolate led to the identification of epicatechin and its metabolites 12 h after ingestion in the HM of mothers obtained at 6 months postpartum. The metabolites were sulfates and glucuronates of epicatechin, metoxy-catechin, and γ-valerolactone [23]. In nursing mothers who consumed a soy beverage containing 55 mg of total isoflavones for 2–4 days, isoflavone contents of their milk increased from 5.1 to 70.7 nmol/L, while amounts in the urine of their infants went from 29.8 to 111.6 nmol/mg creatinine [24]. In addition, the mean isoflavone concentration in the plasma of these infants was 19.7 nmol/L. Data from this research is an indication that isoflavones are available in infants and can potentially protect them from oxidative stress because they are known antioxidant molecules. In a related study, nursing women who received 250 mL of soy drink with an isoflavone content of 12 mg for 6 days had 12 nmol of isoflavone/L in their milks [25]. Compared to the study of Franke et al. [24], 12 nmol of isoflavone/L of HM seems small but this is because the two soy drinks had different amounts of isoflavone (12 mg vs. 55 mg). In another study, breastfeeding women received meals that provided 1 mg of quercetin/kg bodyweight. In milks collected after 12 h, its mean concentration was 68 ± 8 nmol/L and represented about a 1.7-fold increase relative to values before and at 48 h after the supplementation [26].

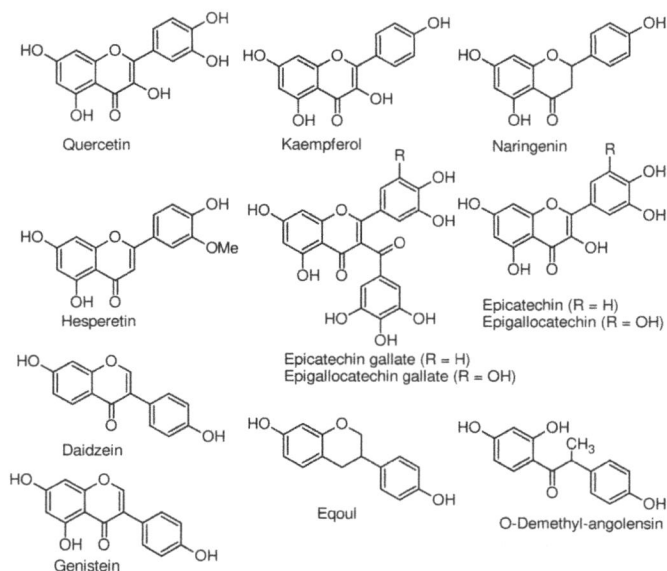

Figure 1. Chemical structures of polyphenols detected in human milk.

2.2. Carotenoids

The other abundant class of phytochemicals in human milk is the carotenoids (Figure 2, Table 1). Dietary supplementation of lactating mothers with antioxidant rich foods has an influence on how much is present in milk and therefore, the exposure of infants to these molecules. In the study conducted by Haftel et al. [27], women took 15 mg β-carotene or 15 mg of lycopene, in the form of carrot puree or mashed tomato, per day. The two carotenoid molecules were detected in HM and their concentrations increased with time to reach maximum values after two or four days, depending on the individual. Lycopene levels rose to a maximum of 130%, and β-carotene to a maximum of 200%, relative to baseline values [27]. In a related work, seven carotenoids were detected in HM collected one to thirteen weeks postpartum from free living mothers (i.e., no diet intervention). Amongst them, β-carotene (164.3–88.0 nmol/L), lutein (121.2–56.4 nmol/L) and lycopene (119.9–49.5 nmol/L) were the most abundant [18]. The concentrations of others were α-cryptoxanthin (30.6–13.5 nmol/L), β-cryptoxanthin (57.4–24.8 nmol/L), and zeaxanthin (46.3–21.4 nmol/L). The amount of each carotenoid decreased from week 1 to week 13 [18]. The variation in the concentration of each of the carotenoid molecules was most likely due to the oxidative status of the mother or to the amount in their diet, although the study did not collect information on the participants' diets. In another study, pregnant women received daily, 6 g of Chlorella, a single-cell green algae rich in carotenoids, from 16–20 weeks of gestation until the day of delivery [28]. There were significant increases of 1.7, 2.6 and 2.7-fold in β-carotene, lutein and zeaxanthin, respectively in HM of the experimental group, compared to the control group, at 0–6 days postpartum. A recent study quantified carotenoids in donors' and lactating mothers' milk and found that concentrations of α-carotene, β-carotene, lycopene and β-cryptoxanthin were 1.9 to 5.7-fold lower in the donors' milk samples [29]. Lower contents of carotenoids in donor milk could be due to the pasteurization of milk necessary to prevent microbial growth and ensure its safety [30], but storage might contribute to the reduction as well. Donor milk is an effective alternative source of nutrition, specifically for preterm infants, when the mother's own milk is not available. Information on whether the amount of antioxidant phytochemicals present in donors' milk has an effect on oxidative stress related outcomes in the preterm infant is not available. Phytochemicals (e.g., flavonoids and carotenoids) have antioxidant properties and their presence in diets might protect pregnant women and their fetuses against oxidative stress induced during pregnancy. The protection can continue after birth because some of the phytochemicals have been detected not only in HM, but also in biological fluids (e.g., blood and urine) [31]. In fact, there are direct correlations between concentrations of HM lutein with its daily intake and this has led to the recommendation by some institutions to increase fruit and vegetable intakes throughout the duration of pregnancy and lactation [32].

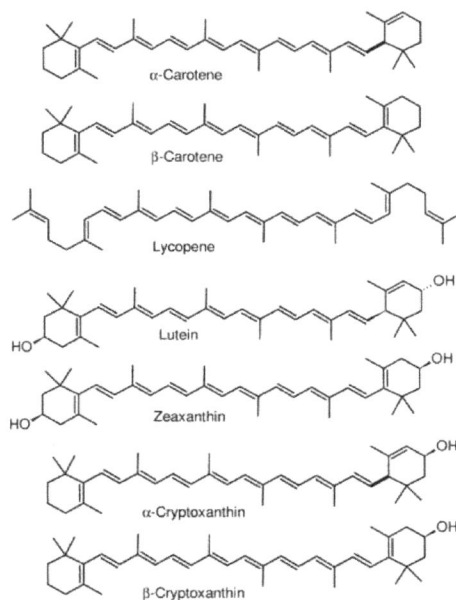

Figure 2. Chemical structures of carotenoids detected in human milk.

Table 1. Concentrations of phytochemicals found in human milk.

Compound	Concentration (nmol/L)	Information on Mothers and Milk
Epicatechin	63.7–828.5	Free living mothers, milk at 1, 4 and 13 week [18]
Epicatechin gallate	55.7–645.6	
Epigallocatechin gallate	215.1–2364.7	
Naringenin	64.1–722.0	
Kaempferol	7.8–71.4	
Hesperetin	74.8–1603.1	
Quercetin	32.5–108.6	Free living mothers, milk at 1, 4 and 13 week [18]
	68 ± 8.44	Diet with 1 mg quercetin/kg of body weight [26]
Lutein	56.4–121.2	Free living mothers, milk analyzed at 1, 4 and 13 weeks [18]
	497–824	Chlorella supplementation, 6 months from gestational week 16–20 until delivery [28]
	280 ± 22	Free living mothers. Milk collected at day 3 [32]
Zeaxanthin	46.3–21.4	Free living mothers, milk at 1, 4 and 13 weeks [18]
	33.2 ± 17.2	Healthy women. Milk collected at days 2–6 [33]
α-Cryptoxanthin	13.5–30.6	Free living mothers, milk at 1, 4 and 13 weeks [18]
β-Cryptoxanthin	24.8–57.4	Free living mothers, milk at 1–14 weeks [18,34]
α-Carotene	23.2–59.0	Free living mothers, milk at 1, 4 and 13 weeks [18]
β-Carotene	88.0–164.3	Free living mothers, milk at 1–14 weeks [18,34]
	75–400	Supplementation, 30 mg β-carotene/d for 28 days [35]
	275–484	Chlorella supplementation 6 months, from gestational week 16–20 until day of delivery [28]
Lycopene	119.9–49.5	Free living mothers, milk analyzed at 1, 4 and 13 weeks [18,34]
	86–244	Chlorella supplementation for 6 months, from gestational week 16–20 until day of delivery. Milk collected at 1–6 days [28]
Isoflavones	70.7 ± 19.2	Soy beverage with 55 mg isoflavones daily for 2–4 days [24]
	12.0	Soy drink, 12 mg isoflavones daily for 6 days [25]

Table 1. *Cont.*

Compound	Concentration (nmol/L)	Information on Mothers and Milk
Epicat-Gluc-4 *	0.0–36.4	
Epicat-Sulf-3 *	0.0–14.5	Free living mothers, milk collected at 1–30 days [23]
MetEpicat-Sulf-3 *	0.0–23.7	
Caffeine **	0.06–0.77	
Theobromine	0.08–0.50 **	Milk of habitual coffee and chocolate mothers [34]
Paraxanthine	0.15–1.68 **	
Theophylline	0.10–0.66 **	

* Epicatechin metabolites; ** Concentrations expressed as µg/mL.

2.3. Other Phytochemicals

Three garlic acid metabolites, known as allyl methyl sulfide, allyl methyl sulfoxide and allyl methyl sulfone, were detected in breast milk 2.5 h after the consumption of garlic [36]. Allyl methyl sulfide affected the odor of milk but showed antioxidant activity, characterized by its ability to reduce the rate of oxidation of cumene [37]. Both odor and antioxidant characteristics of allyl methyl sulfide are due to the presence of sulfur. Caffeine and its catabolic products, theobromine, and xanthine, are key molecules in tea and coffee. Their concentrations and those of related molecules, theophylline and paraxanthine, in HM were determined to vary from 0.06 to 0.77 µg/mL [38]. Caffeine, theobromine and xanthine have been found in model systems to quench hydroxyl radicals, thereby preventing oxidative DNA breakage induced by this radical species [39]. Meanwhile, the effects of caffeine and its congeners at concentrations detected in HM on the biochemistry of HM or on newborn outcomes are unknown.

3. Oxidative Stress in Infants

The higher production of oxygen-derived metabolites, collectively known as reactive oxygen species (ROS) in aerobic organisms, compared to the concentration of available antioxidant molecules and enzymes is termed oxidative stress. The presence of excess ROS is an important mediator of cell and tissue damage [20,40]. Biological molecules susceptible to oxidation include lipids, proteins, and nucleotides [41,42]. In general, organisms prevent oxidative damage by maintaining a critical oxidation–reduction balance, but this is not always the case in the presence of diseases, external stimuli, improper nutrition or exposure to a hyperoxic environment, as encountered at birth. Data exist to show that the transition from an intrauterine to an extrauterine life is characterized by physiological and metabolic changes due, in part, to an increase in the availability of oxygen and a high level of free iron that can enhance the production of highly toxic hydroxyl radicals through the Fenton reaction [40]. Newborns, specifically those who are premature, cannot efficiently deal with oxygen at relatively high concentrations compared with the intrauterine environment because antioxidant enzymes mature during late stage gestation and also, because of inadequate transfer of antioxidants, like vitamins E, C, β-carotene, and ubiquinone, across the placenta [43].

The evaluation of oxidative stress in newborns is based on the quantification of antioxidant molecules, enzyme activities or markers of lipids and proteins, or DNA damage. For example, malondialdehyde (MDA), a marker of lipid peroxidation and 8-hydroxy-2′-deoxyguanosine, a maker of DNA damage, is higher in the cord blood of preterm low birth weight infants [44]. Higher concentrations of protein carbonyls were reported in neonatal lungs of subjects with bronchopulmonary dysplasia [45], while in infants treated with supplemental oxygen, ortho-tyrosine, a marker of protein oxidation, increased with increasing inspired oxygen [46]. Perinatal hypoxia increased the oxidation of lipids in cord blood and also decreased the concentration of the intracellular antioxidant peptide, glutathione [47]. Oxidative stress in newborns has been linked to several conditions. Some of these are chronic lung diseases or bronchopulmonary dysplasia, a condition that usually occurs in preterm infants receiving respiratory support with mechanical ventilation or prolonged oxygen supplementation [48]. Other oxidative stress-associated conditions are necrotizing enterocolitis, an inflammation of the small intestine and bowel surface, with infiltration of epithelial cells by bacteria; and retinopathy of prematurity, a type of oxygen-induced damage to blood vessels in the retina that are undergoing neovascularization [49,50].

There are several strategies for reducing oxidative stress in newborns including supplementation with enzymatic or non-enzymatic antioxidants [51]. Meanwhile, human milk seems to provide better antioxidant protection in early life due, in part, to its ability to scavenge free radicals compared to formulas [52]. This might be due to the presence of the antioxidant enzymes—glutathione peroxidase, catalase, and superoxide dismutase—present in HM but not in formula [53], which, in addition to their antioxidant effects in the gut, may pass through the porous neonatal intestine early in infancy [52]. In addition to enzymes, vitamins E and C, and possibly phytochemicals can contribute to the protection provided by HM.

4. Antioxidant Phytochemicals in Human Milk and Redox Balance in Infants

Secondary plant metabolites, and specifically those with antioxidant and anti-inflammatory properties, play an important role in human health. Human milk (HM) is the optimal food for newborns and is, in many cases, the only source of nutrition for up to six months. The presence of plant antioxidant molecules in HM, like polyphenols and carotenoids, indicates that they might have a role in newborn health outcomes. There are several reviews on the contribution of polyphenols in the management of oxidative stress and related conditions in the adult population [17,54] but not in infants. The effect of the consumption of dietary polyphenols through HM on the health of infants is not entirely understood because only a few studies have attempted to determine the availability of polyphenols in HM of lactating mothers and their potential accessibility to HM-fed infants [23]. The effect can be studied by analyzing phytochemicals in HM and how they affect milk stability or by quantifying the amount of these molecules in infant bio-fluids and relating this to health outcomes in which oxidative stress plays a role. The total concentration of polyphenols in HM, collected three days after parturition, inversely correlated with malondialdehyde, a genotoxic product of lipid peroxidation, indicating an increase stability of milk from mothers with high intake of vegetables that are rich in antioxidant phytochemicals [55]. A recent study found that the carotenoid content of HM samples decreased with an increasing lactation period but, for flavonoids, there was only minimal or, in certain cases, no change in content with the stage of lactation [18]. How this affects the oxidative stability of HM is unknown because it was not part of that study. Other works have been conducted to determine the antioxidant potential of HM collected at various stages of lactation and the information was recently reviewed [56]. Although, in one of the studies, total antioxidant capacity of HM was correlated with α-tocopherol concentration [57], none of the studies looked at the oxidative stability of milk with regard to the content of their antioxidant phytochemicals.

Carotenoids are known for their antioxidant properties and this can enhance the immune system and visual acuity because of their accumulation in the eye. The deposition of lutein and zeaxanthin, for example, in the human retina occurs early in life [58], and their content in HM may then be critical to the development of the infant visual acuity. The macular pigment optical density in the retina of healthy full term infants significantly correlated with concentrations of zeaxanthin in their serum samples ($r = 0.68$) and in their mother's serum ($r = 0.59$) [58]. Additionally, the same work reported mother–infant correlations for total serum carotenoids and skin carotenoids, indicating further potential contribution of this group of phytochemicals to infant development. The retina is exposed to an intense energy source from lens focused light that generates free radicals [59]; the presence of carotenoids in the eye can consequently improve infant visual acuity while also preventing oxidative stress. Lactating mothers with low intakes of carotenoids might possibly expose their infants to less protection from oxidative stress. Fruits and vegetables are recommended throughout the duration of pregnancy and lactation to maintain sufficient amounts of carotenoids [28] and possibly, to better protect infants. In a study by Perrone et al. [60], newborns received lutein at 12 h and 36 h after birth. The quantification of hydroperoxides, a maker of lipid oxidation in the cord blood, at 48 h of life in infants, showed a significant reduction in oxidative stress in the lutein group compared to the control group [60]. This is an indication of a decrease oxidation of lipids in infants due to the antioxidant nature of lutein. In a related work, a combination of lycopene, lutein, and β-carotene given to preterm infants decreased C-reactive protein in plasma and improved rod photoreceptor sensitivity [61]. A possible mechanism for this could be through an antioxidant mechanism that prevented oxidative damage to the photoreceptor.

The exposure of infants to the flavonoid, quercetin, through HM was estimated to be 0.01 mg/day based on the assumption that they consumed 900 mL/day of milk, equivalent to about 45 nmol quercetin/L [26,62]. In a related work, mothers who consumed 20–25 mg of isoflavones daily might have exposed their breastmilk fed infants to 0.005–0.01 mg/day of this group of polyphenols [63]. The contribution of flavonoids to the reduction of oxidative stress in infants is not clear, although genistein, daidzein and glycitein were detected in the urine of 4 to 6 month old infants fed soy products [64]. An increase of 14-fold in isoflavone content was found in the milk of lactating mothers who consumed soy products, concomitantly with an increase of 4-fold in the urine of their babies [24]. The presence of flavonoids in biological fluids of infants is an indication that they might help them cope with oxidative stress, although evidence is needed from future studies.

5. Conclusions

Carotenoids found in human milk may play a role in its oxidative stability and in infant redox balance, inflammatory status and visual acuity. The minimum concentrations needed to provide protective effects are not available. This is due, at least in part, to the limited number of studies that have correlated carotenoid contents in human milk to a specific infant health outcome. The contribution of flavonoids, the other main group of antioxidant phytochemicals in human milk, to infant oxidative status is even less clear. Despite this, the recommendation to consume more fruits and vegetables during both pregnancy and lactation is a key component of dietary guidelines to boost phytochemicals and protect mothers and infants from oxidative damage and related diseases.

Acknowledgments: This work was carried out with the support of the National Science and Engineering Research Council of Canada Discovery Grant No: 371908.

Conflicts of Interest: The author declares that there are no conflicts of interest.

References

1. Fiedor, J.; Burda, K. Potential role of carotenoids as antioxidants in human health and disease. *Nutrients* **2014**, *6*, 466–488. [CrossRef] [PubMed]
2. Griffiths, K.; Aggarwal, B.; Singh, R.; Buttar, H.; Wilson, D.; De Meester, F. Food antioxidants and their anti-inflammatory properties: A potential role in cardiovascular diseases and cancer prevention. *Diseases* **2016**, *4*, e28. [CrossRef] [PubMed]
3. Uchiyama, S.I.; Sekiguchi, K.; Akaishi, M.; Anan, A.; Maeda, T.; Izumi, T. Characterization and chronological changes of preterm human milk gangliosides. *Nutrition* **2011**, *27*, 998–1001. [CrossRef] [PubMed]
4. Lönnerdal, B. Bioactive proteins in human milk: Health, nutrition, and implications for infant formulas. *J. Pediatr.* **2016**, *173*, S4–S9. [CrossRef] [PubMed]
5. Tsopmo, A.; Diehl-Jones, B.W.; Aluko, R.E.; Kitts, D.D.; Elisia, I.; Friel, J.K. Tryptophan released from mother's milk has antioxidant properties. *Pediatr. Res.* **2009**, *66*, 614–618. [CrossRef] [PubMed]
6. Tsopmo, A.; Romanowski, A.; Banda, L.; Lavoie, J.C.; Jenssen, H.; Friel, J.K. Novel anti-oxidative peptides from enzymatic digestion of human milk. *Food Chem.* **2011**, *126*, 1138–1143. [CrossRef]
7. Burrin, D.G.; Stoll, B. Metabolic fate and function of dietary glutamate in the gut. *Am. J. Clin. Nutr.* **2009**, *90*, 850S–856S. [CrossRef] [PubMed]
8. Kunz, C.; Rodriguez-Palmero, M.; Koletzko, B.; Jensen, R. Nutritional and biochemical properties of human milk, part I: General aspects, proteins, and carbohydrates. *Clin. Perinatol.* **1999**, *26*, 307–333. [PubMed]

9.   Jeong, K.; Nguyen, V.; Kim, J. Human milk oligosaccharides: The novel modulator of intestinal microbiota. *BMB Rep.* **2012**, *45*, 433–441. [CrossRef] [PubMed]

10. Smilowitz, J.T.; O'Sullivan, A.; Barile, D.; German, J.B.; Lönnerdal, B.; Slupsky, C.M. The human milk metabolome reveals diverse oligosaccharide profiles. *J. Nutr.* **2013**, *143*, 1709–1718. [CrossRef] [PubMed]

11. Hallman, M.; Bry, K.; Hoppu, K.; Lappi, M.; Pohjavuori, M. Inositol supplementation in premature infants with respiratory distress syndrome. *N. Engl. J. Med.* **1992**, *326*, 1233–1239. [CrossRef] [PubMed]

12. Šantak, B.; Schreiber, M.; Kuen, P.; Lang, D.; Radermacher, P. Prostacyclin aerosol in an infant with pulmonary hypertension. *Eur. J. Pediatr.* **1995**, *154*, 233–235. [CrossRef] [PubMed]

13. Neuringer, M. Infant vision and retinal function in studies of dietary long-chain polyunsaturated fatty acids: Methods, results, and implications. *Am. J. Clin. Nutr.* **2000**, *71*, 256S–267S. [CrossRef] [PubMed]

14. Rodriguez-Palmero, M.; Koletzko, B.; Kunz, C.; Jensen, R. Nutritional and biochemical properties of human milk: II. Lipids, micronutrients, and bioactive factors. *Clin. Perinatol.* **1999**, *26*, 335–359. [PubMed]

15. Ratnasari, N.; Walters, M.; Tsopmo, A. Antioxidant and lipoxygenase activities of polyphenol extracts from oat brans treated with polysaccharide degrading enzymes. *Heliyon* **2017**, *3*. [CrossRef] [PubMed]

16. Du, Y.; Esfandi, R.; Willmore, W.G.; Tsopmo, A. Antioxidant activity of oat proteins derived peptides in stressed hepatic hepg2 cells. *Antioxidants* **2016**, *5*. [CrossRef] [PubMed]

17. Landete, J.M. Updated Knowledge about Polyphenols: Functions, Bioavailability, Metabolism, and Health. *Crit. Rev. Food Sci. Nutr.* **2012**, *52*, 936–948. [CrossRef] [PubMed]

18. Song, B.J.; Jouni, Z.E.; Ferruzzi, M.G. Assessment of phytochemical content in human milk during different stages of lactation. *Nutrition* **2013**, *29*, 195–202. [CrossRef] [PubMed]

19. Hughes, L.A.E.; Arts, I.C.W.; Ambergen, T.; Brants, H.A.M.; Dagnelie, P.C.; Goldbohm, R.A.; Van Den Brandt, P.A.; Weijenberg, M.P. Higher dietary flavone, flavonol, and catechin intakes are associated with less of an increase in BMI over time in women: A longitudinal analysis from The Netherlands Cohort Study. *Am. J. Clin. Nutr.* **2008**, *88*, 1341–1352. [CrossRef] [PubMed]

20. Tsopmo, A.; Friel, J.K. Human milk has anti-oxidant properties to protect premature infants. *Curr. Pediatr. Rev.* **2007**, *3*, 45–51. [CrossRef]

21. Miloudi, K.; Tsopmo, A.; Friel, J.K.; Rouleau, T.; Comte, B.; Lavoie, J.C. Hexapeptides from human milk prevent the induction of oxidative stress from parenteral nutrition in the newborn guinea pig. *Pediatr. Res.* **2012**, *71*, 675–681. [CrossRef] [PubMed]

22. Franke, A.A.; Custer, L.J.; Tanaka, Y. Isoflavones in human breast milk and other biological fluids. *Am. J. Clin. Nutr.* **1998**, *68*, 1466s–1473s. [CrossRef] [PubMed]

23. Khymenets, O.; Rabassa, M.; Rodríguez-Palmero, M.; Rivero-Urgell, M.; Urpi-Sarda, M.; Tulipani, S.; Brandi, P.; Campoy, C.; Santos-Buelga, C.; Andres-Lacueva, C. Dietary epicatechin is available to breastfed infants through human breast milk in the form of host and microbial metabolites. *J. Agric. Food Chem.* **2016**, *64*. [CrossRef] [PubMed]

24. Franke, A.A.; Halm, B.M.; Custer, L.J.; Tatsumura, Y.; Hebshi, S. Isoflavones in breastfed infants after mothers consume soy. *Am. J. Clin. Nutr.* **2006**, *84*, 406–413. [CrossRef] [PubMed]

25. Jochum, F.; Alteheld, B.; Meinardus, P.; Dahlinger, N.; Nomayo, A.; Stehle, P. Mothers' Consumption of Soy Drink but Not Black Tea Increases the Flavonoid Content of Term Breast Milk: A Pilot Randomized, Controlled Intervention Study. *Ann. Nutr. Metab.* **2017**, *70*, 147–153. [CrossRef] [PubMed]

26. Romaszko, E.; Wiczkowski, W.; Romaszko, J.; Honke, J.; Piskula, M.K. Exposure of breastfed infants to quercetin after consumption of a single meal rich in quercetin by their mothers. *Mol. Nutr. Food Res.* **2014**, *58*, 221–228. [CrossRef] [PubMed]

27. Haftel, L.; Berkovich, Z.; Reifen, R. Elevated milk β-carotene and lycopene after carrot and tomato paste supplementation. *Nutrition* **2015**, *31*, 443–445. [CrossRef] [PubMed]

28. Nagayama, J.; Noda, K.; Uchikawa, T.; Maruyama, I.; Shimomura, H.; Miyahara, M. Effect of maternal Chlorella supplementation on carotenoid concentration in breast milk at early lactation. *Int. J. Food Sci. Nutr.* **2014**, *65*, 573–576. [CrossRef] [PubMed]

29. Hanson, C.; Lyden, E.; Furtado, J.; Van Ormer, M.; Anderson-Berry, A. A comparison of nutritional antioxidant content in breast milk, donor milk, and infant formulas. *Nutrients* **2016**, *8*, e681. [CrossRef] [PubMed]

30. O'Connor, D.L.; Ewaschuk, J.B.; Unger, S. Human milk pasteurization: Benefits and risks. *Curr. Opin. Clin. Nutr. Metab. Care* **2015**, *18*, 269–275. [CrossRef] [PubMed]

31. Miyazawa, T.; Nakagawa, K.; Kimura, F.; Nakashima, Y.; Maruyama, I.; Higuchi, O.; Miyazawa, T. Chlorella is an Effective Dietary Source of Lutein for Human Erythrocytes. *J. Oleo Sci.* **2013**, *10*, 905–914. [CrossRef]

32. Cena, H.; Castellazzi, A.M.; Pietri, A.; Roggi, C.; Turconi, G. Lutein concentration in human milk during early lactation and its relationship with dietary lutein intake. *Public Health Nutr.* **2009**, *12*, 1878–1884. [CrossRef] [PubMed]

33. Schweigert, F.J.; Bathe, K.; Chen, F.; Büscher, U.; Dudenhausen, J.W. Effect of the stage of lactation in humans on carotenoid levels in milk, blood plasma and plasma lipoprotein fractions. *Eur. J. Nutr.* **2004**, *43*, 39–44. [CrossRef] [PubMed]

34. Jackson, J.G.; Lien, E.L.; White, S.J.; Bruns, N.J.; Kuhlman, C.F. Major carotenoids in mature human milk: Longitudinal and diurnal patterns. *J. Nutr. Biochem.* **1998**, *9*, 2–7. [CrossRef]

35. Canfield, L.M.; Clandinin, M.T.; Davies, D.P.; Fernandez, M.C.; Jackson, J.; Hawkes, J.; Goldman, W.J.; Pramuk, K.; Reyes, H.; Sablan, B.; et al. Multinational study of major breast milk carotenoids of healthy mothers. *Eur. J. Nutr.* **2003**, *42*, 133–141. [PubMed]

36. Scheffler, L.; Sauermann, Y.; Zeh, G.; Hauf, K.; Heinlein, A.; Sharapa, C.; Buettner, A. Detection of volatile metabolites of garlic in human breast milk. *Metabolites* **2016**, *6*, 18. [CrossRef] [PubMed]

37. Amorati, R.; Pedulli, G.F. Do garlic-derived allyl sulfides scavenge peroxyl radicals? *Org. Biomol. Chem.* **2008**, *6*, 1103–1107. [CrossRef] [PubMed]

38. Aresta, A.; Palmisano, F.; Zambonin, C.G. Simultaneous determination of caffeine, theobromine, theophylline, paraxanthine and nicotine in human milk by liquid chromatography with diode array UV detection. *Food Chem.* **2005**, *93*, 177–181. [CrossRef]

39. Azam, S.; Hadi, N.; Khan, N.U.; Hadi, S.M. Antioxidant and prooxidant properties of caffeine, theobromine and xanthine. *Med. Sci. Monit.* **2003**, *9*, BR325–BR330. [PubMed]

40. Gitto, E.; Pellegrino, S.; Gitto, P.; Barberi, I.; Reiter, R.J. Oxidative stress of the newborn in the pre- and postnatal period and the clinical utility of melatonin. *J. Pineal Res.* **2009**, *46*, 128–139. [CrossRef] [PubMed]

41. Elisia, I.; Tsopmo, A.; Friel, J.K.; Diehl-Jones, W.; Kitts, D.D. Tryptophan from human milk induces oxidative stress and upregulates the Nrf-2-mediated stress response in human intestinal cell lines. *J. Nutr.* **2011**, *141*, 1417–1423. [CrossRef] [PubMed]

42. Friel, J.K.; Diehl-Jones, W.L.; Suh, M.; Tsopmo, A.; Shirwadkar, V.P. Impact of iron and vitamin C-containing supplements on preterm human milk: in vitro. *Free Radic. Biol. Med.* **2007**, *42*, 1591–1598. [CrossRef] [PubMed]

43. Friel, J.K.; Friesen, R.W.; Harding, S.V.; Roberts, L.J. Evidence of oxidative stress in full-term healthy infants. *Pediatr. Res.* **2004**, *56*, 878–882. [CrossRef] [PubMed]

44. Negi, R.; Pande, D.; Kumar, A.; Khanna, R.S.; Khanna, H.D. In vivo oxidative DNA damage and lipid peroxidation as a biomarker of oxidative stress in preterm low-birthweight infants. *J. Trop. Pediatr.* **2012**, *58*, 326–328. [CrossRef] [PubMed]

45. Gladstone, I.M.; Levine, R.L. Oxidation of Proteins in Neonatal Lungs. *Pediatrics* **1994**, *93*, 764–768. [PubMed]

46. Lubec, G.; Widness, J.A.; Hayde, M.; Menzel, D.; Pollak, A. Hydroxyl radical generation in oxygen-treated infants. *Pediatrics* **1997**, *100*, 700–704. [CrossRef] [PubMed]

47. Schmidt, H.; Grune, T.; Muller, R.; Siems, W.G.; Wauer, R.R. Increased levels of lipid peroxidation products malondialdehyde and 4-hydroxynonenal after perinatal hypoxia. *Pediatr. Res.* **1996**, *40*, 15–20. [CrossRef] [PubMed]

48. Ambalavanan, N.; Carlo, W.A. Bronchopulmonary dysplasia: New insights. *Clin. Perinatol.* **2004**, *31*, 613–628. [CrossRef] [PubMed]

49. Aydemir, C.; Dilli, D.; Uras, N.; Ulu, H.O.; Oguz, S.S.; Erdeve, O.; Dilmen, U. Total oxidant status and oxidative stress are increased in infants with necrotizing enterocolitis. *J. Pediatr. Surg.* **2011**, *46*, 2096–2100. [CrossRef] [PubMed]

50. Hellström, A.; Smith, L.E.; Dammann, O. Retinopathy of prematurity. *Lancet* **2013**, *382*, 1445–1457. [CrossRef]

51. Ozsurekci, Y.; Aykac, K. Oxidative stress related diseases in newborns. *Oxid. Med. Cell. Longev.* **2016**, *2016*, 2768365. [CrossRef] [PubMed]

52. Friel, J.K.; Martin, S.M.; Langdon, M.; Herzberg, G.R.; Buettner, G.R. Milk from mothers of both premature and full-term infants provides better antioxidant protection than does infant formula. *Pediatr. Res.* **2002**, *51*, 612–618. [CrossRef] [PubMed]

53. L'Abbe, M.R.; Friel, J.K. Copper status of very low birth weight infants during the first 12 months of infancy. *Pediatr. Res.* **1992**, *32*, 183–188. [CrossRef] [PubMed]

54. Celep, G.S.; Rastmanesh, R.; Marotta, F. Polyphenols in Human Health and Disease. In *Polyphenols in Human Health and Disease*; Watson, R.R., Preedy, V.R., Zibadi, S., Eds.; Academic Press, Elsevier Inc.: Tokyo, Japan, 2014; pp. 577–589, ISBN 9780123984562.

55. Poniedziałek, B.; Rzymski, P.; Pięt, M.; Gąsecka, M.; Stroińska, A.; Niedzielski, P.; Mleczek, M.; Rzymski, P.; Wilczak, M. Relation between polyphenols, malondialdehyde, antioxidant capacity, lactate dehydrogenase and toxic elements in human colostrum milk. *Chemosphere* **2018**, *191*, 548–554. [CrossRef] [PubMed]

56. Matos, C.; Ribeiro, M.; Guerra, A. Breastfeeding: Antioxidative properties of breast milk. *J. Appl. Biomed.* **2015**, *13*, 169–180. [CrossRef]

57. Tijerina-Saenz, A.; Innis, S.M.; Kitts, D.D. Antioxidant capacity of human milk and its association with vitamins A and E and fatty acid composition. *Acta Paediatr.* **2009**. [CrossRef] [PubMed]

58. Henriksen, B.S.; Chan, G.; Hoffman, R.O.; Sharifzadeh, M.; Ermakov, I.V.; Gellermann, W.; Bernstein, P.S. Interrelationships between maternal carotenoid status and newborn infant macular pigment optical density and carotenoid status. *Investig. Ophthalmol. Vis. Sci.* **2013**, *54*, 5568–5578. [CrossRef] [PubMed]

59. Zimmer, J.P.; Hammond, B.R. Possible influences of lutein and zeaxanthin on the developing retina. *Clin. Ophthalmol.* **2007**, *1*, 25–35. [PubMed]

60. Perrone, S.; Longini, M.; Marzocchi, B.; Picardi, A.; Bellieni, C.V.; Proietti, F.; Rodriguez, A.; Turrisi, G.; Buonocore, G. Effects of lutein on oxidative stress in the term newborn: A pilot study. *Neonatology* **2010**, *97*, 36–40. [CrossRef] [PubMed]

61. Rubin, L.P.; Chan, G.M.; Barrett-Reis, B.M.; Fulton, A.B.; Hansen, R.M.; Ashmeade, T.L.; Oliver, J.S.; MacKey, A.D.; Dimmit, R.A.; Hartmann, E.E.; et al. Effect of carotenoid supplementation on plasma carotenoids, inflammation and visual development in preterm infants. *J. Perinatol.* **2012**, *32*, 418–424. [CrossRef] [PubMed]

62. Kent, J.C.; Mitoulas, L.R.; Cregan, M.D.; Ramsay, D.T.; Doherty, D.A.; Hartmann, P.E. Volume and frequency of breastfeedings and fat content of breast milk throughout the day. *Pediatrics* **2006**, *117*, e387–e395. [CrossRef] [PubMed]

63. Setchell, K.D.R.; Zimmer-Nechemias, L.; Cai, J.; Heubi, J.E. Isoflavone content of infant formulas and the metabolic fate of these phytoestrogens in early life. *Am. J. Clin. Nutr.* **1998**, *68*, 1453S–1461S. [CrossRef] [PubMed]

64. Hoey, L.; Rowland, I.R.; Lloyd, A.S.; Clarke, D.B.; Wiseman, H. Influence of soya-based infant formula consumption on isoflavone and gut microflora metabolite concentrations in urine and on faecal microflora composition and metabolic activity in infants and children. *Br. J. Nutr.* **2004**, *91*, 607–616. [CrossRef] [PubMed]

Permissions

All chapters in this book were first published in ANTIOXIDANTS, by MDPI; hereby published with permission under the Creative Commons Attribution License or equivalent. Every chapter published in this book has been scrutinized by our experts. Their significance has been extensively debated. The topics covered herein carry significant findings which will fuel the growth of the discipline. They may even be implemented as practical applications or may be referred to as a beginning point for another development.

The contributors of this book come from diverse backgrounds, making this book a truly international effort. This book will bring forth new frontiers with its revolutionizing research information and detailed analysis of the nascent developments around the world.

We would like to thank all the contributing authors for lending their expertise to make the book truly unique. They have played a crucial role in the development of this book. Without their invaluable contributions this book wouldn't have been possible. They have made vital efforts to compile up to date information on the varied aspects of this subject to make this book a valuable addition to the collection of many professionals and students.

This book was conceptualized with the vision of imparting up-to-date information and advanced data in this field. To ensure the same, a matchless editorial board was set up. Every individual on the board went through rigorous rounds of assessment to prove their worth. After which they invested a large part of their time researching and compiling the most relevant data for our readers.

The editorial board has been involved in producing this book since its inception. They have spent rigorous hours researching and exploring the diverse topics which have resulted in the successful publishing of this book. They have passed on their knowledge of decades through this book. To expedite this challenging task, the publisher supported the team at every step. A small team of assistant editors was also appointed to further simplify the editing procedure and attain best results for the readers.

Apart from the editorial board, the designing team has also invested a significant amount of their time in understanding the subject and creating the most relevant covers. They scrutinized every image to scout for the most suitable representation of the subject and create an appropriate cover for the book.

The publishing team has been an ardent support to the editorial, designing and production team. Their endless efforts to recruit the best for this project, has resulted in the accomplishment of this book. They are a veteran in the field of academics and their pool of knowledge is as vast as their experience in printing. Their expertise and guidance has proved useful at every step. Their uncompromising quality standards have made this book an exceptional effort. Their encouragement from time to time has been an inspiration for everyone.

The publisher and the editorial board hope that this book will prove to be a valuable piece of knowledge for researchers, students, practitioners and scholars across the globe.

List of Contributors

Ruth Edge
Dalton Cumbrian Facility, The University of Manchester, Westlakes Science and Technology Park, Moor Row, Cumbria CA24 3HA, UK

T. George Truscott
School of Chemical and Physical Sciences, Lennard-Jones Building, Keele University, Staffordshire ST5 5BG, UK

Adeola Agnes Afon and Basiru Olaitan Ajiboye
Phytomedicine, Biomedical Toxicology and Diabetes Research Laboratories, Department of Biochemistry, Afe Babalola University, Ado-Ekiti 360001, Nigeria

Oluwafemi Adeleke Ojo
Phytomedicine, Biomedical Toxicology and Diabetes Research Laboratories, Department of Biochemistry, Afe Babalola University, Ado-Ekiti 360001, Nigeria
Department of Biochemistry, University of Ilorin, Ilorin 240222, Nigeria

Adebola Busola Ojo
Department of Medical Biochemistry, Afe Babalola University, Ado-Ekiti 360001, Nigeria

Babatunji Emmanuel Oyinloye
Phytomedicine, Biomedical Toxicology and Diabetes Research Laboratories, Department of Biochemistry, Afe Babalola University, Ado-Ekiti 360001, Nigeria
Biotechnology and Structural Biology (BSB) Group, Department of Biochemistry and Microbiology, University of Zululand, Kwa Dlangezwa 3886, South Africa

Abidemi Paul Kappo
Biotechnology and Structural Biology (BSB) Group, Department of Biochemistry and Microbiology, University of Zululand, Kwa Dlangezwa 3886, South Africa

Shaneice K. Nettleford and K. Sandeep Prabhu
Center for Molecular Immunology and Infectious Disease and Center for Molecular Toxicology and Carcinogenesis, The Pennsylvania State University, University Park, PA 16802, USA
Department of Veterinary and Biomedical Sciences, The Pennsylvania State University, University Park, PA 16802, USA

Sally L. Elshaer, Tahira Lemtalsi and Azza B. El-Remessy
Retinopathy Research, Augusta Biomedical Research Corporation Charlie Norwood VA Medical Center, Augusta, GA 30912, USA

Hongxia Zhang
Department of Food Science, University of Otago, Dunedin 9016, New Zealand

Zheng Feei Ma
Department of Public Health, Xi'an Jiaotong-Liverpool University, Suzhou 215123, China
School of Medical Sciences, Universiti Sains Malaysia, Kota Bharu 15200, Malaysia

Xiaoqin Luo
Department of Nutrition and Food Safety, School of Public Health, Xi'an Jiaotong University Health Science Center, Xi'an 710061, China

Xinli Li
Department of Food Science, University of Otago, Dunedin 9016, New Zealand
Department of Nutrition and Food Hygiene, School of Public Health, Medical College of Soochow University, Suzhou 215123, China

Muhammad Sarfraz, Muhammad Jawad Nasim and Claus Jacob
Division of Bioorganic Chemistry, School of Pharmacy, Saarland University, D-66123 Saarbruecken, Germany

Steffen F. Hartmann, Shashank Reddy Pinnapireddy, Udo Bakowsky and Cornelia M. Keck
Department of Pharmaceutics and Biopharmaceutics, University of Marburg, 35037 Marburg, Germany

Sharoon Griffin
Division of Bioorganic Chemistry, School of Pharmacy, Saarland University, D-66123 Saarbruecken, Germany
Department of Pharmaceutics and Biopharmaceutics, University of Marburg, 35037 Marburg, Germany

Cristina Anna Gallelli, Silvio Calcagnini, Adele Romano, Justyna Barbara Koczwara, Marialuisa de Ceglia, Donatella Dante and Silvana Gaetani
Department of Physiology and Pharmacology "V. Erspamer", Sapienza University of Rome, Piazzale Aldo Moro 5, 00185 Rome, Italy

Rosanna Villani
C.U.R.E. University Centre for Liver Disease Research and Treatment, Department of Medical and Surgical Sciences, Institute of Internal Medicine, University of Foggia, 71122 Foggia, Italy

Anna Maria Giudetti
Department of Biological and Environmental Sciences and Technologies, University of Salento, Via Monteroni, 73100 Lecce, Italy

Tommaso Cassano
Department of Clinical and Experimental Medicine, University of Foggia, Via Luigi Pinto, c/o Ospedali Riuniti, 71122 Foggia, Italy

Caroline Gaucher, Ariane Boudier, Justine Bonetti, Igor Clarot, Pierre Leroy and Marianne Parent
Université de Lorraine, CITHEFOR, F-54000 Nancy, France

Dewald Oosthuizen and Neill J. Goosen
Department of Process Engineering, Stellenbosch University, Stellenbosch 7600, South Africa

Maria A. Stander
Central Analytical Facility, Stellenbosch University, Stellenbosch 7600, South Africa

Aliyu D. Ibrahim
Department of Microbiology, Usmanu Danfodiyo University, Sokoto PMB 2346, Nigeria

Mary-Magdalene Pedavoah
Department of Applied Chemistry and Biochemistry, University for Development Studies, Navrongo, Ghana

Grace O. Usman
Department of Food, Nutrition and Home Sciences, Kogi State University, Anyigba 1008, Nigeria

Taiwo Aderinola
Department of Food Science and Technology, The Federal University of Technology, Akure PMB 704, Nigeria

John B. C. Tan and Danilo S. Boskovic
Division of Biochemistry, Department of Basic Sciences, Loma Linda University, Loma Linda, CA 92350, USA

Danilyn M. Angeles
Division of Physiology, Department of Basic Sciences, Loma Linda University, Loma Linda, CA 92350, USA

Josephine Kschonsek, Theresa Wolfram, Annette Stöckl and Volker Böhm
Institute of Nutrition, Friedrich Schiller University Jena, Dornburger Straße 25-29, 07743 Jena, Germany

Magdalena Timoszuk, Katarzyna Bielawska and Elżbieta Skrzydlewska
Department of Inorganic and Analytical Chemistry, Medical University of Bialystok, 15-089 Bialystok, Poland

Laurie G. Sherlock, Sarah McKenna, Susan Fisher, Clyde J. Wright and Cassidy Delaney
Department of Pediatrics, Section of Neonatology, University of Colorado Anschutz Medical Campus, Aurora, CO 80045, USA

Ashley Trumpie and Laura Hernandez-Lagunas
Cardiovascular Pulmonary Research Laboratories, University of Colorado Anschutz Medical Campus, Aurora, CO 80045, USA

Russell Bowler
Department of Medicine, National Jewish Health, Denver, CO 80206, USA

Eva Nozik-Grayck
Cardiovascular Pulmonary Research Laboratories, University of Colorado Anschutz Medical Campus, Aurora, CO 80045, USA
Pediatric Critical Care Medicine, University of Colorado Anschutz Medical Campus, Aurora, CO 80045, USA

Apollinaire Tsopmo
Food Science and Nutrition Program, Department of Chemistry, Carleton University, 1125 Colonel By Drive, Ottawa, ON K1S 5B6, Canada
Institute of Biochemistry, Carleton University, 1125 Colonel By Drive, Ottawa, ON K1S 5B6, Canada

Index